NO LONGER THE PROPERTY OF THE
CLARKE INSTITUTE OF PSYCHIATRY

THE GERIATRIC PATIENT

Adapted from
Hospital Practice

Illustrated by
Albert Miller

and other contributing artists:
Carol Donner, Nancy Lou Gahan, Neil O. Hardy,
Alan Iselin, Irwin Kuperberg, Lyn Van Eyck
For specific illustrations and for data source credits, see page 233

Designed by
Robert S. Herald

THE GERIATRIC PATIENT

Edited by

William Reichel, M.D.
Chairman, Department of Family Practice
Franklin Square Hospital, Baltimore, Md.

with the collaboration of

Mal Schechter
Contributing Editor, Hospital Practice

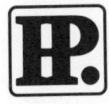

HP Publishing Co., Inc. • Publishers • New York, N.Y.

THE GERIATRIC PATIENT

The material in this book has been updated through June, 1978.
Copyright © 1978 by HP Publishing Co., Inc., New York, N.Y.

Printed in the United States of America

All rights reserved. No part of this book may be reproduced or transmitted in any form or by any means, electronic or mechanical, including photocopying, recording, or storage retrieval system, without written permission from the publisher:

HP Publishing Co., Inc.
575 Lexington Avenue
New York, N.Y. 10022

ISBN 0-913800-09-0

Library of Congress Catalog Card Number 78-60559

Table of Contents

Authors   VIII

Acknowledgments   X

Foreword   XI

PETER P. LAMY *and* ROBERT E. VESTAL   *University of Maryland and University of Washington*
1. Drug Prescribing for the Elderly   1

Many drugs can pose special hazards for the elderly, and drug effects may mimic phenomena associated with old age. Special approaches to prescribing and evaluating medication are described.

DAVID ECKSTEIN   *Meadow Lakes Retirement Community*
2. Common Complaints of the Elderly   9

Geriatric patients having unlimited access to physicians seldom come in without good reason, though not perhaps the ones they give. Common complaints must be taken seriously.

WILLIAM REICHEL   *Franklin Square Hospital*
3. Multiple Problems in the Elderly   17

Guidelines are offered to help the physician avoid "wastebasket diagnoses," to find the treatable problems among the many that beset the aged, and to set priorities for orderly management.

JOY R. JOFFE   *Johns Hopkins University*
4. Functional Psychiatric Disorders   23

Depression or other psychiatric disorder in an elderly person can often be handled best by the primary physician; guidelines are given on counseling, the use of drugs, and seeking referral.

WILLIAM REICHEL   *Franklin Square Hospital*
5. Organic Brain Syndromes   31

Confusion, disorientation, and dementia may be signs of reversible disease rather than untreatable senility. Guidelines are provided for differentiating treatable from untreatable conditions.

KENNETH B. LEWIS   *Johns Hopkins University*
6. Heart Disease in the Elderly   39

Congestive failure, chest pain, and rhythm disorders should not be assumed always to be of degenerative etiology. Often another cause can be identified and the patient helped.

WILLIAM P. CASTELLI   *Framingham Heart Study*
7. CHD Risk Factors   47

The Framingham study has shown that the major cardiovascular risk factors operate throughout life; a method is given for quantifying their impact as an aid in managing the patient.

SOLOMON ROBBINS   *University of Maryland*
8. Stroke in the Geriatric Patient   57

Deciding on treatment poses problems, since intercurrent disease often rules out measures appropriate at younger ages. Prevention of complications and rehabilitation become the goals.

C. ROBERT BAISDEN   *Johns Hopkins University*
9.   Hematologic Problems   65

The elderly tend to have low hemoglobin and hematocrit values, complicating the diagnosis of anemias. Also discussed are leukocytic and thrombocytic disorders.

MARVIN M. SCHUSTER   *Johns Hopkins University*
10.   Disorders of the Aging GI System   73

The patient's socioeconomic and emotional settings are frequent components of gastrointestinal dysfunction in the elderly. In most cases, the physician can intervene on several levels to help.

PAUL J. DAVIS   *State University of New York at Buffalo*
11.   Endocrines and Aging   82

Diagnosis and treatment are discussed for common endocrinopathies, including hyper- and hypothyroidism, adrenocortical diseases, ectopic humoral syndromes, and diabetes mellitus.

A. LEWIS KOLODNY *and* ANDREW R. KLIPPER   *Franklin Square Hospital*
12.   Bone and Joint Diseases   91

In managing patients with rheumatic diseases, it is important to differentiate the varied etiologies so that the most appropriate therapy can be employed. Drug treatment is discussed.

GERALD GLOWACKI   *Johns Hopkins University*
13.   Postmenopausal Gyn Problems   102

The conservative use of estrogens for prevention and treatment of osteoporosis is emphasized, as is the need for meticulous examination for inflammatory processes, prolapses, or neoplasia.

ARTHUR A. SERPICK   *University of Maryland*
14.   Cancer in the Elderly   109

New therapies and a multi-modality approach employing not only surgery but also irradiation and/or chemotherapy offer the hope of cure or amelioration of many cancers of the aged.

ALESSANDRO BASSO   *Johns Hopkins University*
15.   The Prostate in the Elderly Male   118

Surgery for benign hypertrophy rarely endangers sexual function, though psychogenic impotence may follow. Indications for different adenocarcinoma therapeutic techniques are given.

BENJAMIN H. GLOVER   *University of Wisconsin*
16.   Sex Counseling   125

Too often the opportunity for helpful discussion and counseling concerning sexual expression is missed. The first need is for a sympathetic, nonjudgmental approach.

DEREK J. CRIPPS   *University of Wisconsin*
17.   Skin Care and Problems   134

Methods of diagnosis and treatment of actinic keratoses, basal and squamous cell carcinomas, and other malignant and nonmalignant dermatoses are reviewed.

ABRAHAM L. KORNZWEIG *Jewish Home and Hospital for Aged, New York City*
18. Visual Loss in the Elderly   141

Most elderly persons retain useful vision despite the prevalence of cataracts, glaucoma, and diabetic retinopathy. Ocular signs can be clues to neurologic, cardiovascular, and other systemic diseases.

ROBERT J. RUBEN *Albert Einstein College of Medicine*
19. Otolaryngologic Problems   151

Hearing loss may signal trouble not only in the ear but elsewhere, and hearing aids are often not the answer. Guidelines are given for the management of a broad range of conditions.

PHILIP FERRIS *Franklin Square Hospital*
20. Surgical Management of the Elderly   159

The decision to undertake surgery in an aged person is far more complex than for other patients. Principles to guide the decision and specific indications are spelled out.

HOWARD H. CHAUNCEY *and* JAMES E. HOUSE *Harvard School of Dental Medicine*
21. Dental Problems   166

The personal physician may be the first to spot signs of ill-fitting dentures or poor chewing ability, drug effects on the mouth, leukoplakia, and other oral problems needing attention.

T.E. HUNT *University of Saskatchewan*
22. Rehabilitation of the Elderly   172

The family physician can call on many resources in the hospital, family, and community to help restore the disabled aged patient to a degree of functional independence.

JACK KLEH *George Washington University*
23. When to Institutionalize   181

Evaluation of the chronically ill aged patient may show she or he can stay home, with supportive services. Guidelines are given for choosing an appropriate nursing home when necessary.

ISADORE ROSSMAN *Albert Einstein College of Medicine*
24. Options for Care of the Aged Sick   189

Home care may be better than hospitalization even in acute illness; after- or day-care may provide superior long-term therapy. Hospital workups should be done only when necessary.

ROBERT N. BUTLER *National Institute on Aging*
25. The Doctor and the Aged Patient   199

The quality of the doctor-patient relationship is especially critical in caring for geriatric patients, with their frequently multiple problems. Key to a sound relationship is comprehensiveness of evaluation.

Selected References   209

Index   217

Illustration Credits   233

Contributing Authors

C. ROBERT BAISDEN — Assistant Professor (Pathology), Johns Hopkins University School of Medicine, and Deputy Chief, Department of Pathology, U.S. Public Health Service Hospital, Baltimore.

ALESSANDRO BASSO — Assistant Professor of Urology, Johns Hopkins University School of Medicine, Baltimore, and Urologist, Winchester (Va.) Urology Clinic and the Winchester Memorial Hospital.

ROBERT N. BUTLER — Director, National Institute on Aging, Bethesda, and author of "Why Survive? Being Old in America," Pulitzer Prize winner, 1976.

WILLIAM P. CASTELLI — Director of Laboratories of the Framingham Heart Study, National Heart and Lung and Blood Institute, and Lecturer in Preventive and Social Medicine, Harvard Medical School.

HOWARD H. CHAUNCEY — Ph.D., D.M.D., Associate Chief of Staff for Research and Development, VA Outpatient Clinic, Boston, and Associate Professor of Oral Pathology, Department of Oral Medicine and Oral Pathology, Harvard School of Dental Medicine.

DEREK J. CRIPPS — Professor and Head of Dermatology, University of Wisconsin Medical Center, Madison.

PAUL J. DAVIS — Head, Endocrinology Division, Department of Medicine, and Professor of Medicine, State University of New York at Buffalo Medical School.

DAVID ECKSTEIN — Medical Director of Meadow Lakes Retirement Community, Hightstown, N.J.

PHILIP FERRIS — Chairman, Department of Surgery, Franklin Square Hospital, Baltimore, and Clinical Assistant Professor of Surgery, University of Maryland, Baltimore.

BENJAMIN H. GLOVER — Associate Professor of Psychiatry, University of Wisconsin Medical School, Madison.

GERALD GLOWACKI — Assistant Professor, Department of Obstetrics and Gynecology, Johns Hopkins University School of Medicine, and Director, Department of Obstetrics and Gynecology, Franklin Square Hospital, Baltimore.

JAMES E. HOUSE — D.D.S., Chief, Dental Service, VA Outpatient Clinic, Boston, and Assistant Dean, Harvard School of Dental Medicine.

T. E. HUNT — Professor of Geriatric Medicine, University of Saskatchewan College of Medicine, Saskatoon, Canada.

JOY R. JOFFE — Assistant Professor of Psychiatry, Johns Hopkins University School of Medicine, and Director of Clinical Services, Phipps Clinic, Johns Hopkins Hospital, Baltimore.

JACK KLEH	Associate Clinical Professor of Medicine, George Washington University, and Medical Director, Gerontological Treatment Center, Washington, D.C.
ANDREW R. KLIPPER	Co-Chief, Rheumatology Section, Franklin Square Hospital, and Instructor, Health Associate Program, Johns Hopkins School of Health Services, Baltimore.
A. LEWIS KOLODNY	Co-Chief, Rheumatology Section, Franklin Square Hospital and North Charles General Hospital, Baltimore.
ABRAHAM L. KORNZWEIG	Chief Ophthalmologist and Director of Eye Research, Jewish Home and Hospital for Aged; Consultant Ophthalmologist, Mount Sinai Hospital, New York City.
PETER P. LAMY	Professor of Pharmacy and Director, Institutional Pharmacy Programs, University of Maryland School of Pharmacy, Baltimore.
KENNETH B. LEWIS	Assistant Professor of Medicine, Johns Hopkins University School of Medicine, and Chairman, Department of Medicine, Franklin Square Hospital, Baltimore.
WILLIAM REICHEL	Chairman, Department of Family Practice, Franklin Square Hospital, Baltimore.
SOLOMON ROBBINS	Instructor, Department of Neurology, University of Maryland Medical School, Baltimore.
ISADORE ROSSMAN	Medical Director, Home Care and Extended Services Department, Montefiore Hospital and Medical Center, and Associate Professor of Community Medicine, Albert Einstein College of Medicine of Yeshiva University, New York City.
ROBERT J. RUBEN	Professor and Chairman, Department of Otorhinolaryngology, Albert Einstein College of Medicine of Yeshiva University, and Montefiore Hospital and Medical Center, New York City.
MARVIN M. SCHUSTER	Chief, Division of Digestive Diseases, Baltimore City Hospitals, and Professor of Medicine, Johns Hopkins University School of Medicine, Baltimore.
ARTHUR A. SERPICK	Assistant Professor of Medicine, University of Maryland School of Medicine, Baltimore; Head, Division of Hematology and Medical Oncology, Maryland General Hospital.
ROBERT E. VESTAL	Assistant Professor of Medicine, University of Washington School of Medicine, Seattle, and Staff Physician and Coordinator for Research and Development, VA Hospital, Boise, Idaho.

Acknowledgments

"The Geriatric Patient" is based on a series of articles which appeared in *Hospital Practice* (all updated through June, 1978). Thus, many members of our journal staff made important contributions to the book. While space does not allow us to be all-inclusive, this introductory note gratefully acknowledges those contributions and extends special credit where it is due.

Special mention must be made of the work of Gertrude Halpern, Associate Editorial Director, in assisting the editors and individual authors to clarify the texts, and in integrating the illustrations and editorial materials. The design of the articles as well as the book was the contribution of Robert S. Herald, our Art Director, with the aid of his staff.

The extensive index, which we hope will be of value for practitioners seeking precise details for clinical application, is the highly professional work of Theodore Webster of Bethesda, Md.

Herb Cornell, Director of the Book Division of HP Publishing Co., Inc., coordinated the production efforts with the skillful assistance of Katherine Bloch on the editorial side and Carla Netto administratively.

Finally, on behalf of Dr. Reichel as well as ourselves, we want to express our deep gratitude for the support and cooperation of the Franklin Square Medical Foundation in facilitating the work of the book's editor.

David W. Fisher
*Editorial Director
and Co-publisher*
Hospital Practice

New York,
July, 1978

Foreword

The numbers in themselves are instructive. There are 22 million Americans age 65 or older, 10 percent of the U.S. population. By the year 2000, assuming fertility at a replacement rate, there will be approximately 30.6 million persons age 65 or older, 15.5% of the total population. By 2030, there will be 50 million Americans over 65 years of age.

The professional implications of these figures are striking when coupled with the knowledge that the elderly have multiple medical, social, economic, and other problems and that they are heavy users of medical and supportive services. Around the nation, there is suddenly acute awareness that the increasing number of elderly affects all social institutions and therefore demands immediate attention.

For all physicians, there are special aspects in the care of the elderly. The practitioner must understand the elderly, their diagnostic and therapeutic needs, and the methods of meeting these needs in office and institutional practice. There is cognitive information that must be understood, and attitudinal concepts, sensitivities, and skills that are essential.

Universities must begin to pay greater attention within their departments to the special problems of geriatric patients and to long-term care. Medical education that fails to prepare the physician to care for a growing elderly clientele is unrealistic; at the undergraduate, graduate, and postgraduate levels, those concepts, skills, and methods essential to the care of the elderly must be taught.

A premise of this book is that the care of the elderly is overwhelmingly in the domain of primary practice – a nearby, familiar doctor. This is not to say that referral to a subspecialist is irregular, but that the patient who is elderly is not a "heart problem" or a "senility problem" or an "arthritis problem." We are suggesting the use of this book as a handbook or guide for primary physicians in the daily care of the elderly patient.

Family practice, with its clear message of continuity of care and concern for all aspects of the patient and his family, can make a special contribution to care of the elderly. The family physician is especially concerned with care of the *well* elderly and emphasizes prevention, health maintenance, and rehabilitation. And finally, family practice is concerned about the revitalization of the family unit. Strengthening the American family is a critical step in solving the problems that face the elderly, especially in the avoidance of unnecessary institutionalization.

Similarly, the internist is involved on a daily basis with the care of the elderly. In fact, for most internists, the majority of professional time is spent in treating elderly patients and chronic disease. The internist, too, is required to deal with the aging patient as a whole and complex individual in each diagnostic and therapeutic encounter.

The objective of this book is to provide practical, relevant material to the primary physician attending elderly patients. Thus, the special sensitivities necessary in the daily care of the aged are set forth in eight chapters, with details of the multiple disorders these patients are likely to present, their variations in symptoms, and the many emotional and family problems that may affect their complaints.

The diseases and disorders the elderly commonly present with are discussed on a system-by-system basis in 17 additional chapters on the diagnosis and management of bone and joint diseases, brain disorders (both functional and organic), cancer, cardiac diseases, dentistry, dermatology, endocrinology, gastroenterology, gynecology, hematology, ophthalmology, otolaryngology, strokes, surgical management, and urology.

One of my chapters, "Multiple Problems of the Elderly," points out that the physician needs to know how functional capacity declines with time. Reduced glucose tolerance or creatinine clearance, for example, might be physiological or normal. Certain defense mechanisms tend to diminish, and thus, the latency of disease is greater. The elderly may have pneumonia or pyelonephritis without fever or chills, and many serious conditions, such as myocardial infarction, may be present without usual pain. The other characteristic of the elderly population is its burden of multiple diseases and disabilities. Keeping track of these multiple problems makes a problem-oriented record virtually mandatory.

Drs. Peter Lamy and Robert Vestal describe the effects of drugs in the elderly, who often are more vulnerable to toxicity and react more variably than do the young. A number of practical steps in confronting this problem are reviewed.

Dr. David Eckstein of the Meadow Lakes Retirement Community in Hightstown, New Jersey, in his chapter, "Common Complaints of the Elderly," underscores the need for a physician's sensitivity to the complaints – remarkably low-keyed and valid – which are present on a daily basis. When geriatric patients have unlimited access to sympathetic physicians, they seldom come in without a good reason, though perhaps not the ones they initially state.

"Organic Brain Syndromes" warns particularly against "wastebasket" or "scrapbasket" diagnoses. It states that neuropsychiatric disturbance in the elderly is often casually accepted as untreatable, when, in reality, careful examination might reveal a treatable cause in both the acute confusional states and also in the organic dementias. Not all mental disturbance in the elderly represents dementia, and not all dementia is irreversible.

In "Heart Disease in the Elderly," Dr. Kenneth Lewis issues a similar warning: not all congestive heart failure is arteriosclerotic. Congestive heart failure, chest pains, and rhythm disturbances should not always be assumed to be of degenerative etiology in the old. Often, some other cause can be identified and treatment instituted to benefit the patient.

In discussing surgical management of the elderly, Dr. Philip Ferris adapts the age-old adage usually related to drug prescription: first, do no harm. But while it may sometimes be best to leave well enough alone, performing surgery often can be of great benefit to an aged person. Dr. Ferris spells out principles that guide the decision-making process and provide specific indications.

Prevention shares equally with diagnosis and treatment in the book. In "CHD Risk Factors," Dr. William Castelli of the Framingham Heart Study reviews the risk factors revealed in this long-range project, focusing on its elderly subjects. He explains how the physician may quantify the impact of cardiovascular risk factors on individual patients.

Dr. Joy Joffe, in "Functional Psychiatric Disorders," warns against the frequent reluctance to treat emotional disorders in the aged. Such illnesses as depression, grief reactions, sexual maladjustments, paranoid reactions, marital problems, and situational disorders must be recognized and treated, she says. These problems often can be handled best by a primary physician who might ask rhetorically: "If this individual were 40 or 50 years old, would we treat this depression? What is so different about the patient's being 72 years old?"

Although counseling is discussed throughout the book, special attention is given to sex counseling of the aged by Dr. Benjamin Glover. A sympathetic, nonjudgmental approach might reveal sexual dissatisfaction that can cause vague health complaints and might open the way to beneficial counseling, changes in drug regimen, and referrals that can greatly improve the quality of life.

Dr. Jack Kleh discusses institutionalizing the elderly and noninstitutional treatment in "Options for Care of the Aged Sick." He provides guidelines for choosing a nursing home when necessary, but adds that follow-up of the chronically ill may show that the patient can stay at home just as well with support from family and community resources.

Dr. Isadore Rossman, in his chapter "When to Institutionalize," urges every physician to carefully consider any practical alternative to institutionalization. He details his experience at Montefiore Hospital in New York City, where whenever possible home care, after care, and day care are substituted for care in nursing homes or acute general hospitals. Dr. Rossman concludes: "When not to institutionalize? When a rational alternative is available."

In "Rehabilitation of the Elderly," Dr. T.E. Hunt establishes that, short of curing, a family physician can restore a degree of independence to a disabled, aged person by early, delicately managed mobilization, and by calling on hospital, family, and community resources.

Dr. Solomon Robbins, in "Stroke in the Geriatric Patient," reviews when and how to treat stroke in the elderly patient. The entire clinical picture and the list of the patient's problems and diseases weigh heavily in prognosis for any elderly individual and dominate considerations of operability.

Drs. A. Lewis Kolodny and Andrew R. Klipper, in "Bone and Joint Diseases," again stress that it is essential to differentiate the varied etiologies so that the most appropriate therapy can be employed. They emphasize the role of rehabilitation and surgical therapies in the total treatment program, and report that age per se is no contraindication to surgery if the patient is reasonably healthy.

In "Hematologic Problems," Dr. C. Robert Baisden says it is essential to confirm the presence of anemia and establish its etiology. He also discusses such proliferative disorders as chronic lymphocytic leukemia.

Dr. Marvin Schuster, in "Disorders of the Aging GI System," observes that gastrointestinal conditions can be caused by socioeconomic and emotional factors as well as physical deterioration. Whatever the cause, he notes that practical help can be given for most common problems.

In "Endocrines and Aging," Dr. Paul J. Davis reviews diagnosis, treatment, and relevant physiology for endocrinopathies common in the elderly, including hyper- and hypothyroidism, adrenocortical disease, ectopic humoral syndrome, and diabetes mellitus.

In "Postmenopausal Gyn Problems," Dr. Gerald Glowacki evaluates the conservative use of estrogens for prevention and treatment of osteoporosis and urges thorough pelvic examination to detect inflammatory processes, prolapses, and growths.

In "The Prostate in the Elderly Male," Dr. Alessandro Basso examines the indications for treating carcinoma of the prostate by radiotherapy, surgery, and hormones. He also reviews current concepts of benign prostatic hypertrophy, and diagnostic and therapeutic implications.

The skin, eyes, ears, nose, throat, and the teeth reveal much about the total health of the aging individual. Four chapters deal with this:

Dr. Derek Cripps, in "Skin Care and Problems," reviews methods of diagnosis and treatment of actinic keratoses, squamous cell carcinoma, and other malignant dermatoses, as well as nonmalignant skin changes. He observes that some internal malignancies manifest themselves cutaneously. Dr. Abraham L. Kornzweig's "Visual Loss in the Elderly" surveys common ocular problems, including cataracts, degeneration of central vision, glaucoma, and diabetic retinopathy. Ocular signs, he reports, can be clues to neurologic, metabolic, oncologic, nephritic, and other diseases. Dr. Robert J. Ruben similarly stresses in "Otolaryngologic Problems" that hearing loss and dizziness may signal trouble not only in the structures of the ear but elsewhere in the body. Hearing disorders may also trigger withdrawal and other psychiatric problems. Hearing aids are often not the answer to the patient's problem. Dr. Ruben provides guidelines for management of a broad range of conditions. In "Dental Problems," Drs. Howard H. Chauncey and James E. House maintain that the personal physician may be the first to spot oral problems.

In "Cancer in the Elderly," Dr. Arthur Serpick discusses new therapies and a combined modality approach employing surgery, irradiation, and one or more drugs. This approach offers the hope of cure for many cancers or of an amelioration previously unattainable. When death from cancer is imminent, Dr. Serpick points out, the physician is obliged to consider the choice between the impersonal gadgetry at the hospital and the dignity of a less regimented death, preferably at home.

In the final chapter, "The Doctor and the Aged Patient," Dr. Robert N. Butler, Director of the National Institute on Aging, and Pulitzer Prize winner, lists the ingredients of a sound doctor – aged patient relationship. He discusses the problem of ageism in our society and provides examples of the "senile write-off."

A key to building a sound relationship is the comprehensiveness of evaluation. Dr. Butler identifies the following ingredients as crucial to the doctor-patient relationship: 1) knowing the patient through a life history; 2) giving the patient a full hearing; 3) being appropriately frank; 4) viewing the older patient as a participant in making decisions about care; 5) recognizing unconscious prejudice and conflicts; 6) adopting approaches that enhance the patient's independent self-respect and preserve the patient's life style as much as possible; 7) setting realistic treatment goals; 8) recognizing problems referrable to other professionals and to the family; and 9) dealing with the patient's negative attitude towards self and physician.

The book could close with no more meaningful summary.

WILLIAM REICHEL, M.D.

Baltimore, Maryland
July 1978

Drug Prescribing for the Elderly

PETER P. LAMY *and* ROBERT E. VESTAL
University of Maryland and University of Washington

Many valuable drugs are especially hazardous in the old. Digitalis intoxication, potassium depletion from diuretics, paradoxical reaction to barbiturates, extrapyramidal symptoms from phenothiazines, phenylbutazone toxicity, gastrointestinal bleeding from aspirin, hemorrhagic reaction from heparin – all of these effects are more likely to occur in the geriatric patient than in other adults. Steering a safe, effective course between benefit and risk requires understanding of when to give and when not to give drugs.

Ironically, drug-induced illness may go unperceived because it often mimics stereotypes associated with old age: forgetfulness, weakness, confusion, tremor, anorexia, and anxiety.

Caution is the practical byword in geriatric prescribing. Dosages recommended for the "average" patient may not be assumed to be satisfactory for the elderly patient. The older person is an uncertain responder and sometimes the "average dose" may be excessive. There are hazards from age-associated decrements in physiologic function as well as from the effects of illness or trauma. The challenge to the physician is multiple: 1) to determine whether the patient's complaint is justification for medication; 2) if so, to determine what is the preferable agent; 3) to estimate how much of a total drug load may be safely imposed at any one time and therefore to decide whether among various conditions amenable to drugs some may wait until later for therapy; 4) to consider benefits and risks, understanding that they may balance differently for the elderly than for the young; and 5) to keep the total number of drugs in the patient's regimen at a minimum, with the use of any additional drugs deferred if possible. At the same time, while maneuverability often is less in prescribing for the elderly, sometimes the constraints are less too. For example, the currently controversial use of oral hypoglycemic agents may be more readily justified in a 70-year-old than in a 40-year-old person, especially if insulin therapy would be difficult for such a patient.

All of these considerations would seem to fall within the realm of the art rather than the science of medicine. Yet, a good deal has been learned that can be helpful to the office practitioner. Our purpose in this chapter is to offer practical counsel based on pharmacologic concepts and experience. In considering such questions as the pharmacologic significance of some physiologic decrements that accompany aging and the uses and pitfalls of certain drugs, we take the view that the multiple-problem patient is not to be avoided because he or she cannot be cured. The ability to minimize infirmities – to help the patient function the very best he or she can and to be independent for as long as he or she can – can become one of the physician's most gratifying experiences.

Drug Utilization and Adverse Reactions in the Elderly Population

According to the Social Security Administration, the per capita expenditure for prescribed drugs by the elderly is far above that for other age groups. In 1976, spending by the aged on drugs and drug sundries was an estimated $2.78 billion, or almost 25% of the national total in these categories ($11.2 billion), although the elderly comprise only 11% of the population. Averaging more than 13 prescriptions a year (including renewals) per capita, the aged spent over $120 for prescribed and over-the-counter drugs per year.

Even if drugs are given for the right reasons and in the right dosages, the simultaneous use of multiple drugs carries a high risk of toxic reactions. Often, however, prescribing by hospital and office practitioners is inappropriate. A University of Maryland study of the medical records of 33 geriatric cardiac patients in a teaching hospital showed that 13 drugs, accounting for the majority of prescriptions, were given in dosages higher than recommended in their labeling. Another study in the same series showed that the elderly received no general dosage reduction of drugs, whether these were given in the hospital or in the community. Community physicians relied heavily on barbiturates despite the high risk of paradoxical reactions and tended to prescribe potassium supplementation with diuretics less often than hospital physicians.

It is no secret that drug-induced illness is much more frequent among elderly hospitalized patients. In a retrospective study of more than 700 hospitalized patients by Seidl and associates at Johns Hopkins, the proportion of those aged 80 or more with adverse drug reactions was almost 25%, while in the age group 41 to 50 it was about 12%. In a three-year prospective study by Caranasos, Stewart, and Cluff, 3% of 6,000 consecutive admissions to the medical service of the University of Florida Teaching Hospital were attributed to drug-induced illness, and two fifths of these were of patients aged over 60. Eight drugs accounted for one third of the admissions: aspirin, digoxin, warfarin sodium, hydrochlorothiazide, prednisone, vincristine sulfate, norethindrone, and furosemide. Over-the-counter drugs accounted for about a fifth of the admissions for drug-induced illness and included yellow phenolphthalein (Ex-Lax), antacids, and bromides.

Exemplifying the problem is the case of a 75-year-old woman with high blood pressure, congestive heart failure, diabetes, ankle edema, and obesity. Her physician has prescribed a regimen including an oral hypoglycemic agent, a reducing diet, Peritrate, nitroglycerin, a thiazide diuretic, and antacids. The patient takes the diuretic only when she has a headache; despite the label instruction, she takes two or three pills at a time. She keeps the drugs, including the diuretic, in a refrigerator in the belief this preserves them, while in reality the condensation that occurs when the containers are taken out of the cold inactivates the drugs.

In all probability, only two of the drugs in her present regimen are justified. The diuretic is appropriate therapy for both her congestive heart failure and her hypertension but may make treatment of her diabetes more difficult. If diabetic control is significantly impaired by the thiazide diuretic, consideration should be given to the substitution of insulin for the oral hypoglycemic agent. Hyperglycemia might well diminish or disappear altogether if she could lose weight. Alternatively, her physician might attempt to manage the hypertension with another antihypertensive agent and discontinue the diuretic. In

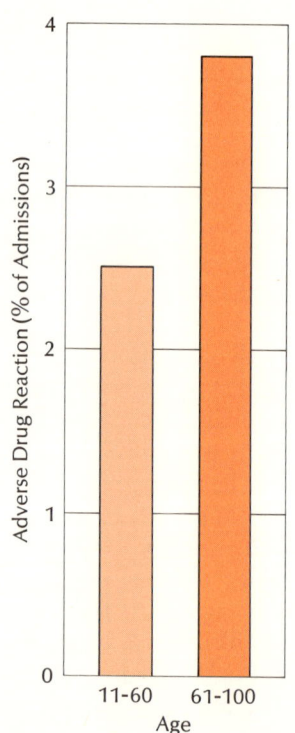

Age Range (yr)	All Admissions (No.)	Adverse Drug Reaction Admissions (No.)
11-20	394	11
21-30	782	19
31-40	746	20
41-50	1,006	21
51-60	1,225	33
61-70	1,213	44
71-80	546	26
81-90	139	3
91-100	12	0
Total	6,063	177

When hospital admissions for drug-induced illness (left) are grouped by age, admission rate in those 61 and over is about 1½ times that of younger persons (Caranasos).

DRUG PRESCRIBING

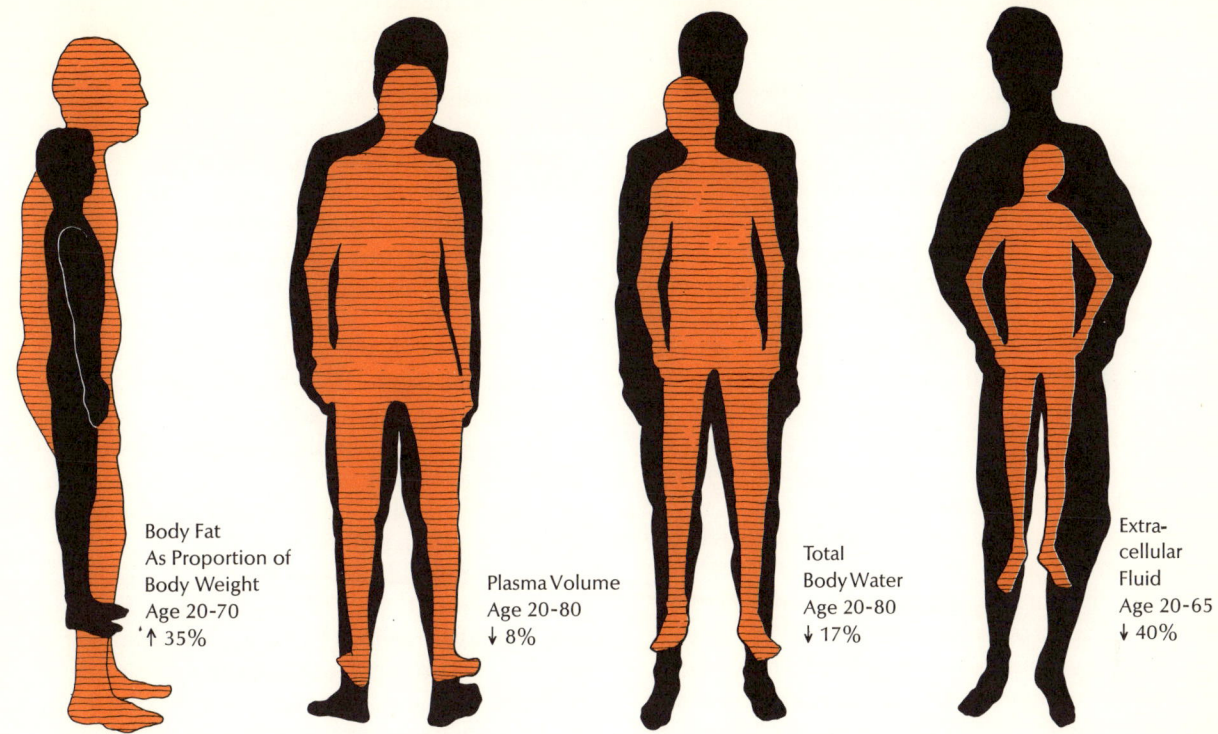

With aging, changes occur in the proportion of body weight accounted for by different parameters of body composition, as the schematic suggests. Thus, as the fluid parameters decrease relative to total weight, the percentage of fat rises. Such changes may significantly affect drug distribution and half-life. Data illustrated are from Blood and Other Body Fluids, Dittmer DS, ed., FASEB, 1961. More recent studies suggest, however, that in healthy elderly individuals, these body-composition changes may not be so pronounced.

addition, this patient probably would benefit from carefully monitored digitalis therapy for the congestive heart failure. If digitalis is added to her regimen, she should be encouraged to eat potassium-containing foods or take potassium supplements and should have periodic measurements of serum potassium levels.

Unfortunately, the patient does not understand the diet and does not follow it. She overeats. Her physician treats her gastric symptoms with antacids. The vasodilators were prescribed only because of the vague complaint that her chest hurt. In 10 years, the physician has not changed the regimen at all, even though lack of success should have prompted review and change. It would have been far better for the physician to have taken the time to explain the need for adhering to the diet, to make sure the diuretic was taken as directed, and to consider whether the chest pains merited any drug therapy at all. Our conclusion is that in this patient drug prescribing has replaced real medical attention.

Altered Physiology and Pharmacology

For drugs to be effective they must be delivered to their sites of action in the body. The process by which this takes place is referred to as drug distribution and depends on physiologic characteristics, such as body composition (body fluid compartments and the masses of bone, muscle, and fat), plasma protein concentration, organ blood flow, and cardiac output. Most drugs are removed from the body by two major routes of elimination: hepatic metabolism and renal excretion.

There is considerable variation among aged individuals in proportions of body water and body fat. While the average older person may have a slightly smaller proportion of intracellular water, the obesity of middle age is not characteristic of aged individuals. On the average, their proportion of fat is similar to the young. For prescribing purposes, obvious water retention and excess fat in subcutaneous and abdominal depots, on the one hand, and emaciation, on the other, must be taken into account. In an obese elderly patient, the capacity to store fat-soluble compounds, such as barbiturates, increases. This enhanced storage capacity may allow for a longer effect and greater risk of toxicity as drugs administered at the usual dosing intervals accumulate. Since high steady-state concentrations would be expected, the usual dose of drugs, such as antipyrine and ethanol, which distribute in total body water, may be more potent (or more toxic) in emaciated, elderly patients.

The lower levels of serum albumin often found in elderly patients means that for drugs that are protein bound the same dose will yield more free drug in the plasma available for delivery to sites of action and sites of elimination. Reduced plasma protein also intensifies competition among drugs for binding sites. For example, aspirin tends to displace warfarin, and excessive free warfarin may produce excessive anticoagulation.

Since the liver and kidney are key sites for metabolism and excretion of drugs, age changes in these organs are of profound pharmacologic importance. Liver microsomal enzymes are responsible for the metabolic degradation of many drugs. Reduction in their activity means that drug elimination would be reduced, leading to drug accumulation and toxicity. There is some evidence for such a reduction in man, and in the rat, microsomal enzyme preparations from old animals have 30% to 40% less enzyme activity than those from young animals.

The decrement in renal function in the relatively healthy older person may range from 20% to 50%. Drugs eliminated from the body primarily by the kidney (notably digoxin and the aminoglycoside antibiotics such as streptomycin, neomycin, kanamycin, and gentamicin) must be used with the awareness that toxic levels may occur unless dosage is reduced in the presence of reduced renal function. With diminished renal and hepatic function, the plasma half-life of drugs may be prolonged, increasing the risk of drug toxicity and drug interactions.

The pharmacologically significant, age-related changes cited above do not necessarily provide quantitative answers to specific problems of dosage and drug selection. To a large extent, this must be individualized. It is not possible to state how much diminution in microsomal activity can be expected in people of different ages and what this means in terms of drug regimens. Present routine tests of liver function detect only major impairment in function such as occurs with hepatitis or cirrhosis. Tests of renal function, however, such as the 24-hour creatinine clearance, are sensitive if carefully done and should be used to guide therapy with renally excreted drugs.

Digoxin is an example of the influence of diminished renal function on drug excretion. G. A. Ewy and coworkers at Georgetown University compared digoxin levels in nine young men (mean age 27) and in five elderly men (mean age 77) after administration of 0.5 mg of tritiated digoxin. Both groups had about the same serum creatinine values, but the rate of creatinine clearance in the elderly was half that of the young. Blood levels of digoxin in the elderly were significantly higher than in the young after the first 24 hours. The same dose had a longer half-life in the old because of diminished renal excretion and smaller body size. The findings support reduction of digoxin dosage because of these physiologic changes with age. An aid to help the physician estimate dosage based on creatinine clearance values is a nomogram recently developed at the Gerontology Research Center that gives normal values for creatinine clearance with aging. Even better would be to make direct measurement of creatinine clearance in the individual patient. In addition to making an educated estimate of the proper maintenance dose based on knowledge of renal function, the physician should utilize plasma digoxin levels to determine the actual steady-state concentration in his patient and modify his therapy accordingly. In the hospitalized, critically ill elderly patient who may require the use of potent, often nephrotoxic, antibiotics, such as gentamicin, which are excreted by the kidney, a similar approach should be adopted.

In addition to physiologic changes, aging brings changes in way of life that may be pharmacologically significant. Nutritional status is likely to be poor. When the price of food goes up, the elderly living on small incomes tend to reduce their consumption. Symptoms of nutritional imbalance may be attributed erroneously to "aging" or may be erroneously "managed" by drugs, e.g., sedatives for nervousness or sleeplessness caused by malnutrition. Apathy, depression after loss of spouse, ill-fitting dentures, and disability also tend to reduce food intake and cause vitamin deficiency, especially of folic acid, ascorbic acid, and vitamins D and B.

Of at least theoretical interest is the fact that such habits as smoking, alcohol and caffeine consumption may influence drug metabolism. These habits differ with age. At the Gerontology Research Center, the half-life of antipyrine was found to be longer in older persons than in younger persons. This age difference in metabolism was in part explained by decreased cigarette smoking in the older group. Alcohol and caffeine consumption did not have a significant effect. Other studies suggest, however, that alcohol and caffeine may either inhibit or stimulate the metabolism of some drugs. Alcohol intensifies the effects of hypoglycemic agents by inhibiting glucose production by the liver. Research on alcohol at the Gerontology Center also showed that although young and old metabolize alcohol similarly, a little alcohol goes a long way in interfering with psychomotor and cognitive functions in subjects of all ages, but most profoundly in the elderly. The importance of considering eating, drinking, and other habits before prescribing drugs should be obvious. Part of a careful drug history in the evaluation of young and old patients alike should include questions concerning habits.

Much research needs to be done to further characterize the effects of aging on pharmacokinetics. As we have illustrated, there is limited information about distribution and elimination. Less is known about drug absorption from the gastrointestinal tract, but a change in absorption patterns may be anticipated in patients with achlorhydria or hypochlorhydria. These conditions are not infrequently encountered in older patients. Water-soluble drugs formulated with dicalcium phosphate or weak organic acids such as barbituric acid derivatives may be affected. The influence of age-related hemodynamic changes, such as reduced cardiac output, has yet to be explored but might lead to impaired drug delivery to renal and hepatic sites of drug removal. It is known, for example, that hepatic clearance of lidocaine from the blood is reduced in congestive heart failure because of reduced blood flow to the liver. Another important aspect of geriatric pharmacology is that of drug sensitivity. Most information currently available is based on anecdotal clinical observations rather than carefully controlled studies. We would hope that in the future, physicians may have improved means of estimating dosages based on multiple parameters: absorption rate, clearance, volume of distribution, half-life (which reflects clearance and distribution volume), and drug sensitivity.

Suggestions for Geriatric Prescribing

In addition to caution based on awareness of the potential age difference in physiology and pharmacology, a careful drug history and periodic review of drug consumption should be basic in caring for the elderly. The wise physician will not take for granted that the patient a) has the prescription filled, b) understands or will remember how to take the drug, c) is on no medication other than that the physician has prescribed, d) continues to take the prescribed drug, and e) is an accurate reporter of intake and adverse reactions.

If experience in a Maryland hospital outpatient service applies elsewhere, many patients fail to have

Aging and Pharmacokinetics in Man	
ABSORPTION	
Acetaminophen	
Phenylbutazone	No age differences in time to peak plasma levels
Sulfamethizole	
DISTRIBUTION	
Diazepam	Increased initial and steady-state volume of distribution giving an increased t½
	No change in protein binding
	No change in plasma clearance
Diphenylhydantoin	Decreased plasma binding capacity because of decreased plasma albumin, giving increased clearance
Warfarin	Decreased plasma binding capacity because of decreased plasma albumin
Antipyrine	Decreased apparent volume of distribution
Morphine	Increased early serum levels at 2 and 5 min after IV administration
	No change in rate of elimination
ELIMINATION	
Renal Excretion	
Digoxin	Decreased clearance (and increased t½)
Antibiotics	
Penicillin	Increased t½
Sulfamethizole	Decreased clearance (and increased t½)
Tetracycline	Increased plasma levels
Dihydrostreptomycin	Increased plasma levels
Hepatic Metabolism	
Antipyrine	Decreased clearance (and increased t½)
Aminopyrine	Increased t½
Amobarbital	Increased peak plasma levels
	Decreased urinary metabolite (3-hydroxyamobarbital)

CHAPTER 1: LAMY AND VESTAL

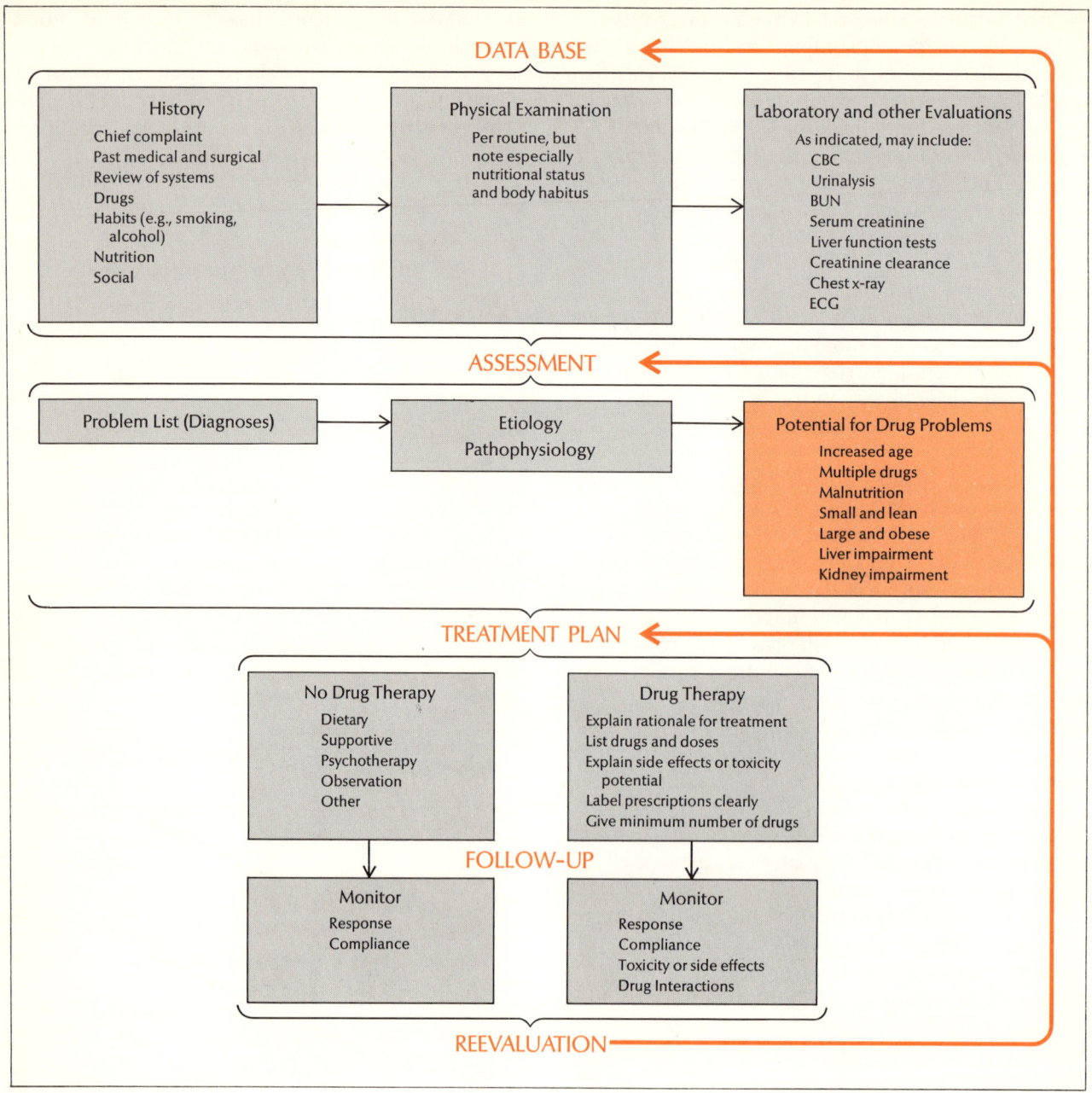

Prescribing for the geriatric patient is greatly aided by a systematic approach like that suggested by flow chart; inputs to "Potential for Drug Problems" may arise from any category within the data base or assessment. Reevaluation as necessary is an integral part of the process; careful records are needed at all stages.

prescriptions filled or refilled. The elderly patient may not have the cash or may prefer to spend it on an OTC preparation. With multiple prescribing, the patient may make his own decisions on which prescription to have filled when. Unless the physician checks, to the extent of asking the patient to bring in drug containers, the physician may increase, substitute, or add to the drug regimen in the belief that prescriptions were followed but failed. Even when the prescription is filled, an elderly patient may not understand or recall what the physician said about administration. Hearing difficulties may be part of the problem. If the label simply says "take as directed," it tells the patient nothing. Nor are instructions such as "take three times a day" sufficient. Does that mean with meals or between meals? At bedtime? Then there is the assumption that the patient can read the label; too often the print is small. The physician should ask that the label instructions be in large type and they should be crystal clear: "Take one pill with a full glass of water at breakfast."

The patient also needs to be told that taking a drug must continue until the physician decides to withdraw it. Some patients stop on their own because they feel better. Medicare, of course, has no outpatient drug benefit, and the tendency to skimp may affect drug prescriptions. Tact should be employed to determine whether the patient can afford a drug or, for that matter, a well-balanced diet.

Even when the physician monitors the intake of prescribed drugs, he may not inquire about OTC drugs. Yet an OTC drug may be a cause of the condition for which the patient sees the physician, or it may interfere with the action of a prescribed drug, or lead to a toxic synergism.

An example is cold remedies containing sympathomimetic amines, which raise blood sugar levels. The product label may contain a long list of contraindications but the elderly patient may not read or understand them. Belladonna alkaloids raise intraocular pressure and are contraindicated for narrow-angle glaucoma. The patient for whom warfarin has been prescribed must be warned against aspirin, which, as mentioned earlier, displaces warfarin from binding sites. If the patient must have aspirin, the warfarin dose should be lowered. A specific inquiry about aspirin in the warfarin candidate is essential.

In addition to inquiring about OTC drug-taking, the physician should try to ascertain whether the patient is taking drugs prescribed by other physicians, or, for that matter, drugs prescribed for a previous illness, or for the spouse. The patient who frequents different physicians may be receiving the same drugs under different names, perhaps in different sizes or forms. The obvious danger is overdosage. When the drugs are different, the danger is adverse interaction. Unfortunately, many old patients do not recall what drugs they take. Whenever possible, family members should be consulted, even though some patients resist for reasons of privacy.

A pharmacy that maintains a drug history, including history of hypersensitivity, can be helpful. A few states, such as New Jersey, require pharmacies to maintain such a record while in others, pharmacies do so voluntarily. But there is always the patient who shops in various pharmacies, including some that keep no record. Certainly the physician can counsel the patient to use a pharmacy that does. In Baltimore, several pharmacies have helped prevent adverse reactions from multiple prescriptions; their procedure is to call one of the physicians about the problem. In some Medicaid programs, consolidated records are kept on drug utilization (as in North Carolina). It is highly desirable that in addition to progress notes in the patient's file, the drug history be set up as a separate patient profile, noting dates of onset and discontinuation of different medications.

Getting the patient's drug history and continually checking on drug intake and nutritional status will take time. There are some indications that the more time a physician spends with the geriatric patient, the fewer the drugs prescribed. Unfortunately, third-party reimbursement methods seem to make it easier to justify the expense of a patient visit that ends with an Rx than one devoted substantially to counseling.

Routine testing of the geriatric patient for hematocrit and fluid and electrolyte balance may be a valuable aid to the physician in avoiding unnecessary drug use. Often, complaints of weakness and fatigue are related to imbalances or deficiencies readily apparent in these tests and readily correctable by diet.

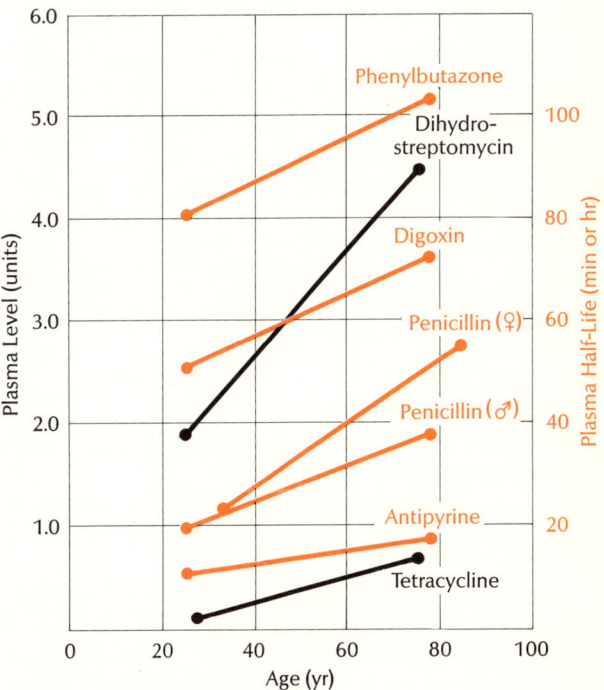

Graphed above are differences between young and old patients in plasma level or half-life of some parenterally given drugs (data summarized by Bender).

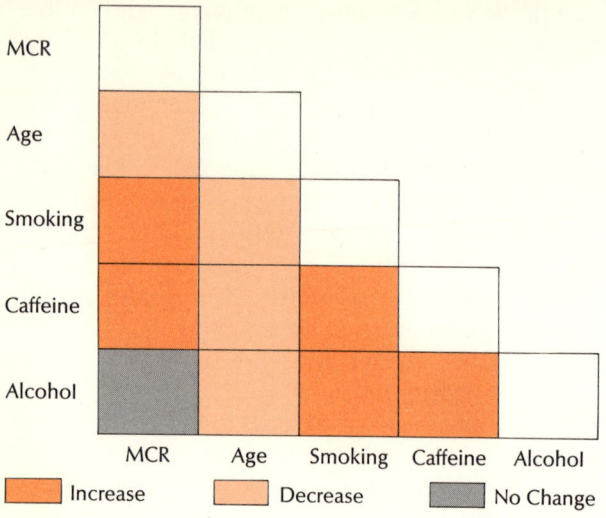

Summary of associations among metabolic clearance rate (MCR) of antipyrines, age, and habits shows age is always a negative factor. By contrast, in the young and middle-aged, smoking and caffeine seem to enhance MCR while alcohol leaves it unaffected. In fact, when all variables are considered together, analysis shows only age and cigarette smoking have a significant effect on MCR.

and prescribed supplements. Using a complete drug record, the physician may be able to warn the patient against habits that nullify these maneuvers. For example, the patient for whom an iron supplement is prescribed can be warned not to take it along with a laxative that would lead to its rapid elimination.

When a patient is admitted to a hospital or a long-term care institution, the physician should make sure that the drug history is sent along. A hospital-based specialist who may not know of the ambulatory regimen may add new drugs to the old. In the nursing home, periodic review of drug regimens sometimes are superficial or careless despite government requirements for monthly endorsement. In the nursing home or any other situation in which the physician's orders are carried out by another health professional, the orders must be crystal clear. It may not be clear to nurses confronted with a thick chart just what a physician means by a cryptic order renewing "drugs 1, 5, 7, and 8." Some drugs may be dispensed PRN, opening up the possibility of unmonitored, injudicious use, especially of tranquilizers. In one Maryland institution, most patients were found to be receiving four or five drugs regularly, with a dozen more ordered PRN. The concern has been expressed that patients may be chemo-manipulated into docility to minimize claims on the staff for attention.

One must scrupulously check that an adverse reaction in an old patient is not routinely passed over as due to "senility" or "aging." An instance of insensitivity to an adverse reaction concerns an old woman in a nursing home. Subject to severe arthritic episodes and incontinence, she medicated herself heavily with aspirin. Embarrassment over having to be helped to the bathroom led her to take the aspirin with very little water. Gastrointestinal bleeding resulted. Since the patient's major complaint remained the arthritis, the physician prescribed increased aspirin. Within two weeks, she was unable to leave her chair. Her weakness was dismissed as "aging" until her bleeding problem was belatedly discovered.

A general principle is to begin with single and 24-hour total doses below the regular adult recommendation, except for antibiotic and replacement therapy. With replacement therapy, the adult dose should be given and care taken to monitor antibiotics closely for side effects and toxicity.

By way of concluding, we would reemphasize the need for caution in geriatric pharmacotherapy, for restricting the number of drugs taken, and for holding dosages to the lowest effective amounts. Such a strategy requires attention to the patient's total intake of drugs, including the over-the-counter variety. The physician's labors do not end with a prescription; rather, they have only just begun. Unfortunately, there are no shortcuts to reliable management of the geriatric patient who may need drugs. One must take the time to get the drug history, check the drug taking, and consider nutritional and other aspects of the patient's condition. Given the fragility of the aged body, the motto for geriatric prescribing is, even more than in other patients, "first do no harm."

Common Complaints of the Elderly

DAVID ECKSTEIN
Meadow Lakes Retirement Community

This discussion of common complaints of the elderly proceeds from what may be an uncommon set of circumstances: I am a primary physician in a retirement community that offers essentially unlimited access to ambulatory care. Neither cost nor distance sets up any barrier. Also, my practice is entirely geriatric. Many physicians have asked me what primary care is like in such a setting. Do the elderly tend to overutilize services and overwhelm the doctor? Is their pattern of complaints radically different from that of other patients?

My response to such questions is no, and I will attempt to show why here. In describing features of my practice and clientele, my objective is not to be encyclopedic about common complaints of the elderly but rather to suggest a philosophy and some of the strategies to which they give rise.

Despite the absence of tangible barriers, my patient population shows no appetite for extravagant physician use. By and large, patients have a good reason for seeing the physician, though the reason may not be the one the patient advances. But there are some *intangible* barriers they must overcome: patients tend to internalize pejorative stereotypes of old people, and they will avoid seeing the physician rather than risk being identified with those stereotypes. Their sensitivity in this area is hardly unusual. Similar reactions are seen in patients on Medicaid.

But the residents of the Meadow Lakes Retirement Community, Hightstown, N.J., are financially secure. They are educated, former business or professional people who have received good medical care all their lives. Medical and skilled nursing services for our 374 residents, who average 81 years of age, are prepaid in their housing contracts. Another full-time physician and I are their primary practitioners. Four surgeons, a urologist, two dermatologists, two ophthalmologists, two podiatrists, and a dentist conduct clinics at the community. We also refer patients to outside specialists. Included on our staff are a registered physiotherapist, a radiology technician, and the nurses and other personnel at our 90-bed nursing facility. We primary physicians have regular office hours and also make emergency calls to apartments and detached dwellings. All in all, the two of us handle about 3,000 patient visits per year.

Complaints referrable to the cardiovascular system account for 13% of our visits. The most common clinical diagnosis is arteriosclerotic heart disease. Ischemic or coronary artery disease underlies about half the congestive failure cases, which are predominantly of the low output kind. Auricular fibrillation and other arrhythmias are often found to be due to too much or too little digitalis, too much diuretic, or too little potassium replacement. Cerebral thrombosis, cerebral hemorrhage, aortic aneurysm, and peripheral vascular insufficiency are seen with some frequency, but the impact in our population is relatively mild. Transient ischemic episodes outnumber the foregoing conditions; they are frightening, frustrating, refractory to specific therapy, and usually prognostic of aggravations. For patients seeking relief of dyspnea, edema, orthopnea, weakness, and angina, we have found that rest is as important as drug and dietary modalities. We tailor patients' activities to cardiac capacities by scheduling bedrest, identifying places where they should stop and wait en route to the centralized dining hall, and prescribing sedentary periods after meals and prior to exercise. Concurrent treatment of anemias and any other oxygen-restricting condition is of course essential, as is diet to maintain a low-normal weight.

Another 13% of visits involve muscles, tendons, joints, and bones. The figure understates the prevalence of these problems inasmuch as it refers only to patients with significant impairments. Most patients have some osteoarthritis; most accept it, if symptomatic, as a fact of long life. But it is upsetting to the person who enjoys the quarter-mile walk to and from the dining room.

In our women patients, osteoporosis frequently presents with pain from compression and overt fracture of dorsal and lumbar vertebrae. Minor falls, with a twisting motion, are disproportionate causes of femoral-neck damage. Sit-down injuries – pelvic fractures with poorly localized pain – are fairly common. In the seventh and eighth decades, men catch up statistically with women in frequency of osteoporosis. More often than with women, the fracture site in men is the femur, not the vertebrae. If the spine is involved, carcinoma of the prostate is considered before we accept a diagnosis of osteoporosis. In men and women with osteoporosis, Paget's disease must be considered.

Not too long ago, a femoral-neck fracture was virtually a ticket to the grave. We refer most patients for immediate surgery and count on having them returned to our skilled nursing facility in 10 days. The guiding word in postoperative therapy is "mobilization." Age is no deterrent if the circumstances are right. We recorded a successful operative result for our oldest resident, who had a femur fracture in her 100th year. She went on to celebrate her 101st birthday. This example does not mean we are complacent about femoral-neck repair. The preconditions for disaster linger on, in poor bone structure and proneness to accidental falls. It has been our experience that refracture produces total disability and accelerates the patient's general deterioration.

About 11% of office visits are for skin problems, generally of three kinds: 1) pruritus associated with dry skin; 2) senile actinic or seborrheic keratosis; and 3) neoplasms, chiefly basal cell carcinoma. The keratotic lesions, which are almost never solitary, are excised if size, number, and locations indicate the need. Basal cell carcinomas often are spread among benign keratoses. Hence the importance of consultation with the dermatologist. The biopsies or excisions required for histologic confirmation are done in our clinic. We are less likely to see squamous cell car-

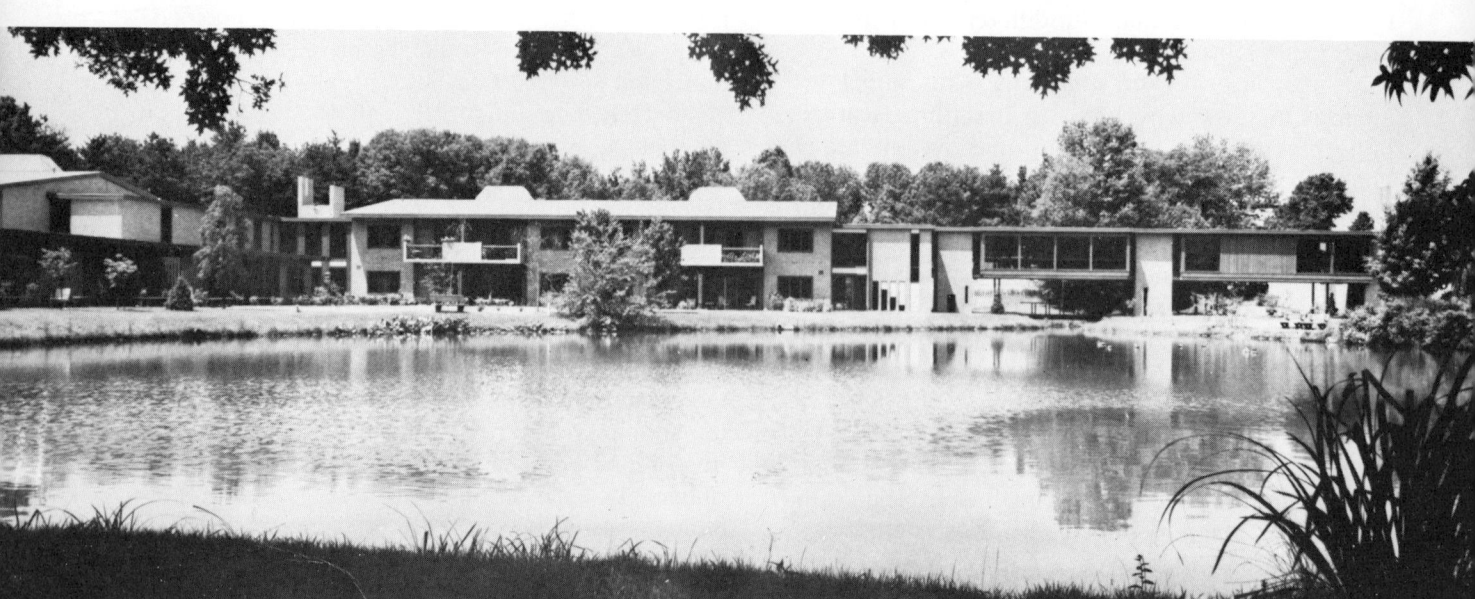

The 40-odd retirement community buildings are connected by enclosed walkways of which bridge seen at right in photo above is part. Residents thus can reach central complex (which includes dining hall and health center) on foot in any weather. Doctors' offices, clinic, and 90-bed skilled nursing facility are grouped in health center.

cinomas, which are of course more dangerous.

The chances of picking up dangerous lesions early are fairly good if they are prominent; concerned for their personal appearance, patients come in quickly to consult about blemishes on the face or hands. The most frequent complaint is itchy, dry, scaly skin; emollients and other compounds may be employed, but it is not easy to control a skin that has lost its lubricants. Pruritus can be set off by underclothes, detergents used in the wash, and even thiazides and other medications. Burns caused by improper use of heating pads are fairly frequent and heal with difficulty. We have found that it is important to provide instruction in the safe use of such devices.

About 8.5% of office visits are for urinary tract diseases. Our consulting urologist makes or confirms most diagnoses and supervises treatment, utilizing measurement of residual urine, cystometry, and cystoscopy. Our investigation of urinary complaints is never casual; it includes microscopic examination of urinary sediment, urine culture, and antibiotic sensitivity tests. In men, obstructive uropathy secondary to prostatic hypertrophy is the single overriding concern. In women, the most frequent problems are incontinence and/or infection. Time and again, we are reminded that atrophic vaginitis must be considered and dealt with (often quite easily with topical estrogen creams), since symptomatic complaints will persist in the absence of adequate hormonal levels.

About 15% of the visits are prompted by annual screenings, which we have found well justified. Aside from overt skin lesions, the greatest yields are breast and colon diseases. For example, one series of screenings produced four cases of right colon carcinoma; two patients are alive without identifiable metastasis two years after surgery. We find two to four cases of breast carcinoma annually, and the survival rate with early identification and treatment appears excellent. Another 5% of the visits are represented by problems of vision and hearing, 5% by respiratory and 10% by gastrointestinal disturbances. The remaining are classified as miscellaneous.

This miscellaneous group includes overt emotional problems, mostly depressive. Chronic alcoholism in our population has about the same prevalence as in any other population of comparable age, background, and affluence. Many have no family; others have been abandoned. This can be disastrous when combined with social rejection and other stresses of group living. My full-time colleague and I do considerable counseling. We have that "luxury" in medical practice that most physicians lack – time to listen and

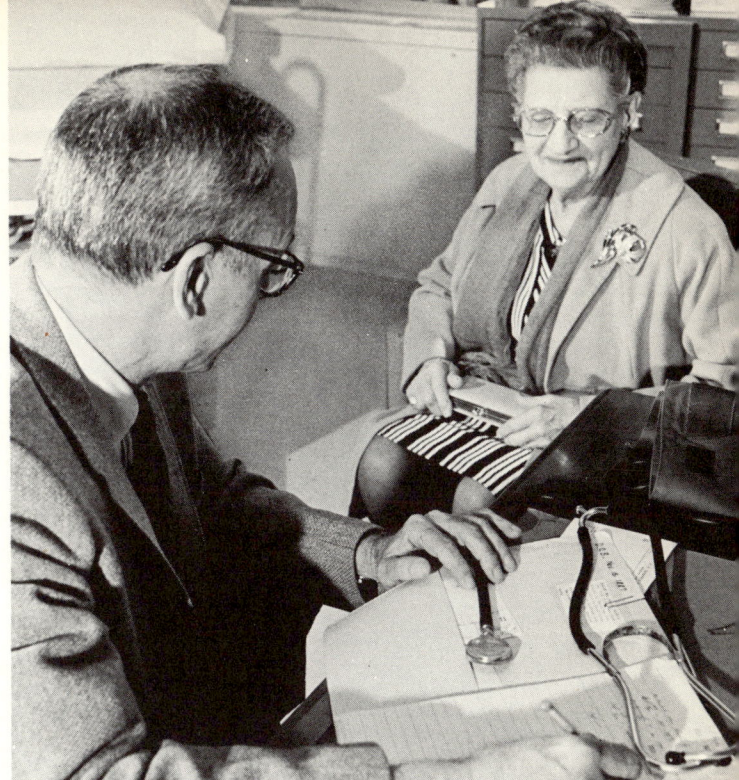

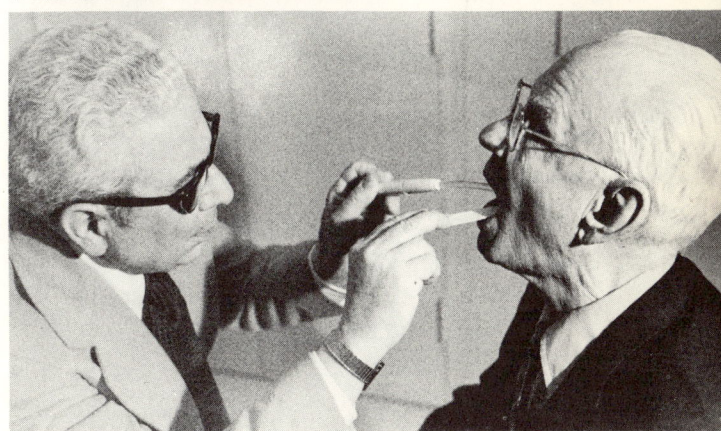

For ambulatory residents a visit to the doctor's office may be for an annual checkup (top), which all are urged to have, or a look at a sore throat (center). For the nursing facility patient (below) rounds may be as important for morale building as for medical problems.

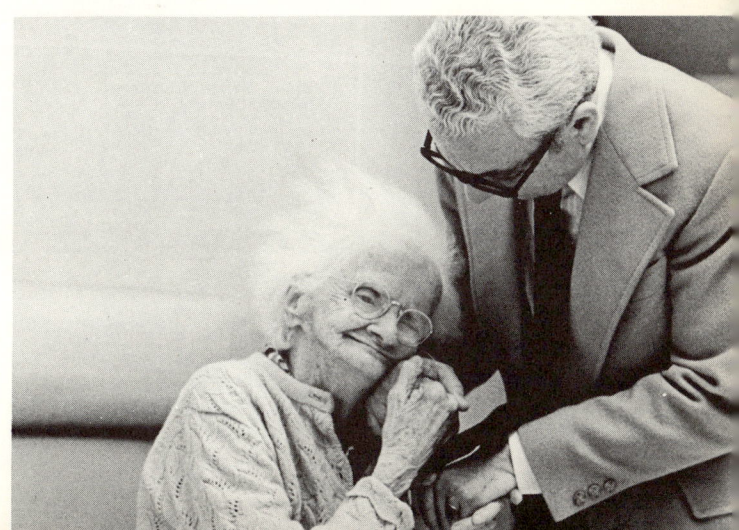

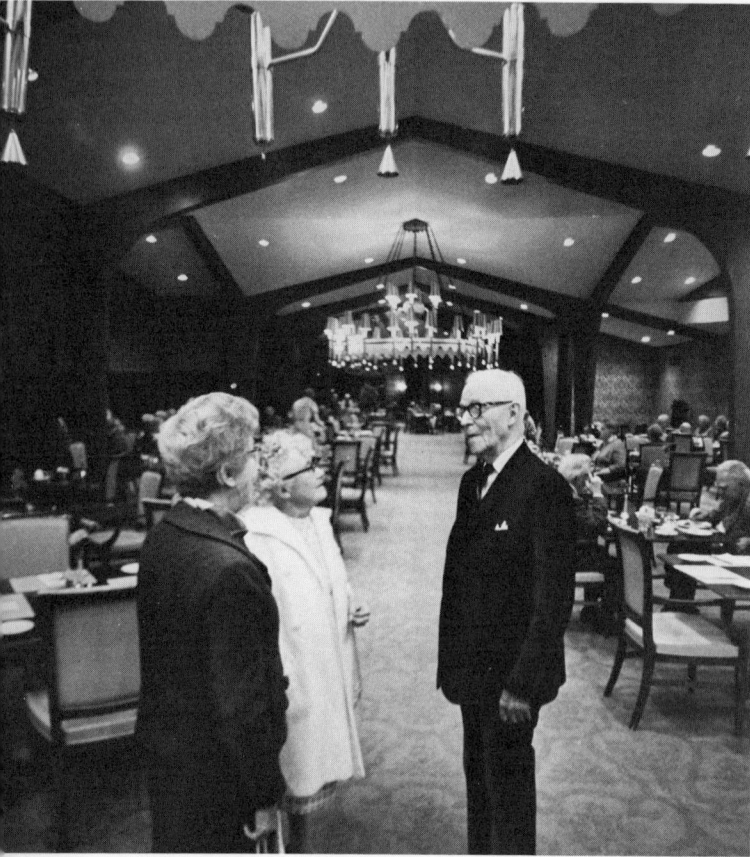

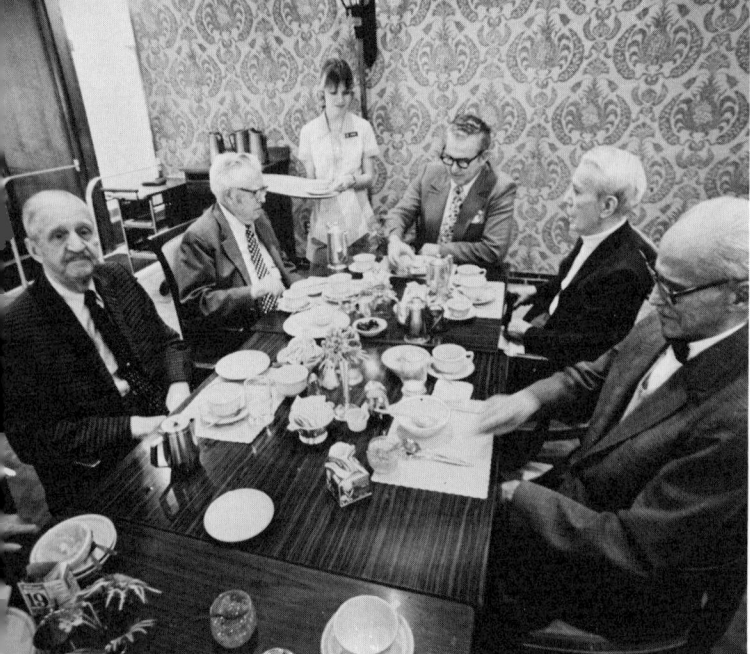

Taking meals in central dining hall (top) gives opportunity for social contact; "breakfast club" for widowers and bachelors (lower photo) helps get day off to good start.

chat with patients. We believe that as a consequence our need to prescribe tranquilizers is minimal.

Depression, agitation, petulance, and aggression may signal serious underlying problems, especially organic senile dementia. This is truly our major problem. As the population's average age rises, the frequency and severity of senile dementia grow. Let me be quite clear: I refer to disorganized, disheveled, frequently slovenly individuals who only recently became that way; hardly a month or year before, they had been well oriented, neat, and capable of independence in activities of daily living (dressing, feeding, walking, etc.). More than half of our 90 nursing beds are occupied by residents unable to function on their own, most of whom have senile dementia.

As I suggested at the outset, when an elderly person comes to see us, the complaint must be taken seriously. Old people do not complain unnecessarily. Their complaints may not be a reasonable interpretation of what is wrong. It's up to the physician to find out. Most of the time, we find that the elderly underplay their symptoms and problems. When I say that the patient nearly always has a good reason for an office visit, I include loneliness as a good reason. The individual may need reassurance that somebody cares. One of the ways in which we convey that we care is to make certain all our residents are well aware that there is medical coverage on weekends. To dramatize my concern, when I first came to Meadow Lakes I would move up and down dining-room waiting lines on the weekend, asking for someone I knew would *not* be there. It was my way of saying: "I'm here if you need me."

During an office visit we encourage patients to talk about their families, vacations, or whatever interests them, so we can know them better. We emphasize touching. We never stand in a doorway and say hello to a bed patient. I instruct the staff to put skin on skin, even to take a pulse unnecessarily. This is our way of encouraging human relationships. One result is that it is easy to spot personality change and recognize the first signs of senile dementia.

There is an emotional price for this policy. It is not easy to watch one's patient-friends disintegrate, nor to be calm in dealing with a difficult person one might prefer to ignore. It is no surprise to me that physicians who are close to the elderly fear what they see, especially the impact of societal attitudes that view the elderly person as expendable, unimportant, or useless. These attitudes have a corrosive effect on the patient. As job, home, and other societal frames are removed, unless the physician is careful he can lose sight of the patient as an individual.

Elderly patients often conceal complaints out of fear of being identified as old and useless. They become apologetic about visiting the physician. "I hate to bother you," they say. The statement bothers *us* very much, because it means they tend to delay obtaining an office consultation that might save them many nights of worry. For example, a woman will suspect breast cancer but will rationalize avoiding the doctor because the lump is "only a little thing"; however, at night, alone, she worries. A man who has rectal bleeding and a 20-pound weight loss will conceal the problem in fear of putting a further strain on the family. Willing to die, the patient resists intervention. One woman delayed seeing us a year so that she would be beyond surgery for breast cancer. She had her wish and died uncomfortably. In my view, when a patient *stops* visiting the doctor, it may signal concealment bordering on martyrdom.

Sometimes the complaint is based on a surrogate symptom. It is up to the physician to probe for the real problem. The patient may tell the doctor, as he tells his wife, that the office visit is occasioned by a wart. Actually, he wants to be examined for chest pains. We are not deterred from exploring possible problems just because the apparent cause of the visit is trivial. We hold fireside conferences for groups of residents to emphasize that they should not trivialize symptoms of potentially serious disease. Five minutes of consultation, we tell them, could prevent weeks of hospitalization. We urge them to articulate their worries, to ask questions about medical care, disease, and aging, to visit or telephone us about minor complaints, and to have an annual review of health status. We tell them that we must know about total drug intake, and we ask them to bring in the contents – often voluminous – of their medicine cabinets every six months; here we often find explanations of, or contributors to, their complaints. We talk about the potential adverse effects of cosmetics, deodorant sprays, and other grooming aids. We go over key points in nutrition, emphasizing how poor diet may be the underlying cause of certain symptoms.

The complaints I regard among the most serious concern mentation. Memory loss, confusion, and personality change are warnings of impending trouble, principally inability to cope with activities of daily living. These conditions may herald the beginning of the end of personal independence. Mental deterioration from cerebral arteriosclerosis or senile dementia progresses implacably, engulfing the individual finally in a dream world.

Some patients realize they are forgetting too many things. If they themselves do not request an office appointment, neighbors may urge them or may call them to our attention. It becomes important to us to

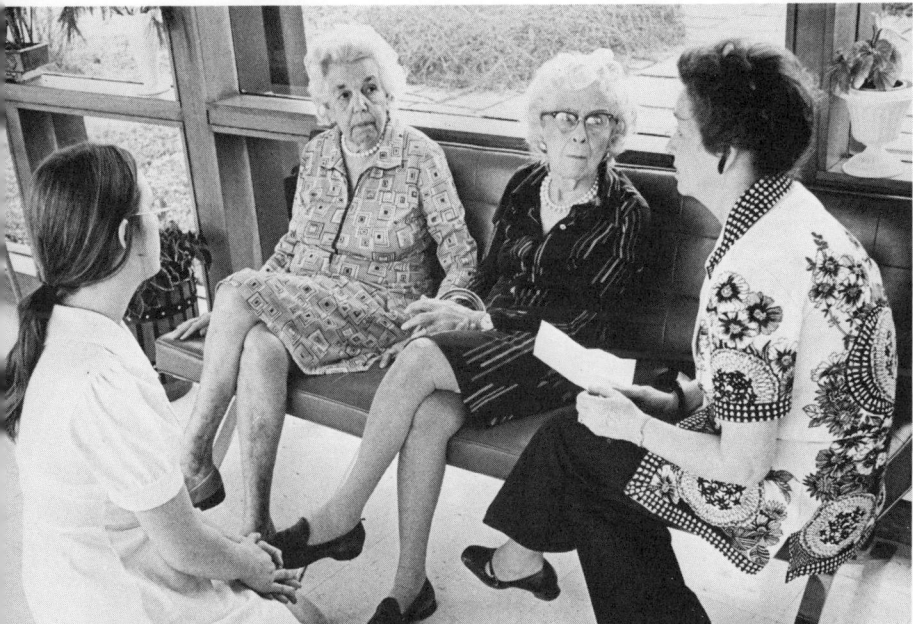
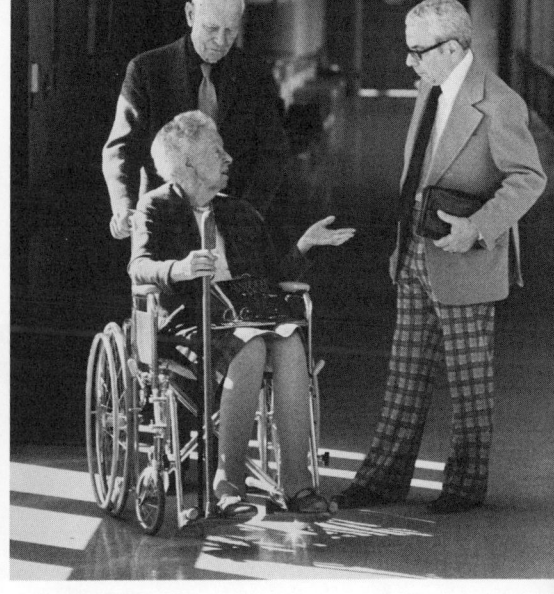

Transfer to the nursing facility is not solely for the bedfast. At left above, two health center staff members discuss food preferences with patients; at right, a corridor conference with physician during daily rounds.

13

know the kinds of social supports an individual may have; the individual who lacks neighbors and family may need closer medical supervision.

Complaints about worsening memory need not be calamitous; this may simply reflect lack of challenge, since memory can also go bad from disuse. In trying to discern the presence of true dementia, it is difficult to distinguish among memory loss, languor, and confusion. The search for a pattern of irrational behavior must be sophisticated, since confusion may not spread uniformly through all areas of activity or cognition. A woman may become well-nigh incompetent in most activities of daily living, but she will still know how to arrange her lipstick. A disheveled elderly woman, on the other hand, must be considered to be seriously ill. By contrast, men tend to become slovenly well in advance of serious mental deterioration, especially widowers who had depended heavily on their wives for self-maintenance. If the widower had already been a liberal user of alcohol, he is likely to begin drinking to excess. Since such individuals resist help, there will be considerable deterioration before the physician knows. At our community, we have a breakfast club of widowers and bachelors in an effort to build peer support.

With good social support, such as neighbors who render comfort and practical assistance, the need for institutionalization may be appreciably delayed. But sometimes neighbors and family have negative effects, which must not be overlooked. For example, we had a patient who was becoming paranoid and violent for no apparent physical reason. The problem turned out to be a domineering wife; it was she who needed counseling. In another instance, a man became depressed because the family exploited the physician's instruction against a dinner highball; it was part of a pattern of depreciating the man. The humiliation was especially profound because others at the dinner table imbibed freely.

In such situations, our experience has been that our own methods of counseling were as effective as referrals for psychiatric care. Finding that recovery from depression took no more time in our own hands, we restricted referrals to the most difficult cases. We learned that patients often simply need a chance to vent their feelings; they may have nobody other than the physician to talk to. At Hightstown, fears of gossip and of being criticized restrain some patients from being intimate with their peers, and individuals with no family visitors depend on the doctor to listen. Our policy is to take the time to do so. In our view, in many instances depression and loneliness reflect an endemic social disease: the stereotyping of the elderly person as "senile" or "peculiar" when he or she acts individualistically.

Fatigue and insomnia, as well as depression, may

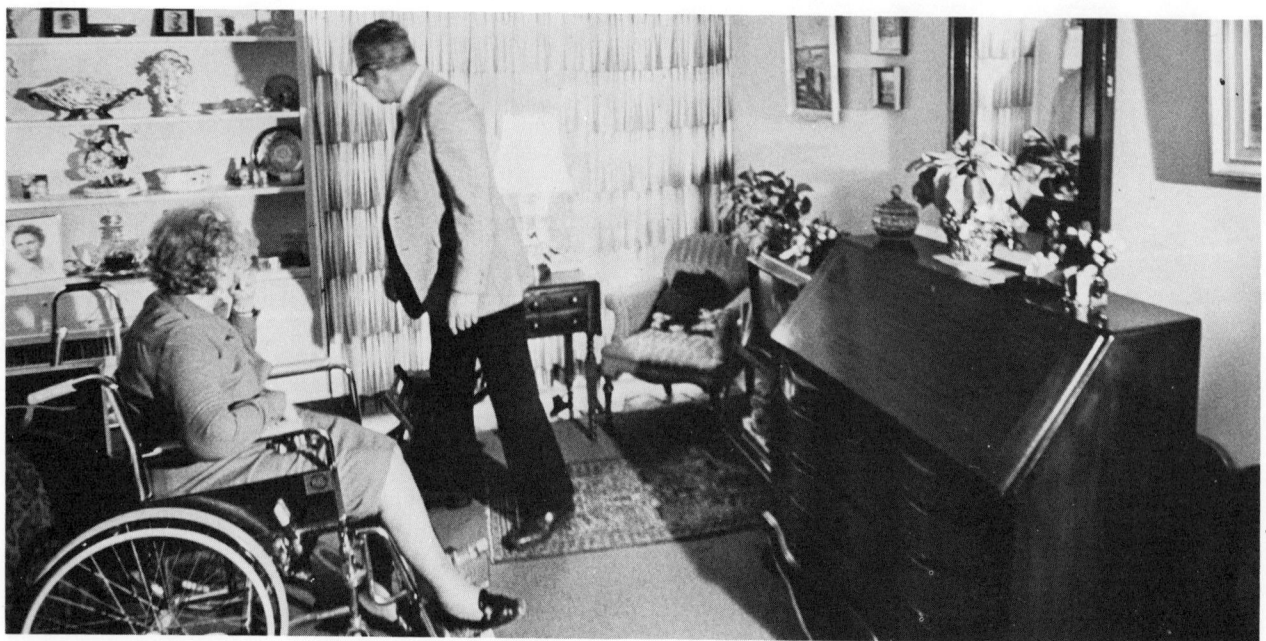

Residents furnish their own dwelling units and when time comes to enter nursing facility, it greatly eases the transition to take along as many as possible of their own possessions, as in the case of the woman seen above.

reflect emotional tensions for which counseling provides a remedy. The complaints *can* be met by prescribing pills. But we do not prescribe until we have tried to identify and resolve the cause of tension. Fatigue may result from apprehension about health, love, disability, dependency, mental deterioration, and rapport with children. In our population of hard-driving achievers, the insecurities of the change in their lives may reinforce a habit of using sedatives and tranquilizers that cause fatigue – another reason for obtaining a thorough drug history.

This is not to say that we have a solution to offer for the functional disorders for which the elderly rely on drug palliation. Rather than sit in judgment, we yield to demands for minor drugs and injections, for example, vitamin B_{12}. If the injection or drug makes the patient feel better, we do not oppose it. It is well-nigh impossible, in our experience, to withdraw the elderly patient from such minor addictions.

Boredom or social withdrawal can also produce fatigue. Abandonment by family promotes withdrawal; it is a matter of embarrassment for the elderly person to be asked by peers why a son or daughter did not visit or why a vacation with one or the other lasted a few days instead of a few weeks. People who cannot cope with emotional crises or unpleasantness want to be left alone with their fatigue.

Fatigue, of course, may have other bases. We do not ascribe fatigue to an emotional cause until physical possibilities have been ruled out. Fatigue, shortness of breath, angina, and edema may originate in cardiac disease or anemia. Besides checking the heart, I routinely ask for a hemoglobin determination for the patient reporting chronic fatigue. In the event of rectal bleeding, my focus goes immediately to the colon and bowel. A surprisingly high number of cancers of the right and ascending colon have been found when this suspicion was followed up. In the man with skeletal pain, urinary difficulty, and bleeding, the seriousness of prostatic possibilities warrants an immediate referral to the urologist.

A patient in the midst of emotional upheaval will present with physical complaints based on genuine disability. Diverticulosis can flare up, complete with diarrhea and cramping. Similarly, existing cardiac disease can worsen because of tension, sleeplessness, and fatigue that are induced by emotional problems. An environmental change – such as change in nursing staff or absence of a friend or a change in residence – may destabilize an elderly person and produce agitation and confusion. Tranquilizers may aggravate the symptoms. (In our nursing facilities, where the staff is stable, we have found little need to tranquilize or restrain most patients.) Change must be viewed as the worst influence on a precariously stabilized or already unstable patient. The traumatic effects can be softened by minimizing environmental change. For example, if a patient must be removed from his apartment to our nursing facility, he is accompanied by a favorite chair, a treasured picture, familiar wardrobe, etc. And there is no medication to rival the support of friends, familiar figures among the nursing staff, and the physician with whom a successful rapport has been built.

The physician may never be sure where a common complaint may lead, of course. As I have pointed out, an emotional complaint may have a physical origin and vice versa. The possible interactions are innumerable and idiosyncratic. That is why I cannot overstress the value of the physician's knowing the patient as a personality rather than as a sequence of problems. The cue to probing for specific physical difficulties often comes from discerning behavioral change. Let me now give some consideration to a few of these difficulties.

Communicative disorders are among the most serious and widely experienced threats to the quality of life. They may present at first as behavioral problems. For example, the patient who develops paranoia may be growing deaf. He cannot make out what others are saying or laughing about and begins to think a conspiracy is afoot. Sometimes a hearing aid will help but sometimes it does not; because it funnels sounds unselectively, the aid may not help the patient focus on what he or she wants to hear. Failure to obtain anticipated results may exacerbate a patient's agitation. We routinely refer patients to a hospital-based audiologist for evaluation and discourage turning to commercial hearing-aid distributors (who have an obvious conflict of interest in making an evaluation and recommendation). Unfortunately, some patients will not accept a professional assessment when the prognosis is unpleasant.

Loss of vision, like loss of hearing, impedes activities our patients thrive on, such as reading, watching television, and writing, and brings out sensitivities to physical symptoms that otherwise might be ignored. The loss may prompt introspection and bitter complaining after the patient is told that little or nothing can be done. In general, patients tend to present earlier with visual than with hearing problems.

If they experience a sharp, severe pain and inflammation of the eye, patients waste no time in visiting us. Our community has been alerted to the possibility of glaucoma. Occasionally surgery can be done the same day a diagnosis is confirmed. Sometimes the surgeon finds the heartbreak of macular degeneration behind a cataract, and what should have been a successful operation becomes an unhappy occasion. By itself, macular degeneration provokes complaints of inability to focus and read, but there is no pain or discomfort, despite loss of central vision. We are frank to tell patients of the hopeless prognosis in order to deter them from a vain round of shopping for specialists and spectacles.

When musculoskeletal problems are combined with vision and hearing deficits, patients are enormously upset. They feel their world brutally contracting. By themselves, musculoskeletal problems are likely to be accepted. The most common complaints are: cervical or lumbosacral pain, difficulty in turning in bed, difficulty in bending to lace shoes, loss of arm strength and pain radiating down the arms, and occasional occipital headache (from cervical degeneration). Ordinarily the patient apologizes for seeing the doctor about these problems. They say they realize it's "old age." We refrain from saying to a complaining patient: "What do you expect at your age?" Nor do we ever categorize musculoskeletal disease by age; I have banished age from our medical charts. What we do attempt, with help of a rheumatology consultant, is to resolve a complaint, and we do not give up until we are certain nothing can be done. Elective surgical intervention and medical therapy have had encouraging results.

We and our patients must be on guard against falls, which can of course be devastating to the patient with fragile bone structure. We pay particular attention to symptoms of poor balance. Staggering, because of slower response by the vestibular mechanism, is a serious cause of accidents. The slower vestibular reaction tends to make the individual pitch or twist too far. Consequently, we try to train patients to compensate. They are advised to turn the whole body, not just the head alone, to sit for a while on the edge of a bed after arising, and to stand for a few seconds before walking away. We teach them to be careful after eating, explaining that the concentration of blood in the abdomen leaves the brain relatively anoxic. We assure worried patients that syncope by itself is not a premonitory sign of stroke. We urge them to report periods of weakness, confusion, or blackout, which in combination with headache, ocular changes, and carotid bruit suggest stroke.

Because muscle tone deteriorates, constipation is a frequent complaint. Patients may complain of constipation when they mean that they are not having the daily bowel movement they consider necessary. The expectation that bowels must move daily is erroneous, and this must be explained. However, even if the patient reports daily bowel movement, a complaint about discomfort in the lower bowel or rectum should be investigated. It is possible to have a bolus of impaction *and* a bypass stool or diarrhea.

Rectal discomfort seems to be well reported; patients apparently have little reluctance to mention problems arising from hemorrhoids and fissures. Even if these are not apparent, we routinely put a finger in the rectum and take a stool specimen to check for blood, a routine that should always be performed; this is especially important in a patient with poor vision, as a negative response to a question about stool color is meaningless from such a patient. (In contrast, patients are likely to report blood in the urine.)

How, then, to summarize our philosophy about the complaining elderly patient? Basically, we view common complaints not as trivia to be dismissed quickly but as opportunities to expand our rapport with patients. I am the first to admit that our retirement community situation gives us considerably more time to do this than the typical primary practitioner may have. But absent this advantage, good medical care of the elderly cannot be accomplished if the effort is not made.

Given the large burden of illnesses and disabilities the elderly endure, the relative paucity of their symptoms, their high threshhold of pain, and their keenness in distinguishing the important from the unimportant symptom, the complaints of the elderly are remarkably low-keyed and valid. They justify compassionate attention. It is a humbling experience to witness the great courage with which so many elderly people meet adversity.

Multiple Problems in the Elderly

WILLIAM REICHEL
Franklin Square Hospital

Five attributes of geriatric patients make diagnosis and treatment in this age group one of the most complex tasks in medicine. The elderly generally show diminutions of physiologic capacities; in fact, the definition of aging is the decline in physiologic capacities or functions in an organism after the period of reproductive maturity. In addition, typical signs and symptoms of disease – such as temperature elevation and pain – may be absent, attenuated, or delayed. The effect of drugs is greater, and so is the potential for adverse reactions and interactions. Physical disease often presents as mental disorder – which is called the acute brain syndrome. Finally, the elderly patient tends to have multiple clinical and other problems, and these bear on the potentials of and approaches to therapy.

Many pitfalls thus stand in the way of correct diagnosis and treatment. Perhaps the greatest of all is stereotyping the elderly patient as the victim of "aging" or arteriosclerosis, obviously irreversible processes. This excuses us from compiling and analyzing the problems about which the patient complains and from considering the differential diagnoses. Somewhere along the line, treatable problems may be passed over. Yet, as I propose to show, there are concepts and methods that the physician can employ to avoid the pitfalls, find the treatable problems, and set priorities for treatment in an orderly way.

Physiologic processes that change with age include kidney and liver function, which undergo decrements that may not be pathologic in themselves. However, decreases in the functional capacity of various organ systems will affect the course of disease elsewhere in the body. An example is the patient with myocardial infarction superimposed on age-associated loss of lung and kidney function. One of the most judgmental aspects of geriatric care is knowing *when* to treat a problem. Some changes with age demonstrable on laboratory tests may or may not be prodromal: decreased glucose tolerance, elevated blood urea nitrogen, or low creatinine-clearance values may be considered normal for age. If youth-based standards of glucose tolerance or other parameters were applied, most of the elderly might be classified as diseased, with a concomitant obligation to treat.

Besides determining when a functional decline has crossed the divide from physiologic to pathologic, we must be able to interpret signs and symptoms of disease that may have a different or more subtle presentation in the elderly. The latency of disease in the aged is exemplified by slower and less intense response to infection. The elderly may have pneumonia or pyelonephritis without a temperature rise. Bronchial pneumonia may appear suddenly as a terminal event with few clinical signs. Indeed, some patients in whom postmortem examination reveals significant bilateral pulmonary infection have been ambulatory until almost the very end.

Leukocyte counts are diminished in the elderly, and pain cannot be counted on to signal disease either. In the elderly, pain may be much less in myocardial infarction and in such acute abdominal crises as perforated appendix, mesenteric infarction, and ruptured abdominal aorta. The older person with subacute bacterial endocarditis may show less evidence of fever and embolic phenomena.

As Drs. Lamy and Vestal pointed out (see Chapter 1, "Drug Prescribing for the Elderly") the elderly are especially prone to adverse reactions from some drugs, particularly tranquilizers, digoxin, and diuretics, at doses generally safe in younger adults. The causes of enhanced drug effect seem to lie in altered metabolic activity, changes in central nervous system responsiveness, and lower rates of elimination because of diminished kidney and hepatic function. Overall, the elderly population shows greater variability in drug response, and adverse drug reaction is among the most common problems observed in daily practice.

I have already mentioned that physical disease often presents as mental disorder. I have dealt with this subject in greater detail in Chapter 5, "Organic Brain Syndromes." However, I would note that because of the compromises in brain function that accompany aging, elderly patients tend to show confusion and disorientation as a first sign of infection, pneumonia, cardiac failure, coronary occlusion, electrolyte imbalance, anemia, or dehydration. The brain changes may have no behavioral expression at all in the absence of major stress. The presumption of senility or "chronic brain syndrome" is unwarranted in the context of sudden behavioral change; rather, we may be dealing with the behavioral concomitants of a reversible medical illness or drug toxicity.

For all the reasons discussed so far, the existence of multiple clinical and pathologic diagnoses in patients aged 70 or more should not be surprising. Postmortem examination may reveal as many as 10 or 20, some of which were asymptomatic. In addition to the elderly patient's multiple problems, he may easily acquire within the hospital or long-term care facility new problems that complicate his total picture. Not uncommonly, a patient may enter a hospital or other institution with cardiac disease or pneumonia and then go on to develop multiple other problems simply because he is in this new and unfamiliar environment with its many potential hazards. Drug reaction, reactions to procedures, accidents and falls, hospital-acquired infections, psychologic decompensation, and medical and nursing errors – including errors of omission – are all potential dangers within an institutional environment. In any environment – the patient's home or an institution – accidents in particular may bring on new problems. If an accident results in immobilization, such physical sequelae as pulmonary emboli may occur. In addition, an accident may precipitate a loss of self-confidence leading to despondency that has a much greater influence on the patient's life-style than the minor physical trauma of the accident itself. For example: an elderly motorist who fails to see a red light and has a collision without physical injury may then refuse to drive again. Loss of mobility because of osteoarthritis and other physical ailments, such as obesity, may also aggravate and intensify the patient's totality of physical and emotional problems. In these ways, multiple problems become compounded and prove as frustrating to the physician as to the patient.

All of these considerations lead us to the essence of geriatrics: the discovery and management of many problems simultaneously. How can the office practitioner cope with these problems systematically? An important tool is the problem-oriented record.

Medical recordkeeping in general has been immensely improved by the problem-oriented approach pioneered by Dr. Lawrence Weed. Among patients, no group can benefit more than the geriatric. The records of geriatric patients are voluminous. Various specialists may have been called into consultation; all report to the primary physician. Without a problem-oriented record, important notes may be ignored, forgotten, or buried, and it would become difficult and tedious to keep track of the patient's multiple problems, to establish treatment pri-

	Attributes of Geriatric Patients
1	Physiologic capacities are diminished; e.g., kidney and liver functions are usually depressed.
2	Typical signs and symptoms of disease may be absent, attenuated, or delayed; e.g., pain may be absent in myocardial infarction or ruptured appendix; fever may be minimal in pneumonia.
3	Drug effects are usually more pronounced and adverse reactions more likely.
4	Physical disease often presents as acute confusional reaction (acute brain syndrome).
5	Multiple clinical, psychological, and social problems are characteristic.

Problem List

S.N. Age: 89
DOB: 12/22/85

Prob. No.	Problem	Date Resolved	Date Onset	Date Recorded
1.	Vertigo		9/73	10/11/73
2.	Osteoarthritis		15 yr	10/11/73
3.	Xerosis of skin		5-12 yr	10/11/73
4.	Cervical spine disease secondary to #2		10 yr	10/11/73
5.	History of orthostatic dizziness		3 yr	10/11/73
6.	History of intermittent dyspnea on exertion		3/73	10/11/73
7.	Bilateral immature cataracts		3 yr	10/11/73
8.	Long history of depression with hypochondriasis		30-40 yr	10/11/73
9.	Arteriosclerotic cardiovascular disease with arteriosclerotic cerebrovascular disease		25 yr	10/11/73
10.	Stress incontinence		10 yr	11/16/73
11.	Nocturnal leg cramps		11/10/73	11/16/73
12.	~~Macular rash chest, back, and legs for 5 days~~	Prior to 3/20/74	2/8/74	2/15/74
13.	Benign gastric ulcer		2/74	3/29/74
14.	Painful gums		10 days	1/29/75
15.	~~Viral upper respiratory infection~~	2/28/75	2/23/75	2/26/75
16.	Calluses on feet		6-12 mo	10/6/75
17.				
18.				

> ### SOAPing' a Problem
>
> In organizing progress notes, the physician refers to the problem list and deals with each problem in a separate note according to the SOAP acronym: Subjective findings, Objective findings, Assessment, and Plan.
> For example:
>
> Date 10/9/75
> Problem #4, hypertension
>
> **S** Occasional frontal headaches, especially with emotional stress. Two episodes of dizziness during the past week.
>
> **O** Blood pressure 190/120, pulse 84, weight 211 lb (loss of 3 lb), grade II retinopathy.
>
> **A** No improvement in control of blood pressure.
>
> **P** Increase methyldopa 250 mg to 2 tablets *t i d;* increase chlorothiazide to 500 mg *t i d*. Continue weight-reduction program. Return in two weeks.

orities, and to follow up the results. I refer not only to medical problems but also to social and psychologic problems as well, including habituation to cigarettes and alcohol, poor diet, loss of spouse and job, and limitations of income and housing.

An essential adjunct to the problem-oriented record is a medication flow sheet covering prescribed and over-the-counter drugs. The per capita drug consumption among the elderly and the potentials for misuse warrant special concern.

The core of the problem-oriented record is the problem list that serves as a table of contents for the patient's chart. Included in the list are the problems derived from diagnoses: isolated or unexplained symptoms, signs, laboratory findings, and social and psychologic information. Based on the data gathering and on the organization of the data into a first approximation of problems, the physician by himself or with specialists will determine which problems merit immediate investigation. With more information and the differential diagnoses in hand, the physician is in an excellent position to formulate treatment priorities. And these, of course, may be changed and supplemented as the patient's condition varies and more information comes in.

Progress notes are organized according to problem. Each note covers subjective findings, objective findings, assessment, and plan (as illustrated on this page). If adhered to by primary physician and specialists, this logical recordkeeping permits progress to be traced with considerable clarity for a single problem over time and for several problems at once.

The approach can be defeated if each problem is not viewed with an open mind. If the elderly patient reports dysuria, the problem should not be presumed out of hand to be benign prostatic hypertrophy; it may be carcinoma of the prostate or obstruction of the bladder neck, among other possibilities. The problem may appear to be dementia, but this is not necessarily arteriosclerotic brain disease; it may be pernicious anemia, myxedema, or normal pressure hydrocephalus, and the list could go on. The physician must be alert to the possibility that a symptom or sign may not represent the entities that he usually sees in daily practice.

If a problem is dismissed cursorily, a treatable condition may be missed. To conclude that congestive heart failure generally represents arteriosclerotic heart disease may be correct, but the individual patient may be among the smaller number who have rheumatic heart disease and may even be a reasonable candidate for surgery.

Geriatrics' major pitfall is the "wastebasket" diagnosis, resulting in unjustified conclusions that dismiss the need for careful evaluation of each elderly patient. The remedy lies in carrying the definition of each problem as far as one possibly can go. Then the physician can consider treatment possibilities.

The decisions concerning any one disease on a

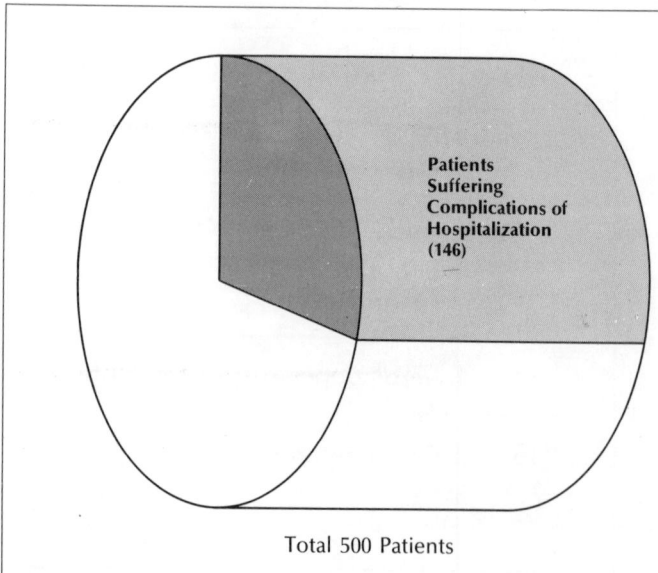

Total 500 Patients

Graphs above are based on study undertaken by the author and demonstrate that the rate of hospital-related

problem list are influenced by all the other diseases and by the patient's physical, psychologic, and social condition. Based on the total picture, it may be proper to elect *not* to treat certain entities. I might be more conservative in treating a stroke victim if the patient has a history of two previous myocardial infarctions and cancer. I may not select certain treatments for less urgent problems when the patient already has received about as large a group of medications as I think he can manage. Similarly, it may be more important to the patient to remain at home with limited therapies available than to reside in an institution where more comprehensive modalities are accessible.

Sometimes, issues posed by the problem list must be left in doubt. Evaluative studies cannot be pushed too far in some frail patients. In an 80-year-old patient with mild anemia that is hypochromic and microcytic, with a history of positive stool guaiacs that have turned negative, and with a normal gastrointestinal series, barium enema, and proctoscopy, I may decline to press beyond these basic hematologic and gastrointestinal studies. It may be desirable to initiate iron therapy and then leave the matter to follow-up and further surveillance. In a younger person, there might be greater pressure to pursue further hematologic tests or endoscopy in order to be more certain of the cause of anemia and blood loss.

In some cases, the problem is identified, but complications deter effective management of it. Let us say that a patient with an ulcer, heart disease, and diabetes develops acute gout, possibly related to the use of thiazide medications for hypertension. Oral colchicine or phenylbutazone may not be used because of the ulcer. Intravenous colchicine is tried but seems to worsen the GI complaints. There are other situations in which the treatment of one problem is complicated by the presence of another. Examples include the stroke patient in rehabilitation who develops serious heart failure or the patient with congestive failure who needs IV fluids or transfusions that aggravate the cardiac condition.

In reviewing the list of problems, the physician may find a physical or mental problem, which, if resolved, would permit the patient to tolerate other infirmities. Relatively minor problems of vision, hearing, dentition, nutrition, and ambulation may precipitate a crisis with respect to self-sufficiency in the patient with multiple disabilities.

A patient's depressive symptoms may have to take priority over physical illness in the management plan. It may be futile to prescribe for the patient's hypertension, gout, psoriasis, or chronic prostatitis if the patient – depressed over recent loss of spouse – does not want to cooperate. The physician may have to wait until the patient's depression is better controlled before other problems are dealt with.

Some elderly patients require multiple types of

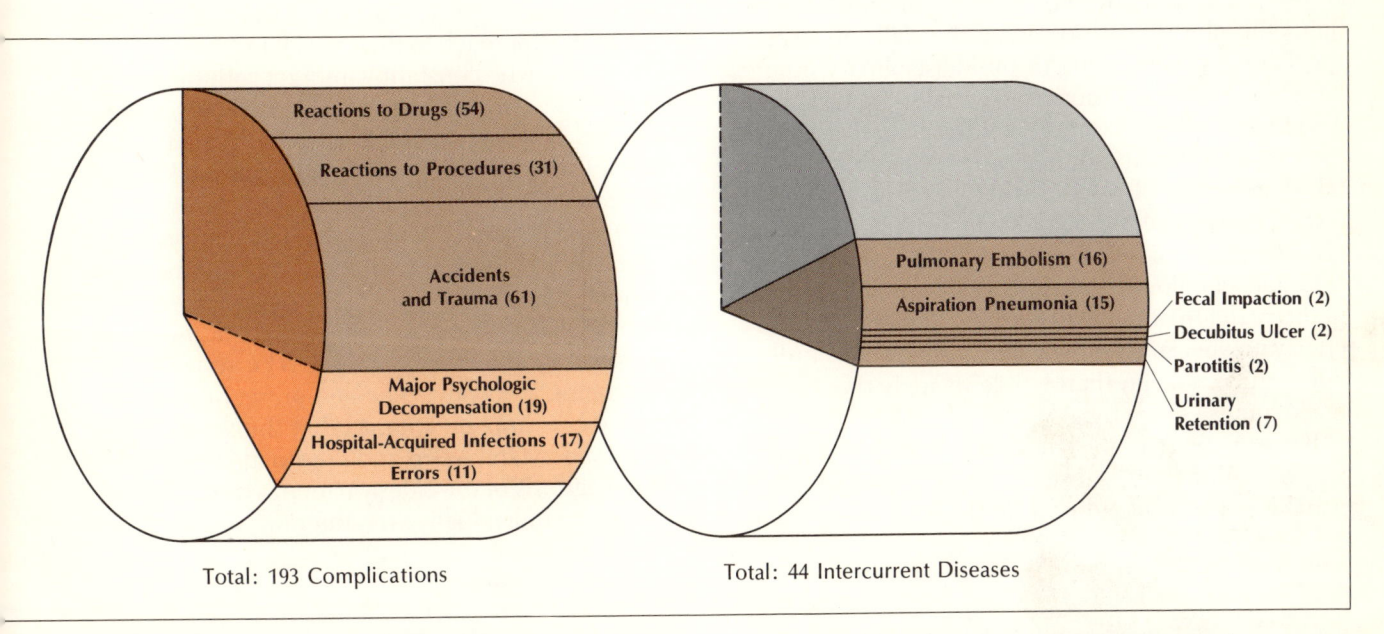

complications in elderly patients is quite high. Among 500 consecutively admitted patients aged 65 or over (average age 77.9 years), 146 experienced 193 adverse reactions and 44 suffered intercurrent diseases.

	Treating The Geriatric Patient
1	Utilize problem-oriented record.
2	Utilize medication flow sheet.
3	View each problem with open mind–consider the full differential diagnosis for the problem.
4	Use as few medications as possible; resist using over two or three medications unless absolutely necessary.
5	Avoid pushing diagnostic studies too far in frail patients.
6	Simplify drug schedules; make instructions very specific; reinforce verbal instructions with written instructions.
7	Resist temptation to treat new symptoms with still more drugs.
8	Involve and communicate with other specialists, counselors, and therapists, such as dieticians, physical therapists, or psychologists.
9	Review patient's problem with patient and/or family.
10	Interact constantly with patient, giving patient sufficient time.

counseling or therapy. The problem-oriented record helps the physician to organize the skills of several specialists. The focusing of multidisciplinary inputs for each problem becomes especially important in deciding whether or not to treat the patient at home, in a day-care facility, or in a nursing home or hospital. The inputs of physical therapist, speech therapist, occupational therapist, social worker, psychologist, dietitian, audiologist, nurse, etc., are most useful when all follow the same format in providing their findings and treatment suggestions. Alone, in conference with specialists one by one, or in a team conference, the physician then is able to apply these organized inputs efficiently.

If the patient is in a hospital or skilled nursing home, the institutional staffs can be drawn on. It is usually not possible to provide the best patient care without multidisciplinary assistance in complex cases; this is especially true in certain problem areas such as stroke. Often, participation by family members in multidisciplinary conferences is valuable in contemplating courses of action, especially in seeking alternatives to institutionalizing the patient.

If the patient's mental status permits, I will review my evaluation of the patient's problems with him or her and, with consent, with family members. In the discussion, problems that require treatment now will be pointed out and others will be noted for treatment later. I present my assessment and my treatment plan in a hopeful manner. It is important to offer positive approaches whenever possible, to help these patients understand their medical status and find meaning and value in old age despite the disabilities. For example, even though a patient is severely restricted by a stroke or a cardiac condition, I believe he or she can appreciate the positive attributes of life – the relationships with children and grandchildren, religious involvement, enjoyment of friends, books, and conversation.

There are, of course, circumstances in which candor is counterproductive. A patient may have to be prepared before he or she can be given information about cancer or severe congestive heart failure. Some patients tell physicians clearly that they do not want to know about cancer. But some show no reluctance; indeed, they go, say, to surgery precisely because they view themselves as partners with the physician in the approach to their problems.

Physicians who constantly interact with the elderly may form a personal view of aging, its multiple problems, and how they would like to be treated if they were in the same situation. Is aging all loss? I don't believe so. There are positive attributes in terms of maturity, experience, insights into truth, expressions of warmth and love, and relationships to others in a new dimension.

A physician's scientific and humanistic resources are tapped by the elderly patient. The response can be medicine at its best. The commitment to providing good care implies, among other things, an obligation to understand when and how to make the differential diagnosis of the elderly patient's multiple problems and to individualize treatment.

4

Functional Psychiatric Disorders

JOY R. JOFFE
Johns Hopkins University

Symptoms of confusion, disorientation, agitation, or disturbances in levels of consciousness in the elderly may have a basis in physical disease and/ or drug toxicity. Such a basis must, of course, be ruled out before a diagnosis of functional behavioral disorder can be entertained, either as a component of the patient's overall condition or by itself. Once the diagnosis of a functional disorder has been made in an elderly person, however, the family or primary physician is often in the best position to manage these emotional problems through counseling, medication, family, friends, and outside community services. (For a discussion of organic dementia and its differential diagnosis, see Chapter 5 by Dr. William Reichel.)

It is essential to recognize that in our culture, aging has physical and socioenvironmental concomitants that often give rise to medical problems. But the belief that emotional illness is a natural attribute of being elderly is a myth. Neither is it true that every aged person who is depressed or paranoid is so seriously or psychotically ill that an office approach is in vain. Actually, relatively few of the nation's 22 million elderly are sufficiently impaired mentally or physically to require long-term institutionalization. Only 5% are in nursing homes, psychiatric hospitals, or similar institutions.

However, there appears to be considerable psychiatric morbidity of a degree that can be handled in office practice. Several community surveys suggest that 10% to 20% of the general U.S. population have some psychiatric morbidity. While some observers might argue that the rate among the elderly is higher, applying the 10% to 20% rate to the estimated elderly population in 1975 would show that 2.1 million to 4.3 million may need help, and that perhaps 430,000 receive institutional services (in hospitals and community mental health centers). A 1973 study by Richard W. Redick and colleagues projected that in 1975 and even in 1980 "about 80% to 84% of those in need of services, among persons of all ages as well as those 65 years and older, would not be receiving services in the defined universe of psychiatric facilities" (i.e., public and private mental hospitals, inpatient psychiatric services of general hospitals, outpatient psychiatric services, and community mental health centers). If nothing else, this study suggests that office practice is encountering, and will continue to encounter, significant mental illness in the aging, and this population segment is growing.

Amid the paucity of epidemiologic data about mental illness, one may find indicators of the seriousness of the problem among the elderly. The highest suicide rates in 1974 (20.5 to 21.5 deaths per 100,000 population) were found in the age groups above 55; they are highest of all among white males, rising progressively from 32.4 in the 50-to-54 age group to 48 plus in the group beyond age 74, and showing a strong correlation with alcoholism.

The physician frequently has to work against a tide of lay misconceptions that contribute to functional disorders. I recall the reaction of a son to my recommendation that his 80-year-old mother be hospitalized so that the proper chemotherapy for depression could be carried out. He resisted. I asked: "If your mother were 40, would you question hospitalization? What is so different about being 80? Isn't her time important to her?" He relented, coming to understand that the persisting depression was destructive not only to his mother but to his family, with whom she lived. Subject to the same kinds of functional disorders as the young, the elderly, regrettably, tend to be abandoned to a degree not only by society but by specialties, such as my own, psychiatry. Some physicians tend to interpret many reversible and treatable functional disorders as irreversible dementia, thus denying the elderly the right to treatment. Such therapeutic pessimism may reflect the difficulty physicians and others have in trying to resolve their own fears of aging, death, and abandonment.

Yet if we look at the facts, we see that the prognosis generally is excellent for elderly patients with depression or another functional disorder. Such depressions are treatable in various ways, provided someone recognizes the problem and is familiar with the modalities.

The primary or family physician who has attended a patient for many years often is in the best position to treat certain functional disorders. Indeed, that physician often has a unique opportunity 1) to estimate the patient's ability to cope with the kinds of stresses expectable in old age; 2) to try to help the patient prepare for them before it is too late and thereby to prevent an emotional crisis; and 3) to treat the troubled patient in the most humanly effective way.

A key to preventing or minimizing functional disorders lies in the fact that people of different temperaments meet adversity in different ways. In Plato's *Republic*, Cephalus responds to Socrates' questioning about old age by noting that "He who is of a calm and happy nature will hardly feel the pressure of age, but to him who is of an opposite disposition youth and age are equally a burden." Life-styles have a timeless character, enduring despite organic impairment. An example is the ex-businessman whose habit of smiling when greeting people continues into senile dementia, or whose gesticulatory pattern persists though he speaks incoherently.

It is imperative for the physician who is first seeing an elderly patient or who is going to follow a patient for years to develop an awareness of how the person meets the stresses of life and what is the person's essential life-style. Rigidity in dealing with stresses – seen in compulsive work activity – may take root early in life and represent behavioral time bombs. When the physical and social losses of old age occur, the effects on the rigid personality may be devastating. An accountant whose meticulousness indicates a

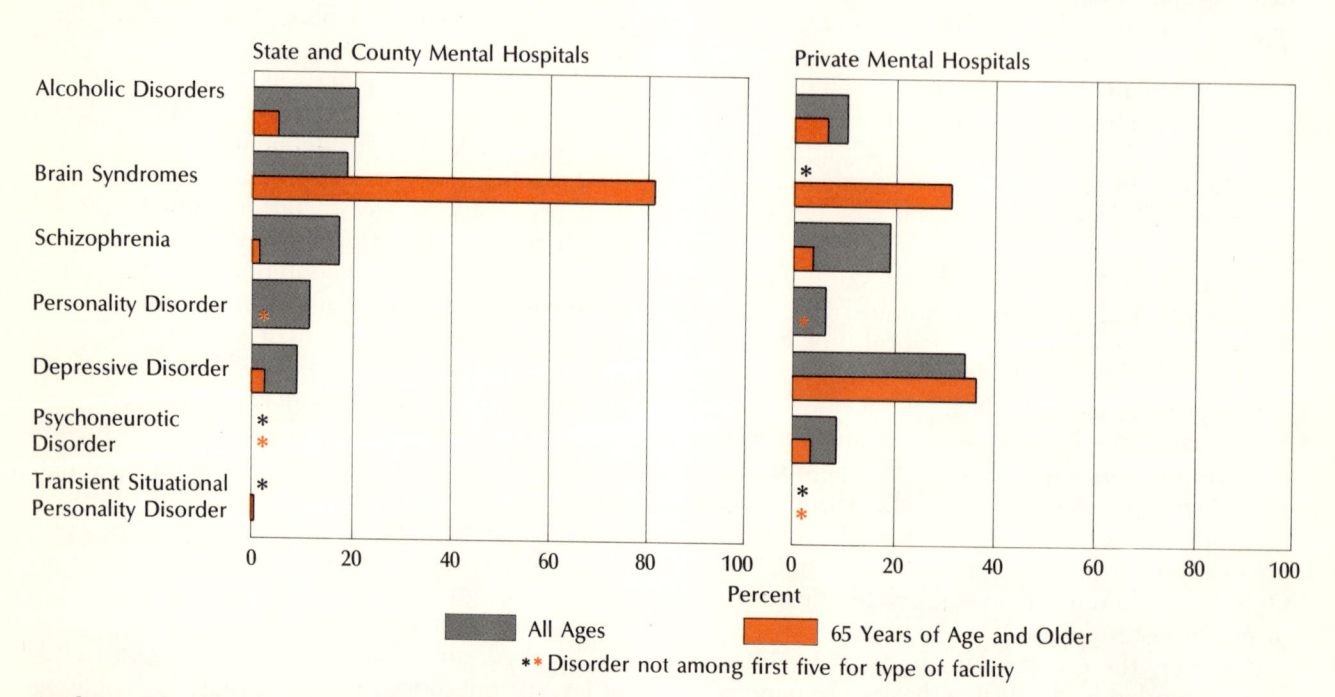

Ranking of five leading causes of first admissions to psychiatric facilities shows significant role of organic brain syndromes in elderly. At all ages, alcoholism disorders are a leading cause; among those who can afford private care, depressive illness is preeminent (data from study by M. Kramer, C. A. Taube, and R. W. Redick).

need to feel "in control" will be particularly depressed by the minor memory loss that accompanies old age. The histrionic woman who exhibits great vanity or depends heavily on sexuality for her sense of self will be depressed when her skin wrinkles and no longer takes makeup as it used to. She may seek attention through a "cleansing hypochondriasis" or an inappropriate seductiveness, neither of which will satisfy her ego. Yet another at-risk life-style is exemplified by the "workaholic"; upon retirement, the individual may become depressed and turn to alcohol. Or the passive-dependent wife, when she becomes a widow or her adult children move away, likewise may have no preparation or emotional resources with which to meet new circumstances; accordingly she may become depressed.

Patients who have had adjustment problems in the past are likely to be at risk of recurrences in later life when circumstances change. A patient who has suffered depressive illness in earlier life because of marital and job problems may have a recurrence in response to retirement, widowhood, etc. Changes of locale or other circumstances may cause serious mental illness to surface for the first time. It is possible for a patient to have the first serious schizophrenic episode in later life; I have in mind a man who functioned acceptably well in a rural area despite schizophrenia but became severely disabled when, in retirement, he moved to a city. Conceivably, if there are indeed genetic predispositions to schizophrenia, manic-depressive illness, or recurrent psychotic depression, these may not be expressed in rare circumstances until old age.

The physician who recognizes maladaptive lifestyle patterns can try to encourage steps aimed at minimizing or preventing later-life consequences. A frank discussion with a middle-aged workaholic to encourage nonwork interests may be productive. Or the passive-dependent wife may be urged to develop interests outside the family. Any adult patient may benefit from a review of current life-style patterns and their relationship to later-life goals.

There are ways to gain insight into styles of stress response, and they can be done unobtrusively. For example, in giving the family history, the patient may mention loss of a son by drowning. Sympathizing, the physician may inquire about how the patient responded, or, pointedly, how the patient showed or disguised his or her anger at the loss. The answer may indicate that the patient tends to go to pieces under stress; or he may hold together during the emergency but later becomes too depressed to func-

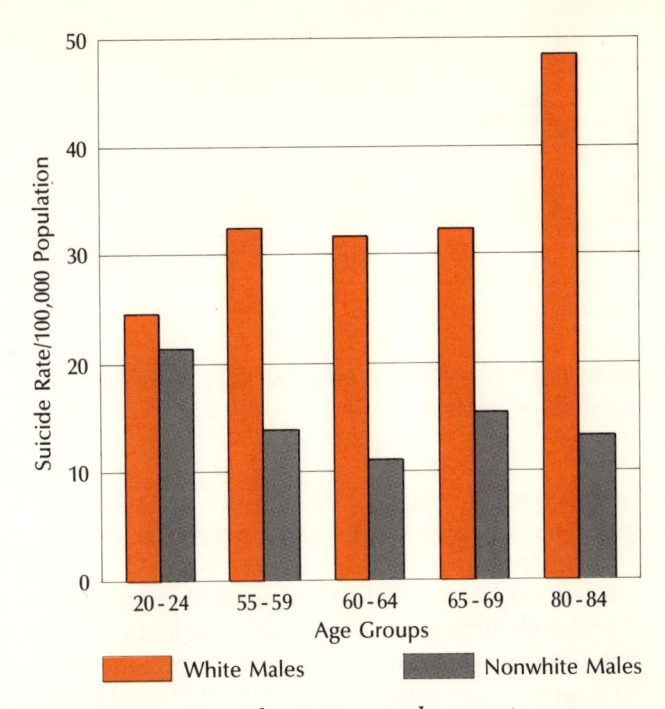

Progressive rise with age in suicide rates is most pronounced among white males. While female rates are always much lower, a rise occurs among white women between ages 55 and 70 that is not seen in nonwhites.

tion well; or he may resist crying or turn to work or prayer. Out of the repertoire of stress responses exhibited in younger days, those still available to the patient in later life may become apparent. A retiree who in the past had relied on religion for comfort in adversity may be less prone to depression than the retiree who used to find consolation through the job. A patient who finds consolation in hobbies, gardening, or volunteer activity may be considered to have defenses against the losses of old age.

In evaluating functional disorder in aged patients, the physician needs to know where and how they live, what they do with their time in contrast to what they did 20 years ago, what they were like when young, what satisfactions life brought them when young, and how aging has affected those satisfactions. Such questions constitute elements of a life-style history.

The answers may be useful in various assessments. A candidate for leg amputation who says he was happy when young because of his love of tennis will probably need considerable emotional support to face the operation. Afterward, if the patient declares that life without participation in sports is not worth living, the history makes the declaration an urgent signal for help. The patient who reports early awak-

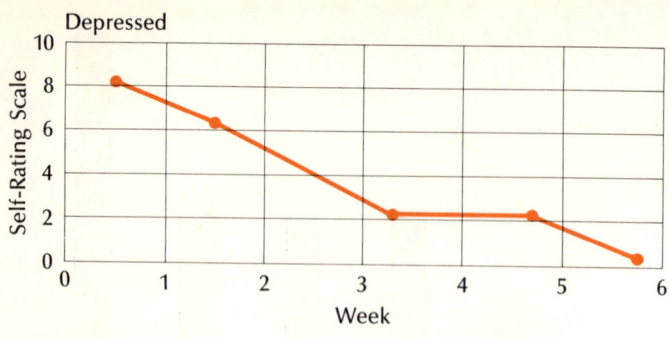

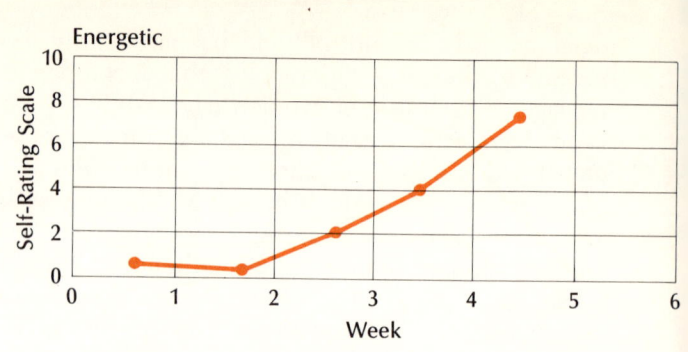

Self-rating scale, with patient asked to evaluate his state of mind, or other parameter, on the basis of a ranking from zero (worst) to 10 (optimal), can be a valuable tool for the primary physician following the patient at regular

ening, a possible sign of depression, actually may have been a farmer; in him this "symptom" may have no diagnostic relevance.

Knowledge of life-style also is important in defining rehabilitation goals for a disabled patient. "Rehabilitation" means an attempt to return a person, insofar as possible, to a life-style the patient used to have, *not* the creation of a new one. A physician may believe that an aged patient should be communicative and participating, but the life-style history may indicate that isolation is more typical. The pattern of isolation may have been chosen, consciously or unconsciously, as a defense against an overwhelming anxiety. No alternative pattern may be in the patient's repertoire. It may be better to leave it alone.

Much of the task of obtaining a life-style history can be done by a nurse or paraprofessional in the office, at least to the extent of alerting the physician to areas for probing. A useful instrument in appraising current emotional status is the Present State Examination of the London Institute of Psychiatry. A shortened version is adaptable for office use. The questionnaire is arranged so that patient responses to a variety of subjects can be elicited systematically, graded, and compared at intervals. For example, the patient is asked such questions as:

Do you keep reasonably cheerful or have you been very depressed or low-spirited recently? Have you cried at all? (When did you last really enjoy doing anything?) How do you see the future? (Has life seemed quite hopeless? Have you given up or does there still seem some reason for trying?) Have you felt that life wasn't worth living? (Did you ever feel like ending it all? What did you think you might do? Did you actually try?)

The Zung scale also can be used with the depressed patient, but even simpler is a self-rating scale that any physician can easily employ. The patient is asked to rate himself on any item – anxiety, sleep, ability to make decisions, etc. – on a scale from zero to 10 (worst to optimal) in terms of his present feelings or of his progress toward recovery. While not as scientific as the Present State Examination or the Zung scale, this simple form of self-rating is surprisingly accurate.

The physician may recognize patients with urgent needs for specialized treatment, such as: 1) conditions involving loss of contact with reality, exemplified by vivid delusions that are depressive or schizophrenic; 2) suicidal threats, which must always be taken seriously; and 3) withdrawal from eating, sleeping, taking vital medications, maintaining cleanliness, or other essential activities. If electing to treat patients with these problems, the primary physician should be prepared for major difficulties in keeping patients on essential medications and in a safe environment pending the outcome of counseling and other therapy. I would recommend referring problems of this magnitude to specialists.

The physician who recognizes behavioral patterns of significantly less gravity can either refer the patient for counseling or try to counsel in the office. For certain conditions, the primary physician is in the best position to treat. Among the objectives of counseling are: 1) to permit verbalization of feelings of helplessness, guilt, and loneliness; 2) to support the patient with assurance, when realistic, that the problem will pass; and 3) to advise the patient on what to do to alleviate the feeling or to tell him when his feelings are unrealistic (for example, he has *not* been abandoned by his children and *does* have enough money to live decently).

To the physician with a busy practice, the recommendation to "just listen" and talk to patients may be exasperating. Physician time must indeed be conserved. How then to reconcile patient needs with the

intervals. The illustrations above are selections from records made by a patient with depression who (objectively also) was much improved after six weeks of counseling that was supplemented by the use of minor tranquilizers.

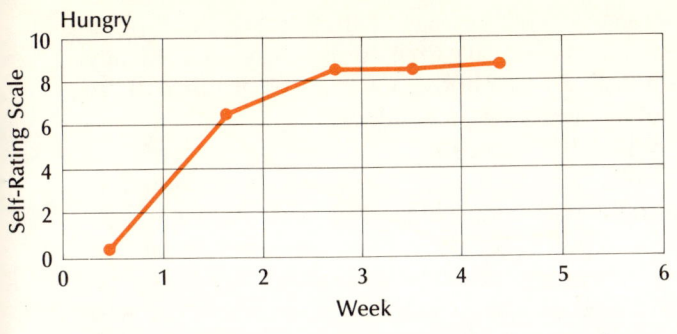

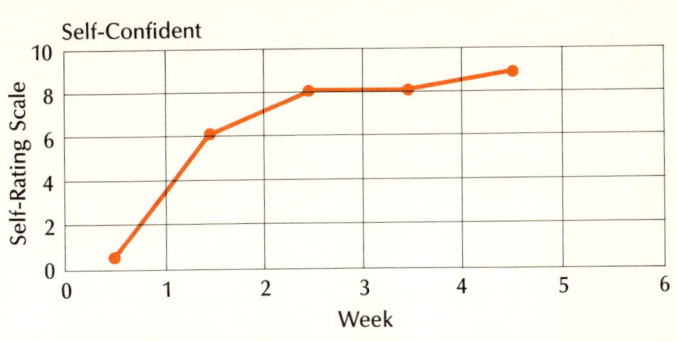

time problem? One way is to schedule the patient to meet with a nurse (or physician extender) who is not as time-pressed. Following general or patient-specific instructions, the nurse can alert the physician to subjects for exploration. The fact that the physician, through the nurse, is in touch with the problem can be made clear simply by (for example) the nurse saying to the patient being ushered into the consulting room: "Remember, Mrs. Brown, I asked you to tell the doctor about your problem with forgetting keys."

Conditions that the primary physician is perhaps in the best position to treat, if he chooses to do so, are grief reactions, sexual maladjustments, marital problems, and situational disorders – especially those arising from physical disease or incapacity. Depression over a myocardial infarction (MI) is an example of the last. A businessman who has had an MI faces the realization that the stresses of his work will require him to retire early. The prospect is suddenly imposed and frightens him. The physician can treat the depression by hearing the patient vent his feelings, by being supportive (give assurances about survival and physical capacity to carry on with non-job interests), and by employing mild ataractics to tide the patient over. The patient can be asked to talk about taboo or sensitive subjects: what having the attack was like and what it meant emotionally, including the fears it generated. Fear of death is common; it may help the patient to know how other MI patients felt and that his fears are not unusual. The patient should be encouraged to talk about these fears with the hope he may try to come to grips with them in terms of a plan for focusing on certain activities and personal relationships.

If the physician has an intimate knowledge of a patient's physical condition and history, he can assist not only the patient emerging from a physical crisis but also one with a depressing but nonemergency problem. From common sense and observation of how patients compensate for disabilities, the physician may be able to suggest a course of action tailored to the individual's capacities. To the patient whose depression relates to constantly mislaying things, the suggestion that a key rack be hung near the front door may be highly beneficial. The patient depressed over forgetting appointments and bills might be able to manage a checklist or a notebook. Simple suggestions may comfort the patient and prevent an exacerbation of the depression. Virtually cost-free therapeutic gains may stem from the physician's getting the patient to talk about what is troubling him or her, including even little things.

Likewise, patients who hint at suicidal thoughts should be encouraged to talk. Whether they should be treated or referred to a specialist may depend on what the physician hears. The physician should ask if the patient has a suicide plan. The patient who has one and tells how it will be accomplished (viz., "I've stored up the sleeping pills") must be considered at high risk. He requires immediate care by a specialist. (Such a patient should never be left alone, even to return home for clothing or to travel to the hospital or psychotherapist.) The patient with suicidal ideas but no plan may not be an emergency. Counseling should be directed toward helping the patient understand the true dimensions of his or her problem and possible means of resolving a predicament.

Like death and suicide, sex is another "taboo" subject that underlies functional disorders. Because of myths about the incapacities of elderly people and the view of sex in old age as lechery ("the dirty old man"), elderly people tend to be treated as if sexless. Depression may result when they react with guilt and shame about "abnormal" drives for their age. They may be as bewildered as the adolescent as to what is normal sexuality for their age. The truth is that sex does not end at 60; when not inhibited, sex life continues well into physical senescence, often beyond the ninth decade, depending not on age but on health status and the availability of a sexual partner.

The well-informed primary physician is in the best position to obtain a sexual history (which is often omitted for geriatric patients), to understand the patient's problems in terms of life-style and physical status, and to offer sex information and advice. Sometimes complaints of anxiety that at first appear related to sex life actually reveal a generalized behavioral pattern. This tends to surface when the discussion broadens to subjects not related specifically to the patient's emotional state; for example, the patient who presents with anxieties about sex may turn out to be a passive-dependent person, unable to cope when some household appliance breaks down, with irritating neighbors, or with money matters. The pattern just described or any other deeply rooted personality disturbance may require referral to a specialist for evaluation and perhaps psychotherapy.

There is an unfortunate professional tendency to rule out psychotherapy for the elderly in the belief that they are poor candidates. Many are. But psychotherapy may well be the right treatment for patients whose functional disorders are refractory to office counseling. The primary physician may have access to a psychiatrist with geriatric interests or to a community mental health center. By and large, mental health resources for the elderly are scarce, and the physician may have to rely on senior-citizen, social-service, and other community facilities to help the patient who is in office counseling.

In dealing with the paranoid patient through counseling, the physician's role is as advocate of reality. The physician may have to tell the patient plainly, "I don't see things that way," or, "We may have to agree to disagree, but I don't think you are being pursued by little people." The paranoid patient may have a delusion of persecution and may also believe he or she is able to do impossible acts (seeing himself, for example, as Christ reborn). Obviously, the severely paranoid patient should be referred to the specialist. Often, however, paranoia in the elderly reflects vision or hearing problems rather than personality changes. If these are corrected with spectacles and hearing aids, the paranoia will disappear.

Hypochondriasis is a difficult functional disorder to manage. Ideally, if counseling exposes the underlying cause, it should be dealt with before the behavior becomes fixed. Often hypochondriasis reflects depression and feelings of inadequacy. The physician can try to deal with it firmly but sympathetically. Referral for psychotherapy may be justified if the problem becomes intractable.

When the source of a situational disorder lies in conflict among family members, they should be brought into counseling along with the elderly patient. Whether the parties are dealt with separately or together, they should be encouraged to articulate to one another what it is that irritates them and what they believe would improve their relationships. Particularly deleterious to family relationships are the tensions adult children create by refusing to let parents talk about weakness and dying. By telling the children that they are not really protecting parents by avoiding these subjects, the physician may help to remove a source of anguish. I tell family members, "You've lived together – why does death, which is part of life, have to be excluded from your shared experience? It's awfully hard for anyone to die alone. Are you sure you are protecting your parents by never allowing them to talk about dying?"

In our culture, individuals find it hard to recognize their anger at someone who is dying or has died. Many have to be assisted in expressing their grief reactions and sense of abandonment. An ability to listen to grief, to help patients understand feelings of abandonment and anger, and to help patients feel able to go on with life is essential in geriatric practice.

For the patient who is depressed over retirement, the approach is the same as I have indicated for other situational disorders: assistance in venting feelings about the loss and in finding ways to go on. The retiree may need advice on finding financial or legal help or things to do in the community that will maintain his self-respect. Some retirees drift into alcoholism in reaction to loss of occupation. They may have to be referred for counseling through such organizations as Alcoholics Anonymous. The most important step in office counseling of such persons is to make them recognize that there *is* a drinking problem.

I have reserved discussion of drugs and hospitalization until last in order to stress counseling, an age-old but often slighted role for physicians. For the types of functional disorder the primary physician may contemplate treating, drugs are useful. But they are not a substitute for counseling, and they carry the risk of deterring the patient from working through the problem responsible for anxiety, disturbed sleep, depression, and other complaints.

Paradoxically, some physicians seem both to overprescribe minor tranquilizers *and* to shy away from

Alternative Approaches to Therapy in Depression: A 'Decision Tree'

Depression

Retarded or agitated	Retarded	Weeping	Agitated
±	+	+	+
Early morning awakening	Weight loss	Difficulty going to sleep	Weight loss
±	+	+	+
Anorexia	Early morning awakening	No weight loss	Insomnia
+	+	+	+
Suicidal plan	Not suicidal	Not suicidal	Not suicidal

Immediate protective hospitalization: do not leave alone until in hospital

Take Detailed Drug History

- **Rule out:** myxedema, carcinoma of pancreas, physical illness with depressive response
- **Rule out:** physical illness
- **Rule out:** thyrotoxicosis, drug reaction (e.g., digitalis toxicity), physical illness

May Try Any or All of the Following

- Drug Therapy Tofranil or Pertofrane, or Norpramin (start low, 10 mg tid)
  - If no response, consider ECT
  - Psychiatric referral
- Counseling in office
  - Minor tranquilizer, (e.g., Valium 2 mg tid)
- Antidepressant and antianxiety drugs (start low, and work up) Triavil, Sinequan, or Elavil
  - Counseling in office
  - Hospitalization
  - Referral to psychiatrist

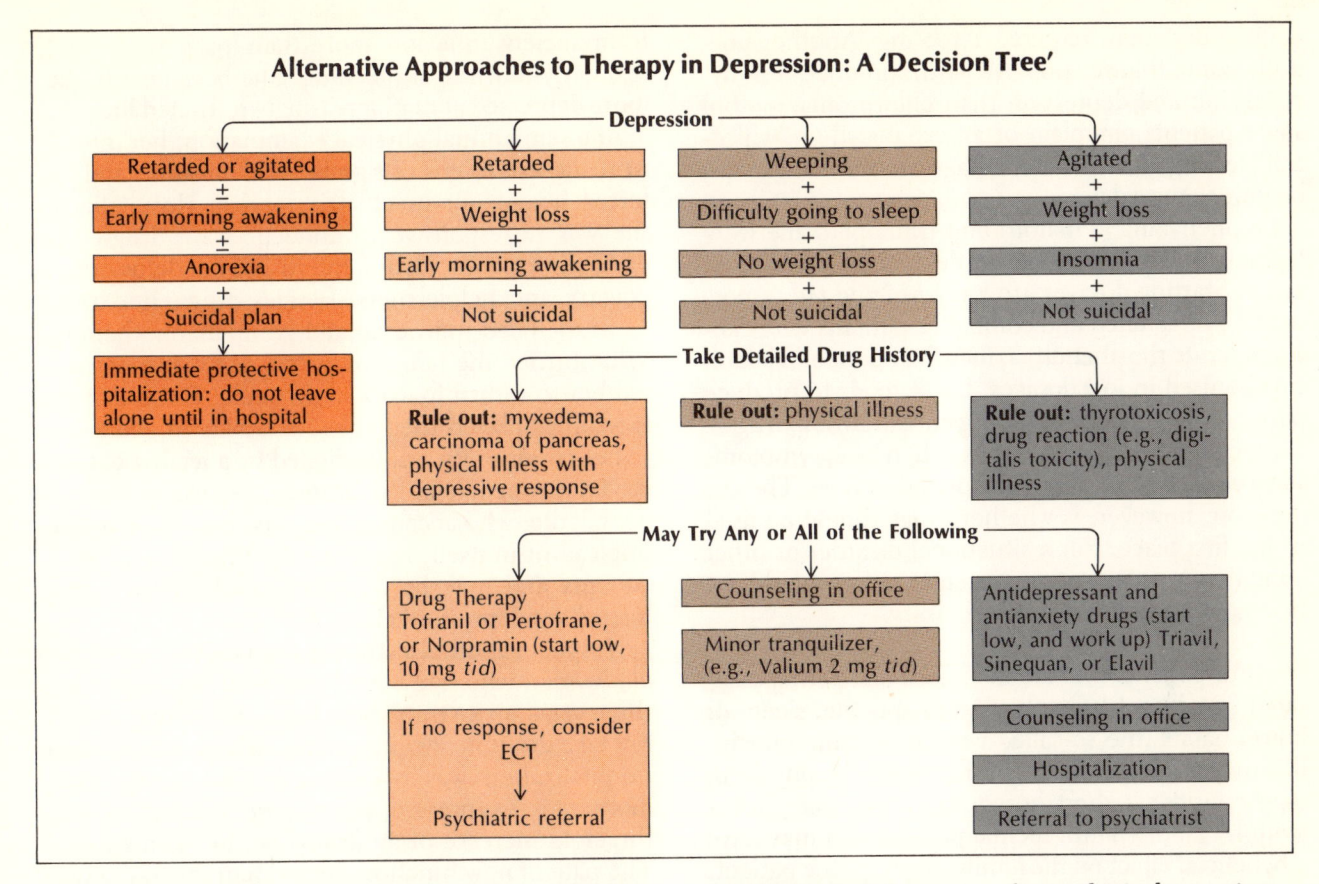

vigorously pursuing a drug regimen. As a general rule, drugs should be prescribed at low starting doses and then increased until they are effective or are found to produce toxicity. As an early chapter in this book showed (see Chapter 1, "Drug Prescribing for the Elderly," by P.P. Lamy and R.E. Vestal), unpredictable drug reactions are more likely among the elderly than younger persons. Moreover, adverse reactions tend to be ignored because they fit stereotypes of "senility." A thoroughgoing drug history is essential when assessing and before prescribing for functional disorders.

For anxiety and sleep disturbance, minor tranquilizers *sometimes* are necessary to tide the patient over, pending the outcome of counseling or other means of resolving a problem. Diazepam (Valium) and chlordiazepoxide (Librium) can be given at bedtime in dosages of 5 and 10 mg, respectively, to promote sleep. For daytime use, starting dosages should be held to 2 and 5 mg, respectively, because release of anger can be a side effect. The dosage should not be raised until the physician is certain it is insufficient for the intended effects. For inducing sleep, diphenhydramine (Benadryl) frequently is effective at a dose of 50 to 100 mg at bedtime. Barbiturates are contraindicated because of paradoxical reactions.

When anxiety and minor sleep disturbance suggest depression, amitriptyline (Elavil) may be helpful, especially (according to some observers) if the patient shows agitation. Another antidepressant drug, imipramine (Tofranil), is favored by some physicians, even though amitriptyline appears to be a bit more sedating. For either drug, the starting 24-hour dose is 30 mg, given entirely at bedtime for inducing sleep. The dosage can be raised fairly rapidly as needed if toxicity does not appear. It must be remembered that full antidepressant effect takes three to four weeks. The patient in a severe depression may need to be maintained for six or more months.

Major tranquilizers, such as the phenothiazines, have been found effective for managing manifestations of psychotic disorders and for control of manic-depressive illness, manic phase. By and large, these are conditions for specialists to manage. The drugs must be used with great care. Patients should be warned against operating a car or machinery because of the drowsiness these drugs produce. They have unpredictable effects; I recall the contrast between a 200-pound hunter who became hypotensive on 30 mg of chlorpromazine (Thorazine) per day, while a

90-pound woman required 1,200 mg. Another phenothiazine, thioridazine (Mellaril), produces less hypotension and depression than chlorpromazine but some patients complain of an exhausted or "wiped-out" feeling. The starting dosage of these drugs must be low, 30 mg a day.

Perphenazine (Trilafon) and trifluoperazine (Stelazine) are two of the least depressing phenothiazines. Starting dosages are 2 mg *bid* and *tid* respectively. For agitated and combative patients who cannot tolerate the phenothiazines, haloperidol (Haldol) can be used in low dosages, but it tends to produce parkinsonian effects, requiring antiparkinson drugs.

Psychochemotherapy stops when the symptoms have cleared for a significant period of time. The key decision, however, is whether drugs should be used in the first place. For a situational disorder or other condition responsive to counseling, drugs should not be employed unless clearly necessary.

For patients who are depressed and perhaps agitated but do not have changes in appetite, sleep, or bowel habits (the so-called vegetative symptoms indicative of more serious disturbances), the physician may consider a short hospitalization to offer relief from social or environmental pressures. It may have a beneficial effect on the family as well as the patient. However, institutionalization can induce confusion and intensify depression.

A short hospitalization offers an opportunity for well-supervised and vigorous chemotherapy for anxiety and depression, for electroconvulsive therapy (ECT) in appropriate patients, and for individual or group psychotherapy. An example of the successful use of ECT and other modalities is the case of a 61-year-old woman who had two previous depressions, one at age 33, at the time of divorce, and another a decade later, when the widowed mother-in-law she attended died after a prolonged illness. In the first depression she received some outpatient care with advice to focus on her work in a store. The second episode went untreated; it lasted six months. At age 61, an employe for 23 years in the same place, the woman recognized her growing inability to cope with the job, became increasingly depressed, asserted helplessness and poverty (untrue), and withdrew from society. She lost more than 15 pounds and had early-morning awakening. She became all the more depressed at her increasingly restricted life.

At a semiannual physical examination, her internist recognized signs of significant depression and referred her to our psychiatric service. Hospitalized, she was unresponsive to antidepressant drugs, became more paranoid, and intensified her delusions of poverty and helplessness. Besides drugs, her treatment included individual and group psychotherapy. What turned the tide, however, was ECT; it permitted her to return to work in six weeks. But the other modalities played their role: her ability to live again in her community was facilitated by a feeling of having known people at the hospital, especially a nurse confidante, who accepted and liked her. ECT, while unpleasant in itself, may turn the tide for depressed patients and may be far less hazardous than prolonged antidepressant chemotherapy.

Hospitalization also turned the tide for a 76-year-old woman who had been treated for depression for three years on an outpatient basis. She simply would not take drugs in adequate doses. When resistance to hospitalization was overcome in the family, chemotherapy was pressed, under close observation, to a threefold increase of amitriptyline, to 150 mg daily. The patient now functions better than she has in several years. She smiles and is more like her old self.

In closing, I would emphasize that symptoms worth treating in the individual aged 20 or 40 are worth treating in the individual at 80. The primary physician's role is to recognize the at-risk and troubled patient, to know the various modalities that may benefit the patient, to capitalize on a rapport with the patient in utilizing counseling, and to refer the problem that deserves specialized attention.

For inspiration, I take note of the exquisite retort of a 74-year-old woman who, when asked by Dr. Martin Berezin of Harvard why she sought psychotherapy, responded: "Doctor, all I have left is my future." This desire to make the most out of life, regardless of age, must be respected. To submerge such a spirit in drugs or indifference not only harms the patient but also, I feel, contributes to the anxieties of professional persons about what awaits us in old age.

5

Organic Brain Syndromes

WILLIAM REICHEL
Franklin Square Hospital

Case A: A 66-year-old woman was brought to the hospital after a few days of worsening confusion and disorientation, dehydration, weakness, depression, and nausea. She was found to have the following daily drug intake: tolbutamide, methenamine mandelate, spironolactone, phenformin hydrochloride, furosemide, nitrofurantoin, reserpine, and prochlorperazine. All drugs were withdrawn. She received intravenous fluids. On discharge to her home, she showed no need for any of the drugs. Her confusion had disappeared completely.

Case B: A 70-year-old woman with striking memory loss for over a year visited her physician, who found her grossly myxedematous. Tests confirmed that she was suffering from hypothyroidism. Several months of thyroid extract treatment improved her intellectual function to the level that existed preceding her memory loss.

Case C: An 80-year-old man presented to his physician with significant intellectual and memory dysfunction, he wandered and was unable to take care of himself, but he refused family assistance. He could not remember from one minute to the next what had been said in an elementary examination. He had no memory of recent events but did recall events of the past, and he appeared pleasant in manner. The family explained that the confusion and inability to care for himself had been progressing for several years. A decision was made to refer the patient to a nursing home for custodial care.

From these three histories, one obtains a glimpse of the variability with which confusion, disorientation, and dementia in the elderly may present. Case A represents a confusional reaction secondary to drug toxicity; the acute brain syndrome, or acute confusional reaction, was reversed easily once the cause was determined. Case B shows elements of a reversible form of dementia, or chronic brain syndrome, secondary to a treatable condition. Case C represents another form of chronic brain syndrome, senile dementia, with a progressive loss of memory and other intellectual functions over an extended period of time.

The focus of our discussion will be on what are widely called "acute brain syndrome" and "chronic brain syndrome," mixtures of the two, and their differentiation from each other and from such functional disorders as depression. We will also consider aspects of these entities that may be overlapping and in some instances reversible.

Armed with concepts for differentiating disorders in which confusion, disorientation, and dementia are prominent signs, the physician in his or her office avoids a major pitfall: casual acceptance of signs of neuropsychiatric disturbance in the elderly as expectable and untreatable results of aging, when in reality a treatable cause may be at issue. True, all of the problems can and do occur in the young as well as in the old, but there is an urgent need to emphasize their relationship in the elderly because they are extremely common in this age group, and other signs and symptoms, which might direct the physician to look beyond the changes in mental status, are often muted or absent.

Acute Brain Syndrome

Acute brain syndrome is characterized by recent onset of confusion, disorientation, excitement, or

CHAPTER 5: REICHEL

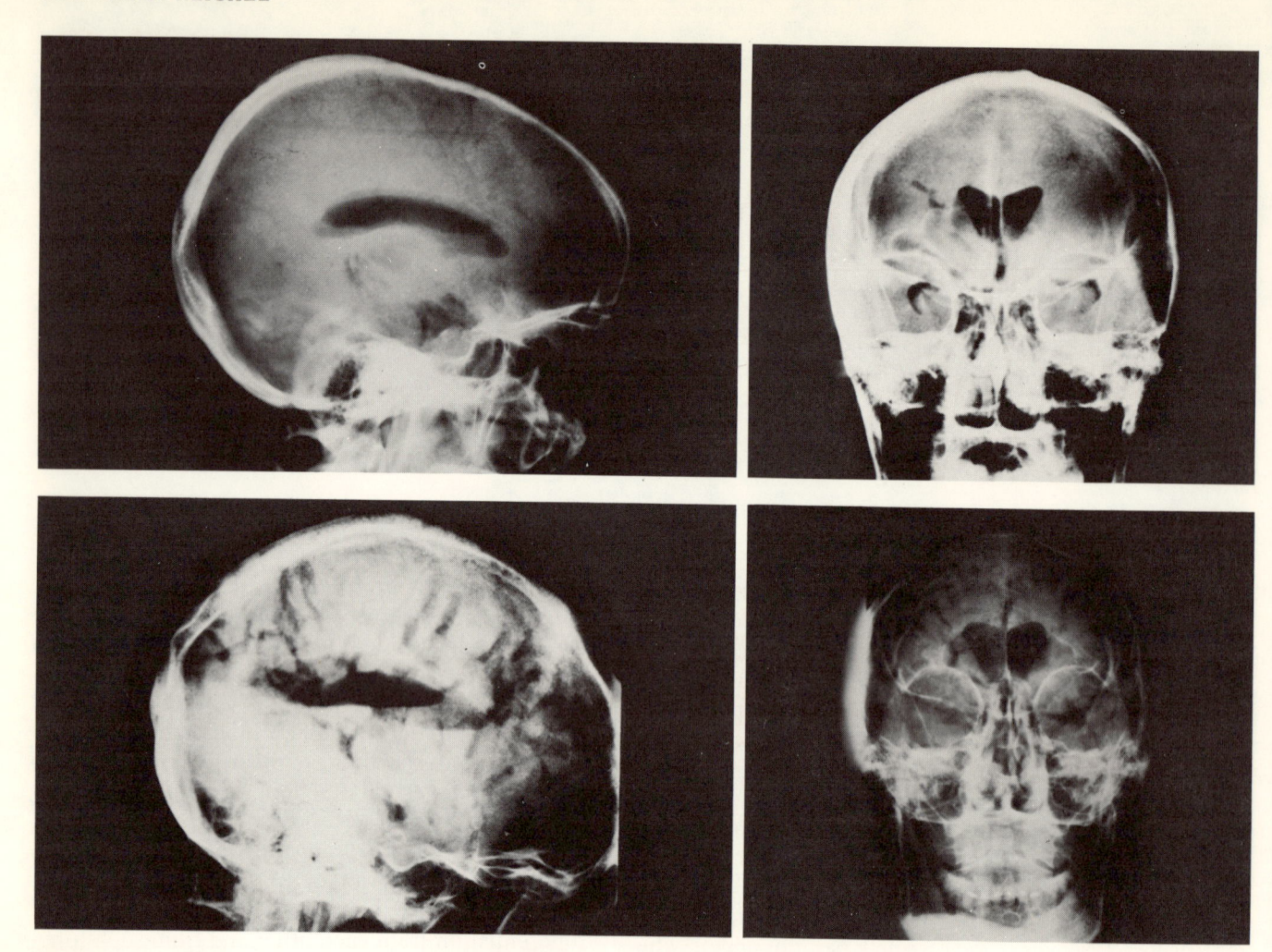

Pathology typical of senile dementia of the Alzheimer type (see lower photos; normal brain in top row) includes atrophy of the frontal and temporal lobes and enlargement of lateral and third ventricles. Considerable air diffuses over cortex. While these anatomic changes are exquisitely delineated by pneumoencephalography,

delirium – mental changes that are among the most common presenting signs or symptoms in any hospital outpatient department, emergency room, or physician's office. The key word in the description is *recent*. In any patient with sudden and unexpected mental change, possible physical causes must be considered and treated. Typically, the elderly patient was well until a few days before he required help. This syndrome may be the first or most prominent sign of a major disease outside the central nervous system. Absence or attenuation of typical signs or syndromes of medical illness should not rule out certain diagnoses. The syndrome may be an indication of myocardial infarction in which the elderly often do not exhibit chest pain; of pneumonia in which they may have little or no temperature rise or leukocytosis; or of pulmonary embolism in which they may not show tachycardia, dyspnea, or chest pain. The differential diagnosis of acute brain syndrome must consider medical illness and drug toxicities in general.

Besides those just mentioned, the illnesses that can produce acute confusional reactions include cardiac failure, mild stroke, hypokalemia, and dehydration. In Case A we see an example of acute brain syndrome due to drug toxicity. "Mr. Jones" is an example of a reversible acute brain syndrome of another sort: an 80-year-old businessman, still active as president of his own corporation, he was hospitalized after several days of increasing confusion, excitability, and unusual ideation. He could not give the physi-

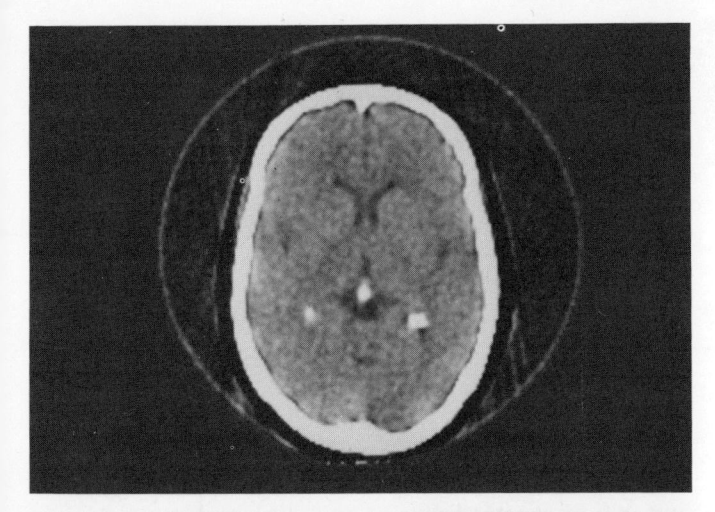

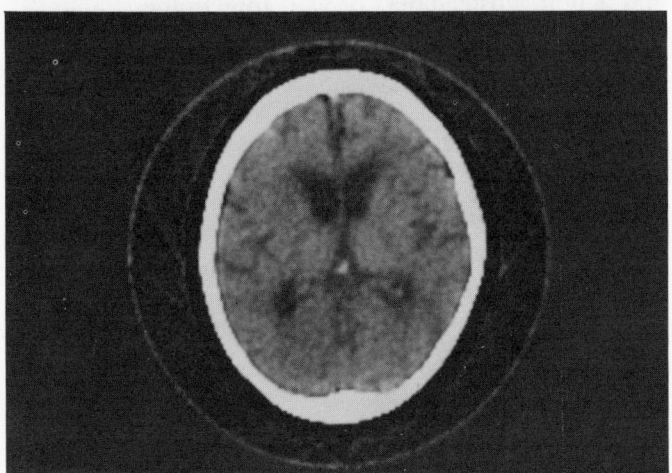

ORGANIC BRAIN SYNDROMES

Chronic Brain Syndrome

If loss of intellectual function is of long standing, roughly defined as six months, we are speaking of a chronic brain syndrome, or organic dementia. Dementia refers to loss of intellectual and cognitive abilities. The major forms of organic dementia include 1) senile dementia of the Alzheimer type, and also 2) arteriosclerotic or multi-infarct dementia. These are not mutually exclusive, but they share the unfortunate attribute of being irreversible, given the current state of medical knowledge.

The chief characteristics of Alzheimer's disease include memory loss, other intellectual impairments, and paucity of voluntary movement (an example of voluntary movement is seen in the vigor of the child bounding up and down the stairs, arms waving). Emotional affect is relatively normal, although there may be depression or anxiety or paranoid features in response to the dementia. Pathologically, atrophy of the frontal and temporal lobes and enlargement of the lateral and third ventricles are present. Microscopically, Alzheimer's neurofibrillary tangles, amyloid-containing senile plaques, and lipofuscin pigment are noted. Little cerebral arteriosclerosis may be present. The diagnosis can be confirmed by pneumoencephalographic demonstration of cortical atrophy and ventricular dilatation. However, the pneumoencephalogram is associated with increased morbidity. At present, computerized axial tomography is preferable for determining the possibility of Alzheimer's dementia.

In the Alzheimer's patient, social responses may appear to be intact despite intellectual failure. The patient may be found looking at a newspaper and seeming to enjoy it; however, the newspaper is upside-down. The patient is courteous but does not retain information sufficiently even to recall that he or she is in a hospital, or to recite three words – such as house, umbrella, boat – a few minutes after they have been presented to him.

Alzheimer's disease refers both to the senile form, which is called senile dementia of the Alzheimer type, and to the presenile form, called Alzheimer's presenile dementia. When appearing in an individual in the fourth or fifth decade of life, the dementia presents explosively as a more exaggerated version of senile dementia of the Alzheimer type. Pathologic findings are the same as in the senile form but also are more exaggerated. Diagnosis, other than by autopsy, is again by computerized axial tomography and pneumoencephalography.

computed axial tomography (normal at top, Alzheimer's below, courtesy Dr. L. Menzer) has become the preferred diagnostic approach as there is no risk of morbidity.

cian a clear history. Blood gas studies revealed arterial hypoxemia, and a lung scan indicated a high probability of pulmonary embolism. After a course of heparin, arterial oxygenation improved, breathing became normal, and mental confusion cleared.

Growing confusion in a 75-year-old retired executive, "Mr. Adams," also proved to be reversible acute brain syndrome. Active as grandfather, sports enthusiast, and churchman, the patient was brought to the physician after three days of intensifying confusion, agitation, and memory loss. He was febrile. A right middle-lobe pneumonia was found on x-ray, and later sputum culture revealed diplococcus. After 10 days of treatment with intravenous and intramuscular penicillin, his mental functions returned to normal as his pneumonia cleared.

Arteriosclerotic (multi-infarct) dementia rarely occurs without a history of recurrent strokes. Strokes are characterized mostly by episodic and focal neurologic disease. There may be focal neurologic signs – motor weakness, sensory loss, or reflex change. There may be evidence of arteriosclerosis elsewhere in the body. Pathologically there must be a history of recurrent cerebral infarction with significant cerebral softening for dementia to be present.

In the hypertensive patient, dementia may be present in the syndrome of pseudobulbar palsy following repeated small strokes. Among the signs are poor emotional control (excessive laughing and crying), difficulty with speech and swallowing, and signs of bilateral upper motor neurone paralysis.

Pathologic studies indicate that the major cause of dementia in the elderly is senile dementia of the Alzheimer type, with vascular or multi-infarct dementia ranking second. The reader is referred to the recent Workshop-Conference on Alzheimer's Disease–Senile Dementia and Related Disorders, convened by the National Institute of Neurological and Communicative Disorders and Stroke, the National Institute on Aging, and the National Institute of Mental Health (Katzman R, Terry RD, and Bick K, in press), for a discussion of recommended terminology, especially in regard to use of the term "senile dementia of the Alzheimer type." The use of this more exact terminology, instead of "chronic brain syndrome" or "senile brain disease," should help focus attention on the very specific pathology underlying this disorder.

There is one form of organic dementia that can be corrected by surgery. This is the syndrome of normal pressure hydrocephalus (first described in 1965 by Hakim, Adams, and associates), which occurs mostly in middle and late life. It is marked by confusion, ataxia, gait disturbance, and progressive dementia. Pneumoencephalography discloses marked dilatation of the ventricles, but no air diffuses over the cortex as in Alzheimer's disease. The brain, so to speak, is plastered against the skull. Today, a cisternal scan and computerized axial tomography offer methods of visualizing the lesions with less risk. A shunt operation has had good results in many reported cases. Normal pressure hydrocephalus, like chronic subdural hematoma, can be a result of head injury in the elderly patient; in fact, both normal pressure hydrocephalus and chronic subdural hematoma should be considered in any elderly patient with history of head injury and deteriorating intellectual functions.

Of course, it is a matter of judgment as to how far the clinician should "push" an evaluation for normal pressure hydrocephalus. If the elderly individual has shown a deteriorated mental capacity for several years and, in fact, functioned poorly and had other health problems prior to that deterioration, then one would certainly be less willing to undertake the effort and expense involved in ruling out normal pressure hydrocephalus. If the individual has been functioning well until relatively recently at his or her business or profession or in his role in the household, and his other physical functions are still in good shape, then the physician in charge would be more inclined to push such a workup as far as possible. In fact, one of the four patients first reported by Hakim, Adams, and associates was a 62-year-old pediatrician with a six-month history of increasing slowness of thought and action, unsteadiness of gait, forgetfulness, and incontinence. He was able to return to practice after a successful ventriculocisternostomy had corrected his partial obstructive hydrocephalus, which was caused by a paraphysial cyst of the third ventricle. Certainly, no physician would argue against the evaluation and management of this individual.

Other treatable causes of chronic brain syndrome or dementia in the elderly include myxedema, as in Case B, and pernicious anemia. Dr. Kenneth B. Lewis in his chapter on cardiac problems in the elderly (see Chapter 6) emphasizes that not all congestive heart failure is arteriosclerotic. Similarly, not all dementia is arteriosclerotic. Proper diagnosis allows us to make specific treatment plans, such as the

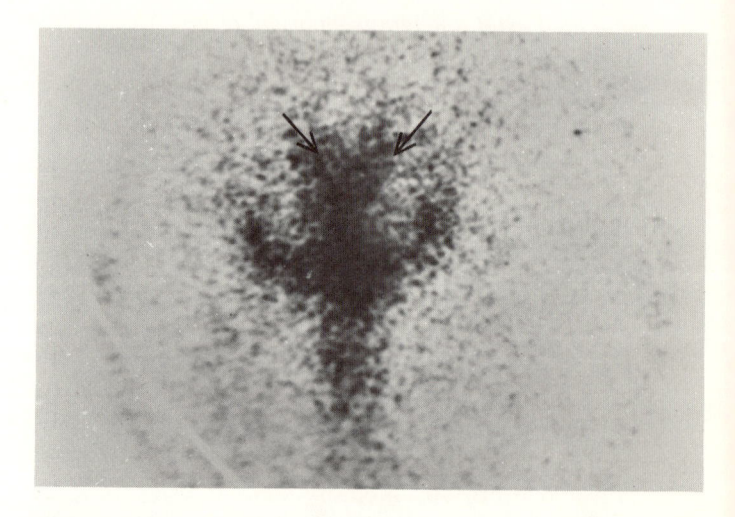

Findings typical of normal pressure hydrocephalus are demonstrated by cisternal scans. Anterior view (left) was obtained six hours after intrathecal administration of indium-111 chloride. Activity in lateral ventricles (arrows) would not be present in normal scan. Other scan is left

treatment of myxedema, pernicious anemia, or normal pressure hydrocephalus in the case of dementia.

The fact that nothing now can be done to reverse most cases of organic dementia must be tempered by the fact that there is still a great deal that the physician can do and should do to help the patient and his family cope with this devastating problem. Years ago, the severely demented patient was sent to a state hospital for the rest of his or her life. Today, the patient can be maintained in the community: at home, in a day-care facility, or in a nursing home. Agitation and combativeness can be ameliorated with judicious use of tranquilizers. However, some patients may require care in a psychiatric facility.

Maintaining the patient at home requires that precautions be taken. Access to firearms, gas ovens, medications, and dangerous implements must be cut off. Patients must be kept from wandering. Children must be guarded against harm from a demented individual. The health of the spouse of a demented patient is a factor that must be considered in attempts to keep the patient in his own home. Supportive services in a home – a visiting nurse, homemaker, friendly visitor – may be necessary. If the patient is unable to handle financial affairs, issues of guardianship may have to be raised with the family. No one is in a better position to aid the family and patient than the family physician.

A caution is indicated concerning the use of psychotropic drugs in dementia. The hazard is that of worsening the patient's mental disturbance, producing chronic oversedation that can lead to additional complications of pneumonia, bedsores, or dehydration. Sedation and restraining devices should be minimized. Social interaction should be stimulated as much as possible. One should make deliberate attempts to help the patient maintain his orientation. In addition to utilizing calendars, newspapers, clocks, radio, and television wherever appropriate, one should use the patient's name in conversation.

Mixed Brain Syndromes

A mixed brain syndrome simply represents a mixture of problems such as those of Case A and Case C. Let us recall Case C, the 80-year-old man with senile dementia who is transferred to a nursing facility for custodial care. He does well there for three and a half months, but then he suddenly develops increased confusion, belligerence, and throws objects at the nursing staff and family members. He appears more confused than ever. He does not complain of chest pain, but electrocardiogram and enzyme changes reveal an acute inferior myocardial infarction. He eventually recovers from this condition at the local community hospital and then returns to the nursing home for further extended care. This example of mixed brain syndrome superimposes an acute confusional reaction secondary to myocardial infarction on the underlying senile dementia.

The Differential Process

As discussed earlier, the patient's history provides a key clue in the recency of the confusion or intellectual decline. Besides probing for medical illness and drug toxicity, the physician also must consider alcoholism in the geriatric patient. Alcoholic syndromes, which must be differentiated, include alcoholic intoxication, withdrawal, nutritional deficiency (Wernicke-Korsakoff syndrome), hepatic encephalopathy, and miscellaneous degenerative disorders such as cerebral and cerebellar atrophy. Of course, functional disorders must also be considered in the appraisal of the elderly patient with seeming confusion, disorientation, or dementia.

In addition to the history and physical examination, the physician can employ tests of intellectual ability for evaluating dementia. The procedures are much like those for testing intelligence, memory, and judgment in children. The physician questions

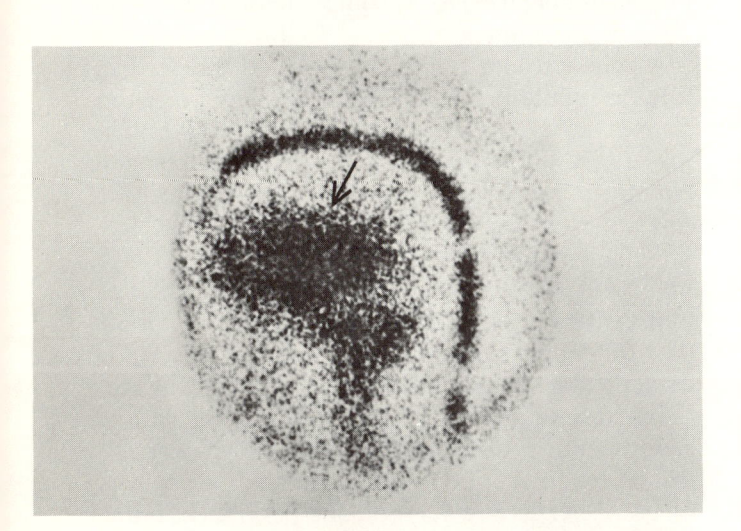

lateral view obtained 24 hours after administration of the radionuclide. Activity persists in the lateral ventricles (arrow), with no progression into the periphery of brain, as would be normal. (Scans are reproduced courtesy of Dr. Pablo E. Dibos, Franklin Square Hospital.)

Acute Confusional State
(Acute Brain Syndrome)

Definition
Confusion, disorientation, or delirium, abrupt and recent in onset, possibly associated with alterations in consciousness and physiologic function. Patient may be inattentive, dazed, stuporous, restless, agitated, or excited.

Differential diagnosis
May be secondary to myocardial infarction, heart failure, pneumonia, pulmonary embolism, drug intoxication, withdrawal state, meningitis, postconvulsive delirium, urinary tract infection, carcinomatosis, or other underlying medical problems.

Treatment
Proper recognition and management of the underlying medical problem and/or drug toxicity.

Dementia
(Chronic Brain Syndromes)

Definition
Generalized loss of intellectual function and memory; onset uncertain; duration usually at least six months. Initial subtle changes in mental function may not be recognized on psychologic examination and may be noted first by family members. Patient experiences difficulty in thinking through projects, comprehending messages, and making decisions. Retention of social behavior patterns at first obscures declining cognitive abilities. Recent memory is impaired first, remote memory last, when patient fails to recognize close friends and relatives.

Differential diagnosis
Senile dementia of Alzheimer type, arteriosclerotic or multi-infarct dementia, normal pressure hydrocephalus, myxedema, pernicious anemia, general paresis, lenticular degeneration (Wilson's disease), Huntington's chorea, chronic subdural hematoma, brain tumor.

Diagnostic tests
Psychologic tests of immediate recall, memory of recent events, memory of events of the remote past. As indicated: computerized axial tomography, cisternal scan, pneumoencephalogram, thyroid function, hematologic evaluation, serology.

Treatment
Proper recognition and prompt management of the underlying disorder.

---

for 1) immediate recall, 2) memory of recent events, and 3) memory of events of the remote past. Broadly speaking, remote events are retained the best as these events are imprinted in the memory system more deeply, recent events are imprinted less well, and milder dementia states will show greater loss pertaining to recent memory.

Ten questions formulated by Kahn and associates help in defining this situation. Where are you now? Where is this place located? What is today's date? What is the month now? What year is it? How old are you? What month were you born? What year? Who is the President of the United States? Who was the President before him?

Other questions can be added about parents, early stages of life, and subjects of interest to the patient. The answers should be verifiable through the family members or other sources. Of course, it is always a problem if this information cannot be verified. Other types of tests may have to be used in such situations. To test judgment, questions about the meaning of well-known axioms or proverbs can be asked (for example, what is the meaning of "a bird in the hand is worth two in a bush"?).

The asking of elementary questions should not embarrass the physician. Such questions are as important in probing dementia as the questions a gynecologist asks about menstrual or marital history. This is not to urge continuing the questioning when or if the patient becomes irritable or belligerent. Then the physician may have to try some other avenues of inquiry to assess intellect.

A patient's poor responsiveness in this type of interview should not be taken for dementia in all instances. Like any other person, the elderly patient may have functional disorders such as depression, paranoia, or anxiety. The diagnosis and treatment of functional disorders are discussed by Dr. Joy R. Joffe in Chapter 4. For the moment, I would simply note that patients with functional disorders (or patients with acute, chronic, or mixed brain syndrome plus functional disorders) may initially appear to be demented or more demented than they actually are.

When functional disorders are interfering with responsiveness, skill in interviewing and observation will be required. The patient depressed over the loss of his or her spouse may respond poorly. His immobile posture and inability to concentrate should not be confused with dementia. The paranoid patient may think the physician is conspiring in a plot against him, and responses may be withheld or falsified. Suddenly, it becomes clear that there is a great deal of paranoid ideation referring to God or some type of conspiracy. The elderly person who has had sensory deprivation – whose eyes have been bandaged for a period after cataract extraction, for example, or who lives alone in a dim apartment and has no visitors, radio, or television set – may only appear to be demented. If such patients with functional disorders can be encouraged to talk, responses characteristic of the specific disorder may appear: the depressed patient suddenly may break silence and cry, asserting that life is not worth living. At this point, questioning is likely to become productive.

The matter of differentiating between senile dementia of the Alzheimer type accompanied by a reactive depression and depression with cognitive dysfunction secondary to it is of great importance. There are certain situations where it is simply too difficult to separate the two entities. Some psychiatrists recommend, when faced with this dilemma, the use of antidepressant medication as a therapeutic trial in order to separate dementia and depression. However, in most cases, with enough probing, the physician should be able to define in which ball park he is playing. The cluster of signs and symptoms should become clear. Either the patient is presenting chiefly with dementia, or with dementia and an overlay of functional components such as depression or anxiety, or a major functional disorder alone, or a functional disorder with some memory loss. The physician's interviewing technique should produce the answer as to whether he is dealing principally with a loss of intellectual function, with a major functional disorder, or with some mixture of both.

Mortality and Brain Syndrome

Without differentiation of acute brain syndrome, chronic brain syndrome or dementia, or functional psychiatric disorders, opportunities for treatment may be missed. As already stated, acute brain syndrome is often a manifestation of a treatable medical problem or drug toxicity. In a study published in 1967, Drs. Leon J. Epstein and Alexander Simon, of San Francisco's Langley-Porter Neuropsychiatric Institute, analyzed the hospital admissions for mental illness of 534 elderly persons who had no prior psychiatric admission. Seventy-one patients came to the hospital with acute brain syndromes. On average, these acute brain syndromes began a week before admission. About one third of these patients died within two years of admission, with most of the mortality occurring during the first month.

Prehospital duration of brain syndromes, and the postadmission mortality patterns were different for patients with chronic brain syndrome (150) and mixed syndrome (177). For the chronic group, the median duration of prehospital illness had been almost three years. Nearly half of these patients died within two years of admission, the mortality curve extending gradually. From the mixed group, prehospital duration of the acute syndrome averaged about two weeks, while their chronic syndrome had been present about two years. About half of the mixed group died within a year of admission. The mortality curve approximated the acute syndrome pattern for the first two months and then leveled off to follow the chronic syndrome pattern. In other words, the curve too was mixed.

The Epstein-Simon study also found that 58 patients had only psychogenic disorders, primarily depressive and paranoid. There were 69 patients with "other organic brain disorder" and nine for whom no diagnosis was given.

These investigators found that the outcome was significantly related to diagnosis. One out of two patients with a diagnosis of chronic brain syndrome had died at the end of two years compared with one out of three with acute brain syndrome and one out of eight with psychogenic diagnoses. In essence, if the patient survived the immediate threat to life signified by the acute syndrome, the chances were good for a return to the community. Patients with acute brain syndrome tend either to die within the first month after admission or to recover. The prognosis for patients suffering from a psychogenic illness is excellent. In those with mixed conditions the decisive factor with regard to retaining the patient in the community vs prolonged institutionalization was the severity of the chronic brain syndrome.

Let me conclude by emphasizing that in any patient, regardless of age, one must first determine what type of neuropsychiatric problem is presenting. Is this an acute confusional reaction with recent onset caused by a medical illness or drug toxicity? Does the history reveal a long-term decline in intellectual function? Or is the presenting disorder chiefly functional or emotional, for example, the elderly patient with recent onset of depression? History, interview, and physical examination are extremely valuable in distinguishing functional disturbance from organic dementias, organic dementia from acute confusional reaction, and mixtures of these presentations. This approach is essential to ensure that treatable neuropsychiatric conditions are not overlooked.

6

Heart Disease in the Elderly

KENNETH B. LEWIS
Johns Hopkins University

Four basic principles should govern the evaluation and treatment of older persons with heart disease: 1) the differential diagnostic possibilities should not be limited by the age factor; 2) as in other areas of medicine, age may modify the individual's response to his disease; 3) nonetheless, age is only one factor in developing an optimal therapeutic regimen, which should be individualized in every case; 4) the physician and the elderly patient with a cardiac problem must set and accept realistic goals as to what can be accomplished in the management of that problem.

These principles may seem so obvious as to require no discussion. But if we are candid with ourselves the realities of clinical practice tell us otherwise. With respect to diagnosis, for example, we would all accept in theory the precept that there is no cardiac condition peculiar to older persons and none from which they are exempt. But it is unusual for an individual past middle age who presents with congestive heart failure and a rapid heart to be given any diagnosis other than arteriosclerotic heart disease unless a predisposing history for another form of cardiac pathology has been established earlier in life. He may in fact have rheumatic heart disease with mitral stenosis, a circumstance in which the murmur very often cannot be heard during the acute failure episode. Only by careful reevaluation after the clinical picture has been stabilized will the true diagnosis emerge. Its therapeutic implications are quite different from and more encouraging than those of degenerative disease, but they will be unrealized unless the possibility of another diagnosis is entertained.

In this context it is worth stressing that no cardiac problem should be labeled until the diagnosis has been established with absolute certainty. Otherwise important diagnostic studies that could clarify the etiology may not be done. For example, if an individual is described as having "chest pain of unknown cause," each time the physician sees the patient he must reconsider what the cause may be. If the patient has simply been described as having "angina pectoris," the label sticks and the matter is considered to have been settled. Yet the diagnosis may be totally incorrect.

Within the framework of the principles stated above, I will discuss three major cardiovascular problems – congestive heart failure, chest pain, and disorders of rhythm – in terms of how they should be approached in the older individual.

Congestive Heart Failure

Congestive failure is, of course, a syndrome or symptom complex secondary to many different etiologies. Some 40 years ago, Dr. Louis Hamman at Johns Hopkins offered a checklist of possible etiologies to help his students avoid missing a diagnosis having important therapeutic implications. Valid at all ages, the approach is especially appropriate in the elderly as a counterweight to the bias favoring a diagnosis of arteriosclerotic heart disease. Dr. Hamman's list, slightly modified, is presented on page 40.

The first item on the list is valvular (rheumatic)

Causes of Congestive Heart Failure

Valvular heart disease	Myocardial disease
Systemic hypertension	Congenital heart disease
Pulmonary hypertension	High output states
Pericardial disease	Traumatic heart disease

heart disease, especially mitral stenosis. While the incidence of acute rheumatic fever in childhood has declined dramatically in the past two or three decades, there is still a large reservoir of rheumatic heart disease among the adult population, and it is not confined, as is generally thought, to adults in the 30- to 50-year age group. The diagnosis had been missed in several elderly patients admitted to our hospital recently. The admitting diagnosis was stroke secondary to arteriosclerotic heart disease; the correct diagnosis proved to be stroke secondary to rheumatic heart disease and systemic embolization.

At Baltimore City Hospital some years ago we followed seven people aged 65 to 73 who had severe, catheterization-proved mitral stenosis. With careful medical management these patients lived four to five more years, an outcome one would not, in a prior epoch, have expected among patients with valvular disease of the severity observed. This would not have been possible of course if the diagnosis had not been considered and appropriate treatment instituted. In most, treatment included chronic anticoagulation to minimize the risk of mural thrombosis and subsequent embolization to the brain. For selected patients in their 70s whose basic health is otherwise good, even valvular surgery can be undertaken with reasonable success.

The second cause of congestive failure on our checklist is systemic hypertension. Unfortunately, by the time heart failure develops secondary to long-standing hypertension, the therapeutic possibilities are limited. The hypertension can be treated and the congestive failure managed with digitalis, drugs, and diet, but there is very little that one can do to reverse the underlying problem.

When the failure is secondary to pulmonary hypertension, however, the implications of correct diagnosis are extremely important for the older patient. The patient may present with failure only, but on physical examination a loud second heart sound may be heard, suggesting high pressure in the pulmonary artery. This is usually secondary to recurrent pulmonary emboli coming from the legs or the pelvic veins. Recurrent arrhythmias, especially recurrent bouts of tachycardia that cannot be explained, are another clue to such embolization. I would stress that these are highly subtle signs: the classic clues of shortness of breath, chest pain, and coughing up of blood are not present. But an orderly review of the possible causes of the failure will alert one to the meaning of these more equivocal clues. It is hardly necessary to emphasize that in this situation institution of anticoagulant therapy, as well as specific treatment for venous disease of the legs when indicated, may well prove lifesaving.

In other patients, congestive failure may reflect pericardial disease. Once one has recognized that the enlargement of the heart is not secondary to arteriosclerotic heart disease, but, say, to compromise of cardiac filling and function by fluid in the pericardial sac, drainage may reverse the failure. The implica-

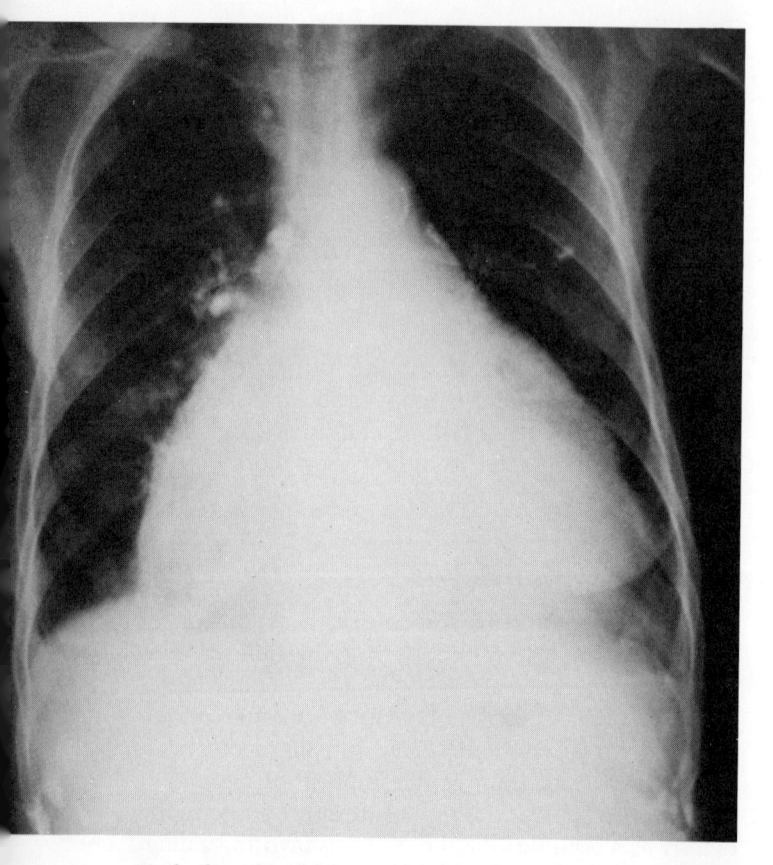

Both chest film above and echogram opposite were made in a 68-year-old woman admitted with acute pulmonary edema. Problem underlying failure was mitral stenosis.

tions here are diagnostic as well as therapeutic, since study of the tapped fluid sometimes reveals metastases from an occult tumor or suggests the presence of some other previously unrecognized disease. Another possibility is that the pericardium has become thickened and fibrotic, perhaps as a consequence of tuberculosis, and the therapeutic implication may be surgery to peel off the constricting layer, enabling the heart to pump more freely.

In myocarditis or myocardopathy, where the heart muscle may have become generally diseased for any one of a number of reasons (chronic alcoholism, recurrent viral infection, recurrent infarction and scarring), treatment cannot do much to overcome the underlying problem. It is of course possible to stabilize the patient's condition by medical management even though the pump will remain compromised.

Previously undiagnosed congenital heart disease would appear to be an even less likely cause of failure in the older person than rheumatic heart disease. Yet it has often been pointed out that people with the milder congenital cardiac anomalies can and do enjoy ordinary good health for many years.

One congenital cardiac anomaly being more readily detected among older people is atrial septal defect (ASD). Patients may have been entirely free of cardiac symptoms prior to the first episode of failure. In many cases, surgery to close the defect can prove totally corrective, as in the patient whose x-ray is shown on page 42. He was a 59-year-old man admitted to Baltimore City Hospital in acute congestive failure. Once the failure had been brought under control, he was reevaluated and a large ASD was discovered. His course has been uneventful in the four years since surgery. But the cardiomegaly at admission might easily have been construed as of degenerative etiology.

Two other items on our list of differential diagnoses are high output failure, which may reflect unrecognized and treatable hyperthyroidism, and traumatic heart disease, e.g., from an auto accident that damaged the aorta or valve structures. If such possibilities are kept in mind, questioning of the patient or his family may elicit supporting data.

The purpose of this chapter is not to review in any detail the therapy to be undertaken once a definitive diagnosis has been achieved; the suggestions made along the way simply illustrate some of the therapeutic implications of the differentiation process. For all elderly people with congestive failure, however, including those whose problem is indeed secondary to atherosclerotic heart disease, one should consider what role their age may play in precipitating the acute episode. The underlying ailment may have been present for quite a while. Why does it surface as congestive failure at the particular time?

The overriding circumstance to be kept in mind is that with age there is a decrease in the heart's ability to respond to demands for higher output. In a person who has previously been under treatment, the first point to check is whether he may have discontinued, consciously or out of forgetfulness, previously prescribed medications such as diuretics or digitalis. Sometimes the individual is not alert enough to tell his physician whether or not he has stopped taking his drugs, and this may make it necessary to proceed very cautiously with the therapy of the acute episode. A drug-forgetful patient may also unwittingly have increased the stresses on his circulation through dietary indiscretion. The physician who asks himself why the episode occurred at this particular time and not before may discover that a family party or some other celebration took place the day before –

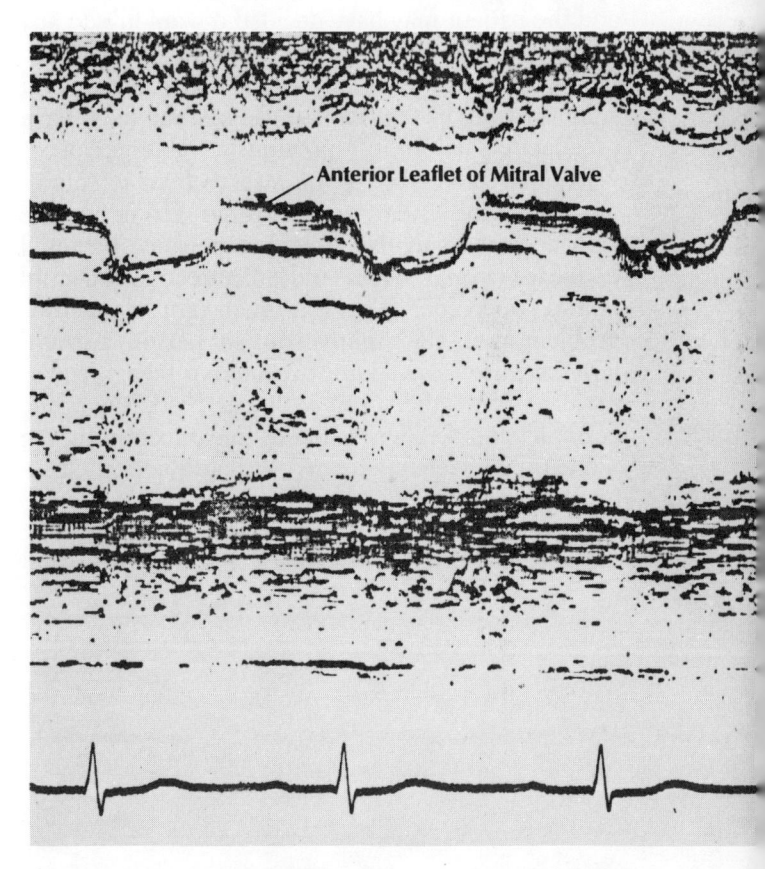

Severity of patient's mitral stenosis is revealed by extreme flattening and decreased amplitude of wave form traced by anterior leaflet during ventricular diastole.

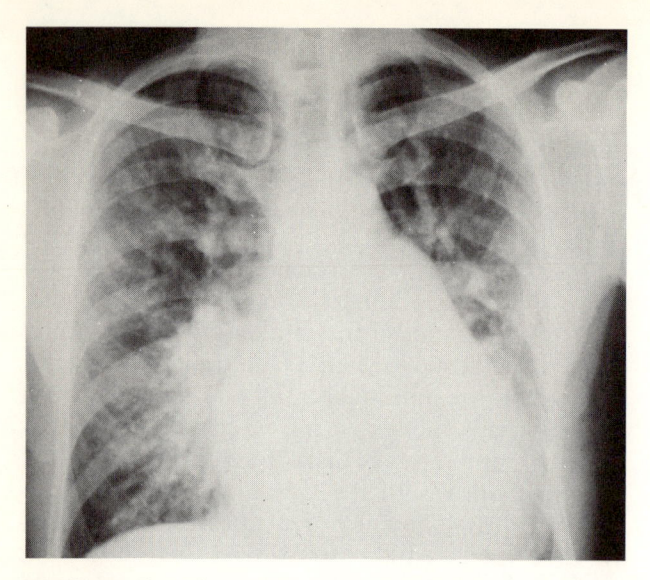

Etiology of cardiomegaly present at admission in a 59-year-old man with acute congestive failure proved to be atrial septal defect, which was corrected surgically.

and the patient may have decided it wouldn't do any harm to forget his salt-restricted diet this one time. Or a spurt of unusual physical activity, perhaps for some reason like putting in a garden, may have precipitated failure in a previously stable person.

Another possibility is the stress of an infection, perhaps of the urinary tract or lungs. Or, in persons with acquired valvular disease, especially, bacterial endocarditis may occur and go unrecognized until failure supervenes. This is a much more dangerous problem in an older than a younger person, particularly because it is seldom suspected or recognized as rapidly. Often the fever is not as high, the white count less markedly elevated. While infections in the old can be effectively treated with antibiotics, efficacy may well depend on how promptly the problem is diagnosed.

Another factor that may precipitate failure is surgical stress, with the hazards of hypervolemia that arise from fluid administration and transfusion. Anemia, whatever its antecedent cause, may also lead to a high-output state and congestive failure.

But there are also times when the way the older patient is treated for acute ventricular failure itself produces problems that can be avoided if the physician remains alert to the fact that he is dealing with an elderly person. *Treatment should always begin with the steps that cost nothing in terms of risk.* Very simply, when we see an individual with marked shortness of breath, bubbling rales in his lungs, and other classic signs of failure and pulmonary edema, elevating the head, putting him at rest to cut down on cardiac work, giving oxygen – none of these steps entails any risk. If we plan to place rotating tourniquets around three of the extremities to cut down on venous return to the heart, we must keep in mind that this procedure (innocuous in younger individuals with large muscles mass) may produce not only venous but even arterial thrombosis in old people with very thin arms and legs.

Advanced age dictates caution in the use of morphine, which is otherwise a fairly standard part of the acute pulmonary edema regimen. In the older person, even a small dose of morphine may produce marked sedation and depression of the respiratory centers. The physician then confronts the much more difficult problem of managing not only the left ventricular failure but also the respiratory failure.

Chest Pain

The four principles noted at the outset of this chapter apply equally to evaluation of chest pain in the older person. Again, the diagnosis may become much more difficult because age modifies the individual's response to his disease. In the younger person, the typical symptoms associated with heart attack – a heavy, squeezing pressure on the sternum

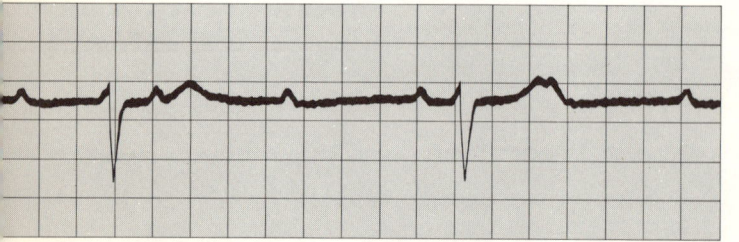

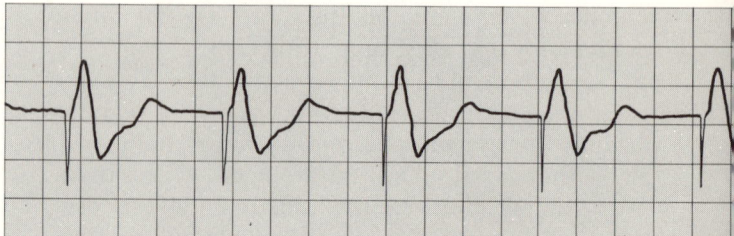

ECG tracings above were made in a 84-year-old woman who suffered frequent episodes of syncope. Tracing at left is representative of complete heart block; the one at right shows improvement following pacemaker insertion.

with sensation radiating to the neck, back, or arm – are usually present. In the older individual, the pain may be very indistinct, either because it is not perceived in the typical fashion or because it is actually not present to the same degree. The aging process may have caused changes within nervous tissue that diminish the intensity of signals reaching the brain.

Another point to be kept in mind is that the incidence of diabetes mellitus increases with age. A number of studies have documented that people with diabetes (a well-known risk factor for coronary disease) often do not experience any pain with a myocardial infarction. In fact, in an elderly diabetic the presenting symptoms may not suggest heart attack at all; they may be those of stroke, failure, or simply a syncopal episode. The incidence of such atypical presentations among diabetics has been reliably estimated at about 25%.

Awareness of such age-related factors will, of course, modify the physician's approach. In an individual who comes in with stroke, especially if he is diabetic, one of the first steps indicated is an electrocardiogram; it may show that the stroke was precipitated by a myocardial infarction. The implications for management are well known. Careful observation for arrhythmias is indicated and fluid therapy would need to be monitored more carefully. Another age-related factor is the probable presence of other diseases; these too must be taken into account in overall management of the cardiac problem. For example, chronic pulmonary disease makes the prognostic index less favorable in MI.

Despite the fact that the prognosis following heart attack declines with age, and despite the high statistical mortality recorded among the oldest age groups, it must not be assumed that the treatment options in the older patient are limited to palliative measures. With an individualized approach, some people – perhaps only a small number – can realistically be considered candidates for a more definitive approach such as coronary bypass surgery. Again, "individualized" is the key word. Recently, we saw a man of 70 who had been having syncopal episodes on minor exertion but otherwise seemed to be in good health. (It was thought he might have heart block and could benefit from a pacemaker.) During an exercise-tolerance test on the treadmill, his systolic blood pressure dropped to 40 mm Hg after 45 seconds and he fainted. Cardiac catheterization disclosed a single lesion that almost totally (90%) occluded the left anterior descending artery. Despite the patient's age – and as noted previously, age is only one factor in developing

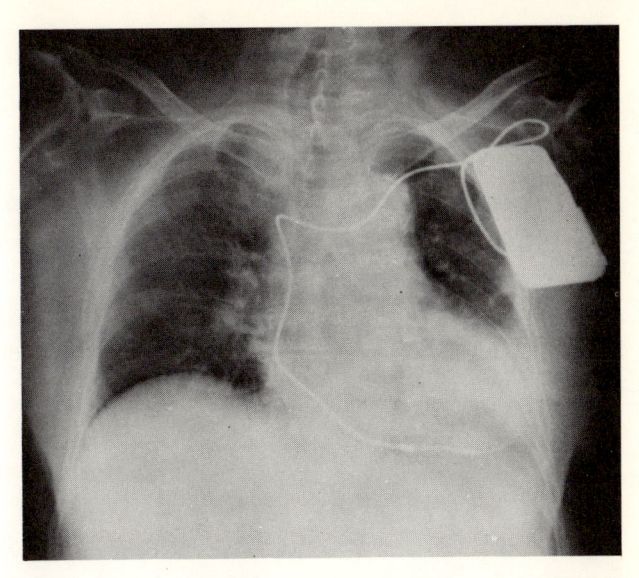

Development of transvenous pacing eliminated thoracotomy and removed age barriers to pacemaker insertion. Shown above is device in 95-year-old woman described in text. Pulse generator is in subcutaneous pocket; pacing wire is passed through cephalic vein into right ventricle. Only local anesthesia is needed.

an optimal therapeutic regimen – we felt there was no alternative to treating him as we would a younger person in the same situation; any significant physical effort was too likely to bring sudden death. Following coronary bypass surgery, he has done well.

Disorders of Rhythm and Conduction

Turning to our third group of problems – cardiac arrhythmias and conduction disturbances – once again we find an increasing incidence with aging; in fact, studies of persons living in homes for the aged suggest that as many as 25% to 35% have disturbances of heart rhythm. The majority of these irregularities are not severe and require no therapy. But it is important to be aware of them and to consider whether, in the particular patient, they signal some significant underlying disease.

An obvious possibility is advancing coronary arteriosclerosis, but the arrhythmia may in fact be the first manifestation of an electrolyte disturbance. If the patient has been on long-term diuretic therapy, we may find that his potassium is now 2 mEq/L instead of 4 mEq/L, and a potassium supplement or dietary change may be indicated. If he has been on digitalis, the dose and the factors that may affect it should be reviewed. It may be that renal function is

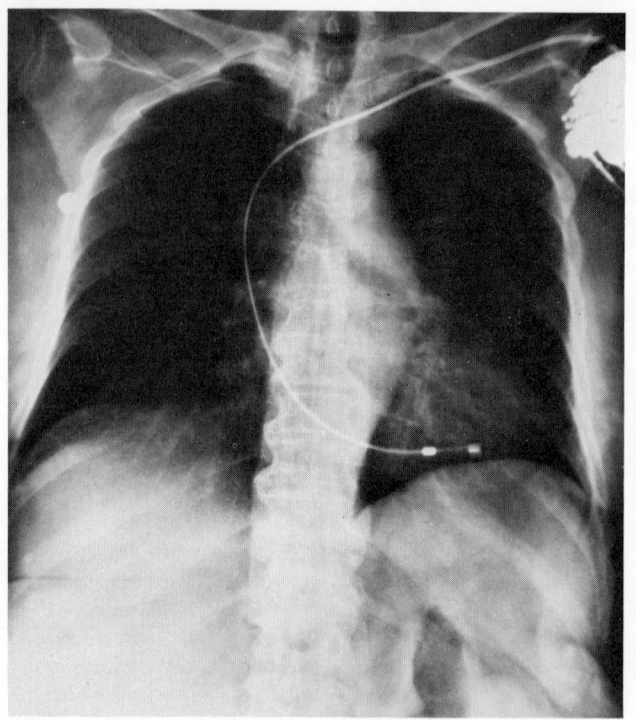

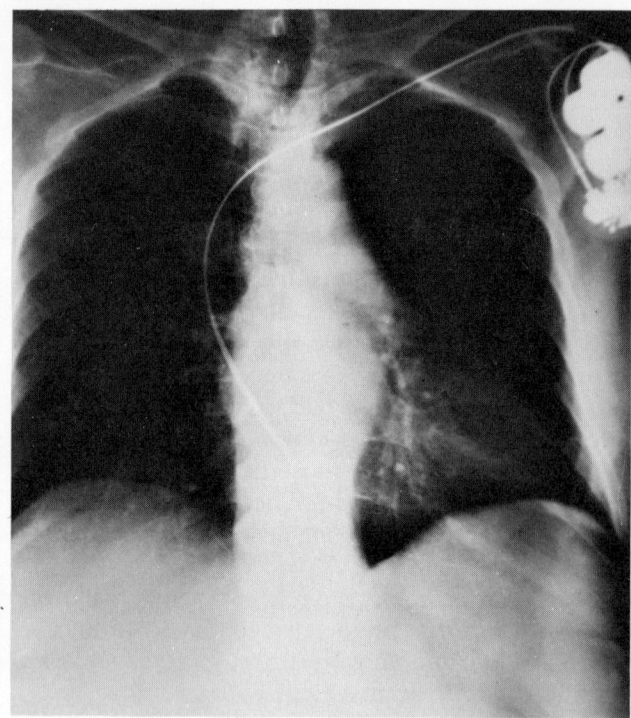

Loose subcutaneous tissue may sometimes cause pulse generators to drift in old people, as illustrated above. Originally, pacing wire was correctly positioned in right ventricle (left) but after six months, generator had descended, catheter was pulled up into atrium and almost out of the heart (right), and patient's symptoms recurred.

diminished and a portion of the dose is not being excreted. Another possibility is that, as noted earlier, the arrhythmia reflects pulmonary embolism; if so, anticoagulation may prevent a disastrous episode.

Evaluating an arrhythmia in an older patient is often a frustrating problem; the patient complains of recurrent fluttering in the chest, yet when the physician sees him, the ECG is totally normal. In this situation, it is often helpful to have the patient wear the 24-hour portable (Holter) tape recorder; review of the tracings, which can be done very quickly, will pick up the intermittent disturbances.

Again, it is important that treatment be individualized, that the patient, not the ECG, become the focus of attention. And age is an important determinant of what treatment is to be given. For example, a supraventricular tachycardia with a heart rate of 180 may be relatively innocuous and require little immediate treatment in a person of 21. In a 70-year-old individual who is also hypotensive and cyanotic, a much more aggressive approach may be required; it may, for example, be desirable to revert the arrhythmia immediately by electroshock, or cardioversion, rather than spend a half hour or more waiting to see whether drugs will have the needed effect. Although I would not recommend use of electroshock routinely as the first intervention in older persons with severe arrhythmias, neither should it be viewed solely or primarily as a last resort, as it so often is. By the time the decision is reached, the patient's capacity to withstand the effects of the arrhythmia may have been exhausted.

Another electrical problem that becomes more common with aging is, of course, heart block. This was formerly considered secondary to coronary atherosclerosis but thanks to the elegant studies of Dr. Maurice Lev and others, we now know that most such abnormalities result from aging within the conductive tissues and not from ischemia as such.

Fainting spells caused by heart block occur very often in the old; fortunately, this is a problem we can often remedy. I refer, of course, to insertion of a cardiac pacemaker. Old age as such is no longer a contraindication to pacemaker implantation. The x-ray on page 43 was made in a 95-year-old woman who was still quite capable of taking care of herself and her household but who was subject to recurrent episodes of fainting. Some 15 years or so ago, when pacemaker implantation required thoracotomy so that the wires could be sewn to the surface of the heart, one might have hesitated to undertake the procedure in a woman of this age, but the development of transvenous pacemakers that are positioned under local anesthesia has eliminated the age barrier. Moreover, present-day pacemakers are mainly "demand" devices that do not pulse unless the patient's heart beat is interrupted for a preset number of seconds. Such devices eliminate the possibility of competition with the heart's intrinsic rhythm.

However, age does complicate some aspects of pacemaker use. The older and heavier devices, especially, tend to drift downward in the very loose subcutaneous tissue typical of some old people and in doing so may actually pull the pacing catheter out of the heart. This problem is illustrated in the x-rays on page 44; six months after her pacemaker was inserted, the patient returned complaining that she was again experiencing fainting spells. While anchorage can be improved by suturing the pulse generator in place or implanting it in a Dacron mesh bag to facilitate anchoring it, the patient should also be seen at regular intervals to check the position of the device. Much of this necessary follow-up can be performed by the office nurse or physician's assistant. Another problem in the older patient with thin skin and very little subcutaneous tissue is the large protuberance the pacemaker creates on the chest wall; a fall may even break open the pocket containing the pulse generator. Patients must be warned of this hazard and helped to avoid it.

Formerly it was recommended that pacemakers be replaced at two-year intervals in anticipation of failure. For devices manufactured before mid-1972 this recommendation remains valid, but most instruments built subsequently are so designed that with the loss of the first of their five cells, the heart rate drops 10 beats per minute. If the patient is being seen frequently, as he should be, the need for replacement will be signaled by the pacemaker itself, obviating automatic "prophylactic" replacement. Efforts are also under way to improve the power sources, and a rechargeable system is now available that permits recharging through the skin. Some 3,000 of these devices have now been implanted.

The Role of Counseling

One of the principles mentioned at the outset of this chapter was the need for physician and patient to set and accept realistic goals in the management of cardiac problems. The pursuit of an individualized diagnosis and therapy is, of course, the ultimate determinant of what those goals will be. But the principle also implies a counseling relation of doctor to patient that may be more important in the older age groups than in any other.

Let me touch briefly on some of the subjects the elderly patient is often most concerned about and that his doctor should be sensitive to. A major one is diet. How necessary is it to institute an aggressively antiatherogenic diet in older people with cardiac problems? This is a debatable point but my answer would be, not very. While I would be aggressive about prescribing a cholesterol-reducing diet for the young person who suffers a heart attack or in whom high serum lipids have been identified, there seems much less point to doing so past the age of 60 to 65.

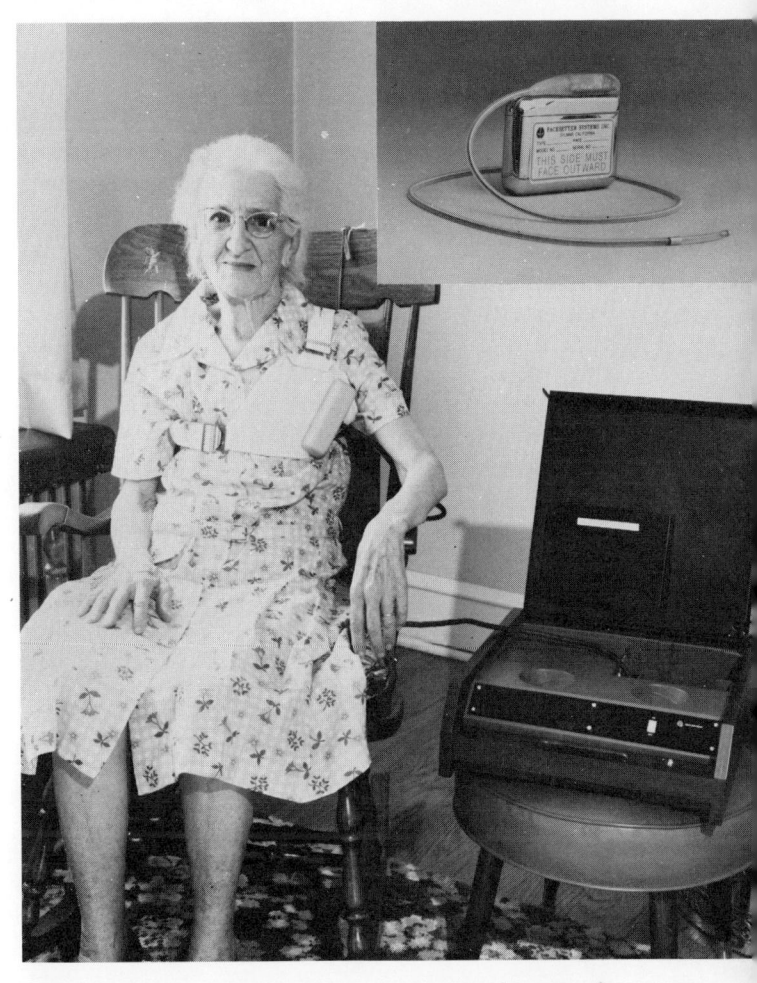

A 76-year-old Baltimore resident is seen recharging the pacemaker she received three years ago at Johns Hopkins, where it was developed. A weekly session of one hour is required to recharge the power cell (inset). Rechargeable feature has made it possible to reduce size and bulk of generator to about 2 fingerbreadths.

There is little evidence that such a diet will affect established atherosclerosis, and many older people get much of their nutrition from foods like milk, cheese, and eggs.

This laissez-faire approach does not apply, however, to salt, which should be restricted if fixed hypertension (several readings above 95 diastolic) or congestive failure are involved. In this situation I have found it extremely helpful to ask patients to weigh themselves every day at home. A small maneuver, to be sure, but useful in more than one way. If the patient who ordinarily puts up with salt restriction falls from grace and eats a salt load, the bathroom scale will disclose a sudden gain of five or more pounds. It has been explained to him initially that a gain of this type cannot be flesh; it must be water. He has also been given a diuretic to take if such an episode occurs. The result, of course, is a rapid return to his previous weight.

After this has happened a couple of times, the patient recognizes the importance of the salt restriction (he has in fact performed a clinical experiment with himself as the subject) and is much more likely to comply. I have also found it feasible, in many patients, to prescribe diuretics on an "as needed only" basis. In turn, this reduces the risk of potassium depletion and often obviates potassium supplements altogether. Moreover, as one would expect, patients who participate this actively in their own care are likely to be much more intelligent and cooperative in all respects than they would be otherwise.

Similarly, it can be helpful for the patient to participate in deciding how much physical exertion is permissible for him. My inclination is to allow patients to continue at whatever level of activity can be undertaken without the appearance of symptoms. Many physicians still tend arbitrarily to tell old people to cut down on activity, though there is little scientific evidence that this is beneficial.

Sometimes patients, or their spouses, are fearful concerning physical exertion. If feasible, a graded exercise tolerance test on a treadmill – with a physician and a technician in attendance in case an arrhythmia develops – can prove to be therapeutic as well as diagnostic. The patient frequently discovers – usually to his great surprise – that he can undertake much more vigorous exercise than he had thought possible. A candid discussion of sexual activity should also take place.

Efforts such as these to involve the patient in his care and to instruct him concerning the nature of his particular problem are a vital element in caring for the old person with cardiac disease. As much information as possible should be provided as to when and what he should report concerning the way he feels. If the problem is angina pectoris, I emphasize, for example, that it is *not* necessary to report every episode but that a change in the pattern of the pain should be communicated: e.g., if it now wakes him at night though it did not do so before, or if it fails to respond to the usual dose of nitroglycerine. If dyspnea has not previously been a problem but episodes of breathlessness or gasping occur, they should be reported; they may be the clue that pulmonary embolism is developing. If edema progresses despite medication, this should be reported; patients (or their families) should not wait until fluid has built up above the knees.

Family members play an especially important role in the communication between patient and doctor, as would be expected in this age group. They should be instructed on how to take the pulse during a syncopal episode, and they should be reassured – in advance – that an episode of pulmonary edema is usually manageable; it is not always as life-threatening as it sometimes appears. They can also be instructed in measures they can take before the physician arrives, such as assisting the patient to sit with his legs dangling over the side of the bed.

Finally, it must be kept in mind that fear is almost always present in the older patient; one must try to sense the implications of a problem to the patient's self-image, while appreciating that cultural backgrounds and supportive resources are highly variable. When such understanding is added to the benefits of precise diagnosis – and the wealth of knowledge physicians already have concerning cardiovascular disease and the treatment possibilities – an optimal job can be done to help the elderly meet and adapt to the problems of an ailing heart.

7

CHD Risk Factors

WILLIAM P. CASTELLI
Framingham Heart Study

When the Framingham study began in 1949, the 5,127 men and women aged 30 to 62 who were entered into its ranks were free of cardiovascular disease. They have been followed up at two-year intervals for the last 26 years in order to establish correlations between antecedent personal attributes and living habits and the development of atherosclerotic illness. As the reader is well aware, the findings at these biennial examinations have been subjected to detailed, continuing analysis, and the effects of the "risk factors" so identified have been studied minutely in terms of how they promote disease. It is not too much to suggest that the epidemiologic approach to the natural history of cardiovascular disease, including not only the Framingham study but many others in both the United States and abroad, has since paid off handsomely in understanding how to prevent heart attacks and strokes.

But as the study's findings were being translated into clinical applications among young and middle-aged adults, with correction or abolition of risk factors emphasized as the key to reducing "premature" cardiovascular disease (generally defined as occurring prior to age 65), the Framingham cohort itself was, of course, growing older. Many of its members are now approaching or already fall within so-called geriatric age groupings. One major aspect of the older population is that not all the people are the same. Some have stayed remarkably healthy, others have suffered heart attacks and strokes. Yet the people who developed heart attacks or strokes differed years in advance from those who have remained healthy. Whatever one's feelings about "you can't live forever" or "the patients lived a good life, now it's time to leave them alone," it is abundantly clear in Framingham that many of the major risk factors appear to be operative in the geriatric age groups, and it is not outside the realm of possibility that better management of these factors in the older persons will result in a better life. Also, as Dr. Weldon J. Walker recently pointed out, the decrease in cardiovascular death rates observed over the last 10 years has occured right up to age 85, and to only a somewhat lesser degree in the elderly than in younger age groups. Are there some risk factors that one can never outgrow? What can be gleaned from the most recent Framingham experience to assist the primary and/or family physician in the care of his elderly patients? Or, to put it another way, how should the doctor assess risk in an older person, and what should he do about it?

We will return to these questions in the course of this discussion, but let us begin by recalling the risk factors defined by the Framingham study and some of the interactions among them. Those about which the individual can do relatively little are age, sex, and heredity; those subject to intervention are hypertension, elevated blood lipids, cigarette smoking, diabetes mellitus, left ventricular hypertrophy (as evidenced on the ECG) and hyperuricemia. Most of this chapter will be concerned with the latter group, but let us say briefly about age that it must be considered the most potent risk factor of all, since the incidence of cardiovascular mortality and morbidity (hereafter CHD) advances with age no matter what interventions are undertaken. (Yet, as we all know, there are people who show few atherosclerotic

CHAPTER 7: CASTELLI

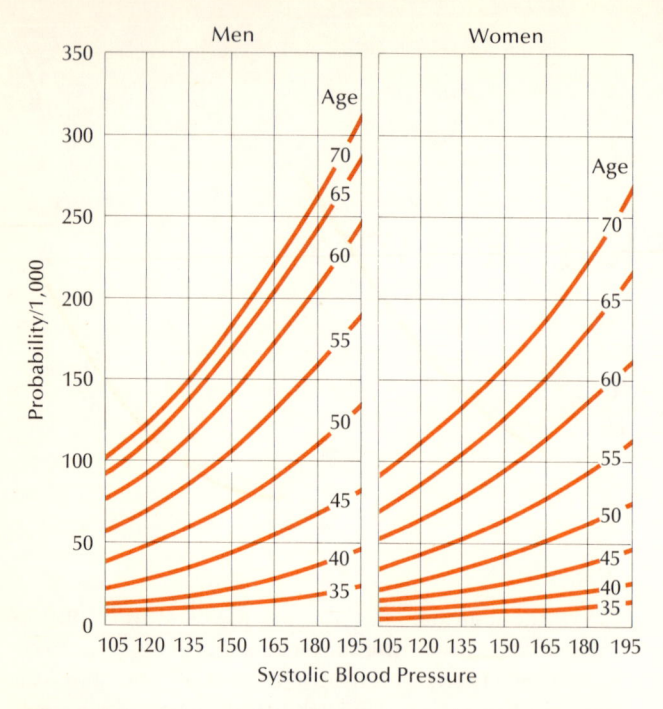

That gradient of risk from hypertension becomes steeper with age is shown by graph of probability of cardiovascular disease within eight years among low-risk subjects in Framingham study. Data reflect 18 years of follow-up.

changes even at an advanced age, and it would be interesting to know what makes them more resistant – even as it would be interesting to know what makes others more susceptible – to the disease process.) As for heredity, the only factor of consequence established by the Framingham data applies to men: if a father died of coronary heart disease before age 60, his son's risk is double the standard risk. The effects of male or female sex will be discussed in the context of the various parameters making up the "risk profile." As for some other factors often considered to raise CHD risk, the Framingham study did *not* find that intake of alcohol and coffee, number of hours of sleep, and educational, emotional, or socioeconomic status are positively correlated with CHD incidence.

At any time in life, including old age, the most potent of the controllable risk factors is hypertension, and this applies to both sexes. Even trivial elevations of blood pressure raise the incidence of coronary heart disease and atherosclerotic brain infarction. The misconception that older people "tolerate" hypertension well may have arisen because the young person with hypertension does in fact have a poor prognosis. But such young individuals are rare, relatively speaking, and their hypertensive disease is simply not comparable to the age-associated disease that becomes manifest in so many people later in life. It does not follow that age-associated hypertension in the elderly is a benign condition. In reality, the Framingham data show that the gradient of risk from hypertension becomes *higher* with age. On the average, then, the elderly tolerate higher pressures not better but much less well than younger people.

If the old saw has been discredited that "normal" systolic blood pressure in millimeters of mercury equals 100 plus one's age, so too has the view that it is only the diastolic pressure that counts. An important finding in the Framingham study is that systolic pressure is as predictive as diastolic of CHD (see graph on page 49). Disproportionate rises in systolic pressure, such as are seen in aging, are also far from innocuous. Actuarial studies have in fact shown that at *any* diastolic pressure (low or high), CHD risk is proportional to systolic pressure. Nor is there any evidence, as another old saw holds, that women – especially postmenopausal women – are tolerant of hypertension. The Framingham data show that women with normal diastolic pressure but borderline or definitely hypertensive systolic pressure have a CHD risk that is 50% above standard. This is little better than that of comparable men and cannot be considered evidence of "tolerance." Indeed, at any level of pressure, men and women run about equal risk of stroke. Rather, age-associated hypertension probably holds at least part of the explanation as to why the male-female CHD gap narrows with advancing age.

One of the earliest and clearest "messages" delivered by the Framingham study was that there is no blood-pressure threshold of safety, i.e., that there is a steady increment of risk at all blood pressure levels. We now know that this is as true of systolic as of diastolic pressure, that it is true at all ages, and that it is true in the absence of distressing symptoms. We would, accordingly, urge the physician who says "I treat symptoms, not blood pressure measurements" to reconsider his position. True, it may take skill and tact to convince an asymptomatic patient that inconvenient or uncomfortable actions are necessary, such as changing his or her diet, losing weight, or taking drugs. But the task should not be blinked at in a society where every fifth man will undergo a coronary episode prior to age 60!

In managing hypertension, the goal should be a reduction at least to 140/90. Drug regimens should be preceded by a trial of diet to lose weight and/or reduce salt intake. This failing, the general rule is to move from less to more potent drug interventions, beginning with a diuretic trial and progressing, if necessary, to drugs such as reserpine, methyldopa, propranolol, guanethidine, and others, using low doses of several drugs rather than multiple doses of one drug. The details of such regimens are well known.

To conclude our discussion of hypertension as a risk factor, we would note that the physician caring for older people will find it extremely helpful to control the condition as a means of limiting the incidence of congestive heart failure. About 75% of congestive failure patients can be identified as having uncontrolled hypertension by the simple maneuver of taking their blood pressure. If these hypertensives are identified in advance and aggressively treated, the number of congestive heart failure cases is assuredly going to be reduced. In the classic Veterans Administration studies by Freis et al, which conclusively laid to rest the idea that hypertension did not necessarily require treatment, no cases of congestive failure at all developed in the treated group as compared with 20 among the controls.

Blood Lipids

With respect to intervention to lower blood lipids, the evidence is less strong than with hypertension. And indeed, as an epidemiologist, I must concede that clinical experience has not yet provided a picture of the value of reducing blood lipids clear-cut enough to render recommendations in this respect noncontroversial. Be that as it may, evidence is not lacking. Of especial interest in connection with the geriatric age group is a Veterans Administration study conducted by Dayton and Pearce at an old soldiers' home in San Francisco. In this study 846 residents (mostly men, of course) were followed for some seven years. At the beginning of the study the average age of the subjects was 67 and the age range 54 to 88. Dietary control of blood lipids was pursued by using a diet enriched with polyunsaturates as compared with a control group who ate the usual diet. There was a 25% reduction below the expected CHD death rate in the treated vs the control group, with the bulk of the improvement occurring at the younger (54 to 64) end of the age range. Unfortunately, no diet study has been done in which the blood lipids were lowered to those levels seen in developing countries where the disease is unknown. Yet adoption of a typical Asian or Mediterranean diet would do this.

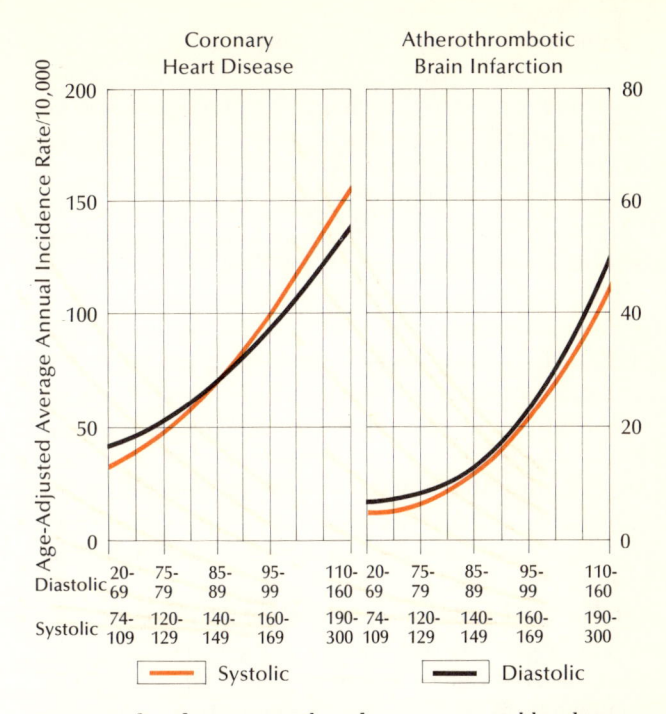

Increased risk associated with increases in blood pressure is as clearly demonstrated by systolic as by diastolic measurements, Framingham data show. Graph is based on experience of women aged 45 to 74.

Ordinarily one assesses the blood lipids as a CHD risk factor in terms of elevation above some standard considered normal for the particular population. Positive correlations have been found between risk and elevations of total cholesterol, low-density lipoproteins, very-low-density lipoproteins, and triglycerides; i.e., the higher the concentration of any of these in the blood, the higher the risk. Since 1951, it had also been appreciated that there is a lipoprotein class that has an inverse, or negative, relationship to cardiovascular risk — the high-density lipoproteins (HDL), or alpha cholesterol. In this case, the *lower* the concentration, the higher the risk.

Now the Framingham study is providing evidence that of *all* the lipoproteins and lipids measured, HDL has the largest actual impact on risk in the older age groups. Starting in 1969, or 20 years after the initiation of the study, 1,025 men and 1,445 women still free of cardiovascular disease and now aged 49 to 82 were enlisted into an effort to explore this subject. Some 142 new cases of CHD have since developed among this subset. At what was generally their eleventh biennial examination, the subjects gave fasting blood specimens that were then analyzed by various techniques to permit correlations of antecedent lipoprotein levels with subsequent CHD risk.

The graph on page 51 summarizes the strong negative correlation between HDL value in these individuals and CHD incidence. The inverse correlation is present in both sexes, even though women tend to have substantially higher values. This is, of course, consistent with their lifelong (if narrowing) advantage with respect to CHD, yet at any level of HDL, women and men run comparable risks.

As noted above, the negative correlation of HDL with CHD risk has been known for some time. Recently Glueck's group in Cincinnati, who have been studying families of notable longevity, showed that one characteristic of these people who live into their late eighties and nineties in very good health is an unusually high HDL level. In addition, other epidemiologic study groups – in Albany, Hawaii, Evans County (Georgia), and San Francisco – have found the HDL relationship operative in CHD risk.

The suggestion of metabolic workers seeking a possible mechanism of action is that HDL may serve somewhat as a "scavenger" lipoprotein, sweeping cholesterol out of deposits in various parts of the body and delivering it to the liver for excretion. It is also conjectured that HDL interferes with cellular uptake of cholesterol.

What is the significance of these developments for the practitioner caring for the geriatric group? First of all, one should appreciate that the HDL determination is a very simple one, requiring only a colorimeter and centrifuge, and can be made by any laboratory that can test for serum cholesterol. When heparin manganese is added to the usual cholesterol preparation, all the lighter lipoproteins are precipitated. An aliquot of the supernatant is then processed through the usual methods for cholesterol to produce the HDL value.

By requesting an HDL as well as a cholesterol determination, the physician adds considerable specificity to the assessment of his patient. A cholesterol value between 200 and 250 might be considered normal or borderline for an American, but in combination, say, with an HDL value below 45, a strong alarm is sounded for CHD risk. If the usual dietary changes do not suffice to bring the cholesterol values down substantially, one would then consider instituting drugs such as cholestyramine or nicotinic acid, or clofibrate or nicotinic acid if the problem is primarily hypertriglyceridemia. Long-distance runners tend to have much higher levels of HDL, and this adds weight to the introduction of a better physical activity training program for older patients.

An HDL determination may provide specificity in other ways as well. For example, in older women, cholesterol values are sometimes deceptively high. Let us say that in such a patient the total cholesterol determination is given as 260. If the HDL value proves to be 100, the patient does not need treatment, since so substantial a share of the total is in the alpha or HDL fraction. She is also at relatively low risk because her HDL value is high.

What dietary recommendations can be made to the elderly to aid them in controlling blood lipids? As suggested by the VA study in San Francisco it still appears to be highly desirable to keep the proportion of saturated fats in the diet low and to emphasize cooking with polyunsaturates. Although many old people get a good deal of their protein requirements from eggs and dairy products, and one should therefore proceed cautiously so as not to deprive them of nutrition while trying to correct hyperlipidemia, they *can* be advised to substitute skim milk for whole milk, margarine for butter, and cottage cheese for hard cheeses. Eggs should be used only sparingly; a two-egg-a-day habit elevates serum cholesterol by 25 mg/dl. It is better to call upon the services of a dietitian, so that a proper mix, for example, of weight reduction, lipid reduction, and nutritional balance can be attained. Nutrition as a genuine medical therapy is neglected in this country. Yet most of us with a little study could learn the basis of good nutrition; medical schools should begin teaching it seriously and so should house officer training programs. While physicians do not have the time to do all the patient training, they will be better able to coordinate these therapies through stronger dietetic services that they helped to foster in their own practice areas.

With age, as we have all observed, women tend to fatten and men to slim down, and while obesity has not been shown to be directly atherogenic, it has indirect effects on risk via hypertension and cholesterol elevation. In fact, weight reduction, together with restrictions on salt intake, may make it possible to control hypertension in some individuals without drugs or with fewer drugs. Indeed, weight loss in Framingham is associated with a fall in cholesterol, blood pressure, blood glucose, and uric acid. The reverse of the obesity coin is physical inactivity and even in the elderly, reduced activity is associated with greater CHD risk (though less so than in younger people). Depending on their musculoskeletal status, a graduated walking program is the obvious recommendation for improving physical activity and assisting weight reduction in the elderly.

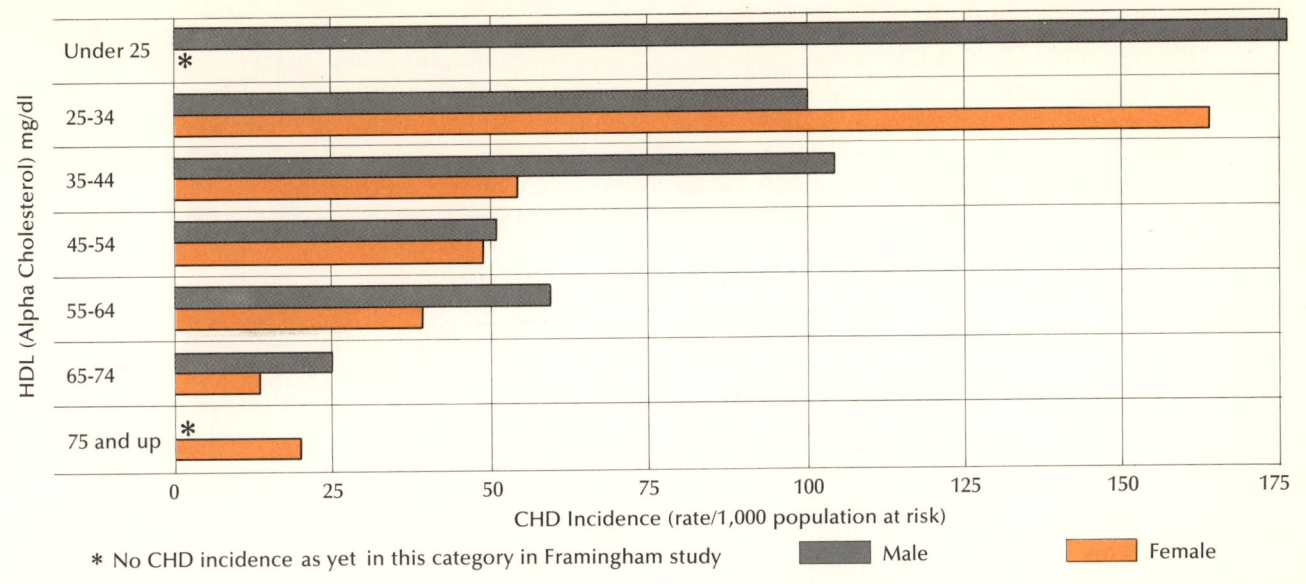

The strong negative correlation between high-density lipoprotein (HDL) values and CHD risk is apparent in graph based on data from 11th biennial examination of 1,025 men and 1,445 women of Framingham study. Among the older age groups (50 to 80), HDL is now considered the most risk-predictive of the lipoproteins.

The Other Risk Factors

Left ventricular hypertrophy as seen on the electrocardiogram must be viewed as placing the individual in a high-risk category. A patient with such an ECG change has the same prognosis as a person who has already had a myocardial infarction. The changes observed are a nonspecific ST-T wave change, in conjunction with an R or an S wave change (greater than 20 mv in standard leads, 11 mv in augmented limb leads, or 25 mv in precordial leads, or a combined R plus S change of 35 mv in the precordial leads). There may also be evidence of bundle-branch or intraventricular blocks. Even nonspecific ST-T changes increase the risk of a subsequent cardiovascular episode. Besides searching for left ventricular hypertrophy, bundle-branch blocks, and other nonspecific changes, the doctor should use his ECG routinely in this age group to look for unrecognized and "silent" myocardial infarctions – heart attacks occurring in people without the usual symptoms. The Framingham study identified this "silent MI" problem as considerable, accounting for a fourth of the total incidence of myocardial infarction. If the asymptomatic MI patient has a frank infarction later, he or she may not be recognized as having the poorer prognosis attached to a second attack. Statistics show that within five years after a first infarction, about half the patients have a second, and about half of these die of it.

Detecting the small changes indicative of the silent MI is facilitated if the physician already has a baseline tracing of the patient. A strict lead-by-lead comparison of baseline and fresh tracing is the key to diagnosis. If the baseline ECG shows no Q wave, the appearance of one with a 0.02- or 0.03-second duration supports the diagnosis of an asymptomatic unrecognized infarction. Such a small abnormality generally tends to be overlooked. A Q wave of 0.04-second duration in AVF, AVL, or any precordial V lead is reasonably good evidence by itself of an old infarction; this finding plus nonspecific ST-T changes would constitute strong evidence.

The risk of cardiovascular disease also increases with blood glucose value, whether or not it falls into the diabetic range. In the study, anyone with a casual value over 110 was strongly suspected of being diabetic and was given a glucose tolerance test, following which he or she was classified according to standard glucose tolerance criteria.

In the first 16 years of follow-up, 55 diabetics in the Framingham study population died, 42 of them of cardiovascular causes, resulting in a mortality rate almost three times higher than that of the general population. The impact on women was especially severe, raising their risk to the same as that of men in comparable age groups – in other words, a very substantial jump. In both sexes, the diabetes effect is primarily expressed through death from coronary heart disease. Although other CHD risk factors (e.g., hypertension, hyperlipidemia) are also elevated in diabetics, the diabetes effect is not solely secondary to this phenomenon. Statistical analysis shows there is an increment, especially in women, that cannot be accounted for by the other CHD risk factors alone.

Lacking prospective data based on controlled intervention trials, one may logically assume that controlling blood sugar would reduce CHD incidence. But it is also logical to do so in context. Dietary manipulation in diabetics thus should consider the effects not only on blood sugar but also on blood pressure and blood lipids. Yet a recent major new diabetic diet allows bacon and eggs for breakfast, ignoring the probable impact on hypertension and hypercholesterolemia.

Except in the geriatric ages, cigarette smoking is one of the three most important CHD risk factors. In the elderly, however, its impact is slight. It may be that by old age the persons most vulnerable to the CHD effects of cigarettes have already perished; the Framingham data identify smoking as a contributor to the sudden death of apparently healthy people.

Does this mean that the physician should look with equanimity on the heavy smoker among his geriatric patients? The impact in terms of coronary heart disease in the elderly may be low (and it has always been known to be modest in terms of stroke), but cigarette smoking is an extremely important factor in the chronic bronchitis, emphysema, and cancer problems so important among the geriatric age groups. Our advice would thus not be to condone smoking because its CHD relevance has diminished but to continue to encourage cessation of smoking, if anything, more vigorously than before.

Let us conclude this section on the risk factors as such with a word or two about hyperuricemia and gout, which have been found in the Framingham data to be associated with a twofold increase risk of CHD. The excess risk appears to be accounted for by the tendency of patients with hyperuricemia, including those without overt gout, to have higher lipid values, hypertension, and obesity. Why the association with atherogenic traits exists is not yet known.

Assessing CHD Risk

To some extent, the foregoing discussion of risk factors in the special context of the elderly has had a certain artificiality. There should be no discontinuity in approach between the middle-aged and the old so far as attention to risk factors is concerned. Sufficient data, from Framingham and other epidemiologic studies, have now been analyzed to permit persons at high risk to be identified at a time when appropriate treatment or modification of living habits can still have great impact on their long-term health and survival. CHD risk profiles have been developed that now make it possible to identify the one fifth of the population that will eventually develop 40% of the coronary heart disease, 58% of the peripheral arterial disease, 81% of the strokes, and 73% of the congestive heart failure. Moreover, only very simple office-based procedures are adequate to accomplish identification of these people: a cholesterol test, an alpha-cholesterol (HDL) test among older age groups, a blood pressure reading, blood sugar determination, and ECG. These parameters suffice to launch the necessary interventions.

For those who consider these statements excessively sweeping, we would cite the fact that the Framingham data have now been analyzed in sufficient detail not only to delineate the CHD risk factors but also to quantify the impact of each, individually and compositely over a broad range of ages. It is now possible to take an individual patient with a given risk-factor constellation and estimate concretely his personal probability of experiencing various types of cardiovascular events. (The method is demonstrated in the tables on pages 53, 54, and 55.) By permitting a single risk factor to be assessed in context, the analysis focuses attention on undesirable characteristics and prevents overreaction to a single minor problem.

To show how these tables apply to treatment strategy, let us take the example of a man who is 70 years old, has a systolic blood pressure of 195, serum cholesterol of 310 mg/ml, smokes a pack of cigarettes a day, is positive for left ventricular hypertrophy on ECG, and has glucose intolerance. All of us would recognize this as a rather poor risk profile but hardly an unusual one. The table states this man's chances of CHD within eight years as 815 out of 1,000.

Yet had he not smoked but otherwise remained the same, his risk would drop to 716/1,000; if the only change had been a systolic pressure reduction to 120, the risk would go down to 576. If both parameters had changed, the risk would be reduced to 437. If, in addition, he had no ECG changes his risk would improve to 213. In any of these situations, the impact of serum cholesterol appears to be minor, in part, perhaps, because the cholesterol elevation was of such long standing. In contrast, compare the risk of several 50-year-old men having the same profiles: such a

CHD RISK FACTORS

series of risk would range from 789 to 187.

Indeed, if he has data like those shown in the tables, a physician can ascertain any patient's relative risk by simply making a toll-free call (in New Jersey, 800-452-9146; elsewhere in the U.S., 800-631-8690) between the hours of 9 A.M. and 5 P.M. He will be connected with "Cardiodial," a service of Ciba-Geigy, which will give him the answer appropriate to the patient's age, sex, and risk-factor profile.

Let us conclude this chapter with the true story of an elderly patient whose motivation did indeed prove adequate to the difficult task of cooperating with her physician to reduce her risk. Obviously, the story is anecdotal, so that the caution recommended with respect to epidemiologic data must be reiterated.

This is the story of a 70-year-old former dancing teacher, a woman with a great appetite for life and a leading spirit at a local senior citizens' club. She had

Probability (per 1,000) of Developing Cardiovascular Disease in Eight Years According to Specified Characteristics: 70-Year-Old Man

LVH-ECG NEGATIVE

Does Not Smoke Cigarettes

	SBP→	105	120	135	150	165	180	195
Glucose Intolerance Absent	Cholesterol 185	100	123	150	183	221	264	312
	210	101	124	152	185	223	266	315
	235	102	125	153	187	225	269	317
	260	103	127	155	188	227	271	320
	285	104	128	157	190	229	273	323
	310	105	129	158	192	231	276	325
	335	106	131	160	194	233	278	328

Smokes Cigarettes

	SBP→	105	120	135	150	165	180	195
Glucose Intolerance Absent	Cholesterol 185	162	196	236	281	331	385	442
	210	164	198	238	284	334	388	445
	235	165	200	241	286	337	391	448
	260	167	202	243	389	339	394	451
	285	168	204	245	291	342	397	454
	310	170	206	247	294	345	400	457
	335	172	208	249	296	347	402	460

	SBP→	105	**120**	135	150	165	180	195
Glucose Intolerance Present	Cholesterol 185	168	203	244	290	341	396	453
	210	170	205	246	293	344	399	456
	235	171	207	249	295	346	401	459
	260	173	209	251	298	349	404	462
	285	175	211	253	300	352	407	465
	310	176	**213**	255	303	355	410	468
	335	178	215	258	305	357	413	471

	SBP→	105	120	135	150	165	180	195
Glucose Intolerance Present	Cholesterol 185	261	309	361	417	475	534	592
	210	263	311	364	420	478	537	594
	235	265	314	366	423	481	540	597
	260	268	316	369	426	484	543	600
	285	270	319	372	428	487	546	603
	310	272	321	375	431	490	549	606
	335	275	324	378	434	493	551	609

LVH-ECG POSITIVE

	SBP→	105	120	135	150	165	180	195
Glucose Intolerance Absent	Cholesterol 185	241	286	337	391	448	507	565
	210	243	289	339	394	451	510	568
	235	245	291	342	397	454	513	571
	260	247	294	345	400	457	516	574
	285	249	296	347	402	460	519	577
	310	252	299	350	405	463	522	580
	335	254	301	353	408	466	525	583

	SBP→	105	120	135	150	165	180	195
Glucose Intolerance Absent	Cholesterol 185	356	412	470	529	587	642	695
	210	359	415	473	532	590	645	697
	235	362	418	476	535	593	648	700
	260	365	421	479	538	595	651	702
	285	367	424	482	541	598	653	705
	310	370	427	485	544	601	656	707
	335	373	429	488	547	604	659	710

	SBP→	105	**120**	135	150	165	180	**195**
Glucose Intolerance Present	Cholesterol 185	366	423	481	540	597	652	704
	210	369	426	484	543	600	655	706
	235	372	428	487	546	603	658	709
	260	375	431	490	549	606	661	711
	285	378	434	493	551	609	663	714
	310	380	**437**	496	554	612	666	**716**
	335	383	440	499	557	614	668	718

	SBP→	105	**120**	135	150	165	180	**195**
Glucose Intolerance Present	Cholesterol 185	503	561	618	672	722	766	806
	210	506	564	621	675	724	769	808
	235	509	567	624	677	726	771	810
	260	512	570	627	680	729	773	811
	285	515	573	629	682	731	775	813
	310	518	**576**	632	685	733	777	**815**
	335	521	579	635	688	736	779	817

Framingham men age 70 years have an average SBP of 145 mm Hg and an average serum cholesterol of 231mg%; 37% smoke cigarettes, 4.0% have definite LVH by ECG, and 15.2% have glucose intolerance. At these average values, the probability of developing cardiovascular disease in eight years is 229/1,000.

Framingham data have made it possible to quantify the impact of CHD risk factors, alone or in combination, on the individual patient. Color highlights changes in risk of 70-year-old man described in text with alterations in his risk-factor values. Similar tables for the man and woman aged 50 are presented on pages 54 and 55.

53

Probability (per 1,000) of Developing Cardiovascular Disease in Eight Years According to Specified Characteristics: 50-Year-Old Man

LVH-ECG NEGATIVE

Does Not Smoke Cigarettes

Glucose Intolerance Absent

Cholesterol \ SBP	105	120	135	150	165	180	195
185	37	46	57	71	89	110	135
210	44	55	69	85	106	130	159
235	53	66	82	102	125	153	187
260	63	79	98	121	148	180	218
285	76	94	116	143	174	211	252
310	91	112	138	168	204	244	290
335	108	133	162	197	237	282	332

Smokes Cigarettes

Cholesterol \ SBP	105	120	135	150	165	180	195
185	62	78	96	119	146	177	214
210	75	92	114	140	171	207	249
235	89	110	135	165	200	241	286
260	106	130	159	194	233	278	327
285	126	154	187	225	269	318	371
310	148	181	218	261	309	361	417
335	174	211	253	300	351	407	465

Glucose Intolerance Present — Does Not Smoke Cigarettes

Cholesterol \ SBP	105	120	135	150	165	180	195
185	65	81	100	123	151	184	222
210	78	96	119	146	177	214	257
235	93	114	140	171	207	249	295
260	110	135	165	200	241	286	337
285	130	160	194	233	278	327	381
310	154	187	226	269	318	371	428
335	181	218	261	309	361	417	475

Glucose Intolerance Present — Smokes Cigarettes

Cholesterol \ SBP	105	120	135	150	165	180	195
185	108	133	163	197	237	282	332
210	128	157	191	230	274	323	376
235	151	184	222	265	314	367	423
260	178	215	257	305	357	412	470
285	208	249	296	347	402	460	519
310	241	287	337	392	449	508	566
335	278	328	382	439	497	556	613

LVH-ECG POSITIVE

Glucose Intolerance Absent — Does Not Smoke Cigarettes

Cholesterol \ SBP	105	120	135	150	165	180	195
185	98	121	148	181	218	261	309
210	117	143	175	211	253	300	352
235	138	169	204	245	291	342	397
260	163	197	237	282	332	387	444
285	191	230	274	323	377	433	492
310	222	266	314	367	423	481	540
335	257	305	357	412	470	529	587

Glucose Intolerance Absent — Smokes Cigarettes

Cholesterol \ SBP	105	120	135	150	165	180	195
185	160	194	234	278	328	382	439
210	188	226	270	319	372	428	487
235	219	262	309	362	418	476	535
260	253	300	352	408	465	524	582
285	292	343	397	455	514	572	628
310	333	387	444	503	561	618	672
335	377	434	492	551	608	663	713

Glucose Intolerance Present — Does Not Smoke Cigarettes

Cholesterol \ SBP	105	120	135	150	165	180	195
185	166	201	241	287	338	392	449
210	194	234	279	328	382	439	498
235	226	270	319	372	429	487	546
260	262	310	362	418	476	535	593
285	301	352	408	466	524	583	638
310	343	398	455	514	572	629	682
335	387	445	503	562	619	672	722

Glucose Intolerance Present — Smokes Cigarettes

Cholesterol \ SBP	105	120	135	150	165	180	195
185	258	305	358	413	471	530	588
210	296	348	403	461	519	578	634
235	338	393	450	509	567	624	677
260	383	440	498	557	614	668	718
285	429	487	546	604	658	709	755
310	477	536	593	649	700	747	789
335	525	583	639	691	739	782	819

Framingham men aged 50 years have an average SBP of 133 mm Hg and an average serum cholesterol of 236 mg%; 62% smoke cigarettes, 1.5% have definite LVH by ECG, and 6.5% have glucose intolerance. At these average values, the probability of developing cardiovascular disease in eight years is 115/1,000.

a history of angina pectoris and was being maintained on propranolol and digoxin but began sleeping poorly at night because of the angina and dyspnea, eventually resulting in congestive heart failure. At examination, her blood pressure was found to be 190/110, serum cholesterol 348, alpha-cholesterol 35.

Her physician gave immediate priority to control of the hypertension, prescribing hydrochlorothiazide (50 mg/day) with potassium supplementation, and removing the propranolol. The patient did not tolerate this regimen well; accordingly the thiazide-potassium combination was cut back to three times a week, and four tablets per day of methyldopa were added. This regimen also did not produce complete control of the hypertension and angina occurred frequently; accordingly, propranolol, which had been discontinued because of the congestive failure, was reinstituted. Isosorbide dinitrate was also added to counter the chest pain. Blood pressure came down to 128/80, where it was maintained.

In addition, the patient was counseled concerning diet. Typing studies were carried out and indicated that she had familial hyperlipidemia, type II. She cut back her intake of all meats, used only polyunsaturated margarines, and avoided other cholesterol and saturated fat-rich foods. Nonetheless, cholesterol fell only to 300 mg/ml. Cholestyramine (4 gm/day) was then prescribed and serum cholesterol fell to 225. Although her physician would have preferred a lower value still, she could not tolerate more drug.

CHD RISK FACTORS

Probability (per 1,000) of Developing Cardiovascular Disease in Eight Years According to Specified Characteristics: 50-Year-Old Woman

LVH-ECG NEGATIVE

Does Not Smoke Cigarettes

	SBP→	105	120	135	150	165	180	195
Glucose Intolerance Absent	Cholesterol 185	22	27	33	41	50	62	75
	210	25	31	38	46	57	70	85
	235	28	35	43	53	64	79	96
	260	32	39	49	60	73	89	108
	285	36	45	55	67	82	100	121
	310	41	51	62	76	93	113	136
	335	47	57	70	86	105	127	153

Smokes Cigarettes

	SBP→	105	120	135	150	165	180	195
	185	23	28	34	42	52	64	78
	210	26	32	39	48	59	72	88
	235	29	36	44	55	67	82	99
	260	33	41	50	62	76	92	112
	285	38	46	57	70	85	104	126
	310	43	53	65	79	96	117	141
	335	49	60	73	89	108	131	158

	SBP→	105	120	135	150	165	180	195
Glucose Intolerance Present	185	42	52	64	78	95	115	139
	210	48	59	72	88	107	129	155
	235	54	66	81	99	120	145	174
	260	61	75	92	111	135	162	193
	285	69	85	103	125	151	180	215
	310	78	96	116	140	168	201	238
	335	89	108	130	157	188	223	263

	SBP→	105	120	135	150	165	180	195
	185	44	54	66	81	98	119	144
	210	50	61	75	91	111	134	161
	235	56	69	84	102	124	150	179
	260	64	78	95	115	139	167	200
	285	72	88	107	129	156	186	221
	310	81	99	120	145	174	207	245
	335	92	112	135	162	194	230	270

LVH-ECG POSITIVE

	SBP→	105	120	135	150	165	180	195
Glucose Intolerance Absent	185	51	62	76	93	113	136	164
	210	57	70	86	104	126	152	182
	235	65	79	97	117	142	170	203
	260	73	90	109	132	159	190	225
	285	83	101	122	148	177	211	249
	310	94	114	137	165	197	233	274
	335	105	128	154	184	219	258	301

	SBP→	105	120	135	150	165	180	195
	185	53	65	79	96	117	141	169
	210	60	73	89	108	131	158	188
	235	67	82	100	122	147	176	209
	260	76	93	113	136	164	196	232
	285	86	105	127	153	183	217	256
	310	97	118	142	171	203	241	282
	335	109	132	159	190	226	266	310

	SBP→	105	120	135	150	165	180	195
Glucose Intolerance Present	185	96	116	140	168	201	238	279
	210	108	130	157	187	223	262	306
	235	121	146	175	208	246	289	335
	260	136	163	195	231	272	316	365
	285	152	182	216	255	298	346	396
	310	170	202	239	281	327	376	428
	335	189	224	264	308	356	407	460

	SBP→	105	120	135	150	165	180	195
	185	99	120	145	174	207	245	287
	210	111	135	162	194	230	270	315
	235	125	151	181	215	254	297	344
	260	140	168	201	238	279	325	374
	285	157	188	223	263	307	355	405
	310	175	209	247	289	335	385	438
	335	195	231	272	317	365	417	470

Framingham women aged 50 years have an average SBP of 136 mm Hg and an average serum cholesterol of 246 mg%; 41% smoke cigarettes, 0.2% have definite LVH by ECG, and 2.9% have glucose intolerance. At these average values, the probability of developing cardiovascular disease in eight years is 48/1,000.

Indeed, the physician regarded her drug load as uncomfortably heavy and tried to eliminate some of it, but invariably it became clear that blood pressure would rise unacceptably or angina recur. Eventually, some improvement in left ventricular hypertrophy was observed on the ECG.

It is now four years since the effort began, and this is how her physician sums up the present situation: "She's like a new woman, the way she gets around! She just got back from a vacation in the Berkshires and is planning to go to Hong Kong. When she first came to me I thought she had a 95% chance of being dead within a year. My job now is arguing with her to slow down."

8

Stroke in the Geriatric Patient

SOLOMON ROBBINS
University of Maryland

By and large, the treatment of stroke in the elderly, and of its possible precursor, the transient ischemic attack, is likely to be the responsibility of the primary physician rather than the neurologic specialist. Opportunities for surgery or chemotherapy are limited. Treatment for stroke per se is chancy and is usually not feasible in the old because of the presence of collateral disease. Management essentially is oriented toward minimizing or preventing pulmonary, cardiac, and other complications. During the acute phase, expert medical and nursing care in the hospital can improve stroke survival, and further increments depend principally on the quality of posthospital care – by the family physician or internist, nursing home, home health service, and family.

By understanding the general characteristics of stroke and the limitations of its treatment, the physician may be able to pick out the minority of elderly patients for whom more aggressive intervention may be worthwhile. But, just as important, the physician also may be able to spare elderly patients the rigors and risks of fruitless maneuvers and false hopes. Since a fair degree of function returns spontaneously in many, and risks attach to drugs and surgery, I feel that conservatism in managing the elderly stroke patient is indicated.

As the term implies, a "stroke" is a sudden striking down of the patient. One moment well, the patient suddenly is unable to move a limb and/or loses sensation in an extremity or entire side. If restoration does not occur within 24 hours, the stroke is termed a "completed stroke." If the deficit is temporary, it is considered a "transient ischemic attack," or TIA. The terms "stroke in evolution" or "progressing stroke" are applied to patients who display increasing weakness after sudden onset, and both evolving and permanent deficits may be present simultaneously.

In the main, strokes are of thrombotic, embolic, or hemorrhagic origin. A rarer etiology, almost entirely limited to the geriatric population, is temporal arteritis. This disease is worth mention because effective treatment *is* possible, with steroids. Little can be done as yet for most intracerebral hemorrhages, which carry a very high morbidity and mortality. The principal focus of this chapter will be on stroke and TIA of thrombotic or embolic origin.

The immediate mortality of completed stroke is up to 30% in the first month and up to 45% within five years, according to selected data. Between a quarter and a half of survivors of a first stroke have further episodes. The sequels carry the poorest prognoses. However, if the stroke patient survives five to seven years without a stroke, chances are fair that he will not have further episodes.

Completed stroke as a sequel is reported to occur in 12% to 62% or more of TIA cases. The higher estimates fit with the longer duration of focal neurologic deficit, i.e., loss of function or sensation related to ischemia of a specific brain site. One study showed that about 25% of TIA patients followed for 40 months experienced a completed stroke. A 24-hour period of sensory and/or motor loss is reported to precede a completed stroke 30% of the time. Over

CHAPTER 8: ROBBINS

Intracranial and Extracranial Vascular Lesions Producing Strokes

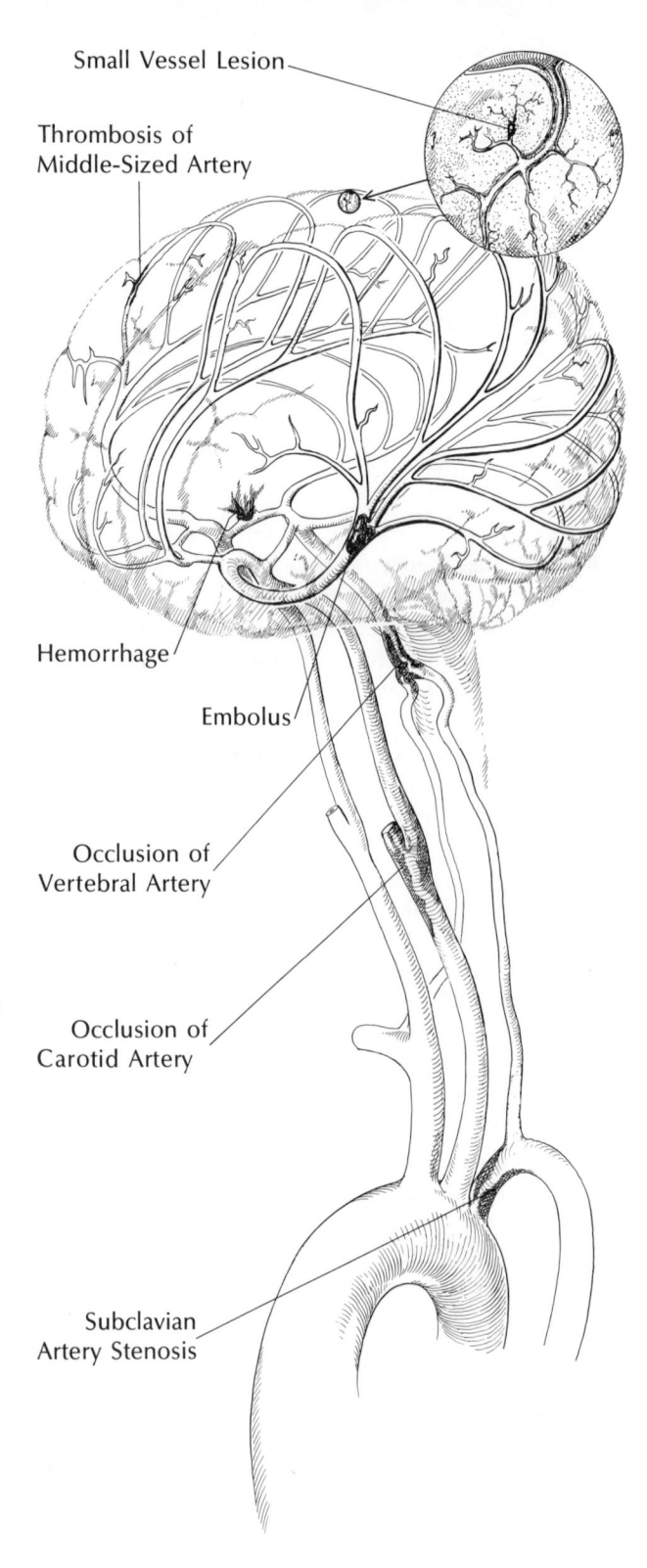

Small Vessel Lesion

Thrombosis of Middle-Sized Artery

Hemorrhage

Embolus

Occlusion of Vertebral Artery

Occlusion of Carotid Artery

Subclavian Artery Stenosis

60% of TIA patients who later have a completed stroke are said to recover enough function eventually to return to normal activities. As a 15-year follow-up of 73 TIA patients by the Mayo Clinic showed, half went on to die of documented or presumed cardiac disease and 36% died of stroke. In other words, 86% of the deaths involved vascular causes.

Given the difficulties of defining, identifying, measuring, and reporting TIAs and strokes, it is no wonder that the data are fuzzy. Yet experience and statistics seem to suggest that many TIA patients have no more TIAs, that many will not have a completed stroke or will not survive heart or other ailments to live long enough to have stroke, and that many stroke patients experience significant recovery of function or sensation if they survive the first month.

Obviously, it would be highly beneficial to have a means of preventing TIA or completed stroke, or, better yet, of identifying patients at most risk of having them in the first place. If this could be done early enough in the life span, perhaps preventive measures could be taken against cerebrovascular disease. Risk factors are discussed in Chapter 7 by Dr. Castelli, so I will simply mention here that hypertension, diabetes, and serum lipid abnormalities are associated with increased risk of cerebrovascular disease. The influence of hypertension is such that stroke appears much earlier in hypertensive patients than in others; by the fifth decade of life, the greater frequency is strikingly apparent. As the graph on page 60 shows, the incidence rate of stroke rises steeply with age; it is more than ten times greater in the age group 75 to 84 than in the group 55 to 64, for example.

The keystone in the diagnosis of stroke is a clear history of sudden, acute neurologic deficit. The patient or family may have to be questioned painstakingly to make sure in completed stroke that onset was sudden and that, in what appears on report to have been a TIA, a genuine neurologic deficit occurred. A simple report of "numbness" in an elderly patient

While there is considerable overlap of signs and symptoms of strokes secondary to disease in different vessels (drawing at left), some frequent associations can be cited. These include: for carotid artery disease, unilateral weakness and sensory loss, hemianopsia, dysphasia with major hemisphere involvement; for vertebral-basilar disease, hemianopsia (may be partial or bilateral), crossed syndrome (involvement of ipsilateral cranial nerves and contralateral motor and sensory loss), ataxia and incoordination, nystagmus, diplopia, and vertigo.

Aspects of Presentation of Stroke by Etiology

	Thrombotic	Embolic	Hemorrhagic
Previous history of TIAs	Frequent	Occasional	Rare
Onset	Acute or stepwise over hours to a couple of days	Acute	Acute, usually with progressive worsening or coma
Associated headache	Occasional, usually not severe	More often, moderate degree	Frequent, severe
Stiff neck	Rare	Rare	Frequent
Coma (loss of consciousness)	Occasional, usually not at onset	Occasional, usually brief at onset	Frequent

should be pursued; the meaning may vary from a "tingling sensation" to true loss of sensation, which is the important symptom. Likewise, terms such as "dizziness" or "weakness" should be explored. By dizziness, does the patient mean true vertigo, a spinning sensation? Vertigo is critical to the diagnosis of stroke *only* in combination with other symptoms, which may include diplopia, dysphagia, stammer, and partial loss of vision. Such findings are highly relevant to a stroke diagnosis when the history of sudden, acute deficit is clear.

When the history is muddled – especially if the deficit could have had a gradual onset – consideration should be more of a mass lesion than a stroke. Brain scanning by computed tomography or by radioisotope uptake, to visualize a mass and to search for abnormal vascularity, is a key approach. If the results are negative, tumor is usually ruled out. When scans are not obtainable, a skull film may show pineal displacement suggestive of a mass. Although sometimes helpful, an electroencephalogram is not completely discriminating, since the cortical activity it measures may have been compromised by *either* tumor or stroke. Lumbar puncture in stroke patients is indicated if hemorrhage or syphilis is suspected. If there is a question of increased intracranial pressure, it is usually best to avoid the lumbar puncture because of the possibility of herniation. An elevated sedimentation rate may raise the possibility of temporal arteritis as the cause of stroke. These patients usually also have a history of headache and visual symptoms. Confirmation of this disease is by biopsy of the temporal artery, and treatment with steroids, as previously noted, is indicated.

An electrocardiogram should be made routinely in cases of suspected stroke or TIA. The ECG may relate the episode to an embolus secondary to myocardial infarction or ischemia produced by cardiac arrhythmia.

The clinical profile usually indicates whether the stroke involves the carotid or vertebrobasilar arteries, a distinction important to possible management. Supplying the cerebrum and ophthalmic region, the carotid system includes extracranial arteries readily accessible to the surgeon and intracranial arteries that are not yet generally approached in most areas. The vertebrobasilar arteries, supplying the brainstem, are for all practical purposes inapproachable. Abnormalities involving subclavian arteries should be considered in patients with findings suggesting vertebrobasilar distribution.

In carotid occlusion, the focal neurologic deficit occurs in the side of the body opposite the affected artery and may be accompanied by aphasia if circulation to the dominant cerebral hemisphere is compromised. Motor or sensory loss of one or both limbs on the contralateral side and loss of vision in the ipsilateral eye constitute a clear profile of carotid occlusion. Other signs are diminished carotid pulses; bruit over the carotid artery or eye; emboli in the retinal vessels; relative hypotension, as determined by ophthalmodynamometer; and relative hypothermia, as determined by thermometry of the ipsilateral medial aspect of the forehead.

If the stroke is related to ischemia in the brainstem, any combination of limbs – even all four – may be affected. Facial paresthesia may be present. Although I have cautioned against the pitfall of presuming that an elderly patient has had a TIA simply on the basis of vertigo, vertigo *in combination with focal deficits* is a key finding in brainstem ischemia. Light-headedness or dizziness alone or with vertigo may be associated with cardiac arrhythmia, postural hypotension, or vestibular disease. (These signs may appear after head trauma and during middle ear infection as well as after stroke.) Benign positional vertigo or transient vertigo after sudden head movements indicates some vestibular system involvement, probably old and nonprogressive, and not transient ischemia.

Ischemia in the posterior distribution, as noted above, may result from a surgically approachable lesion in the subclavian artery, producing the subclavian steal syndrome. In this condition, blood flow to the brain is altered by occlusion or stenosis of the subclavian artery, causing blood to flow in a retrograde fashion through one vertebral artery to fill the subclavian. This "steals" blood from the brain after producing clinically recognizable ischemic episodes in the vertebrobasilar distribution. These patients often have a difference in blood pressures of the arms. The diagnosis is confirmed by arteriography.

While arteriography is indispensable if one wishes to evaluate the feasibility of carotid or subclavian endarterectomy, even in the best hands it carries some risk. Accordingly it should be employed *only* if the clinical profile indicates an approachable lesion and the patient is considered operable. The history and physical examination are more important considerations when contemplating surgery than morphologic evidence of impaired blood flow. For example, angiographic evidence of an occluded carotid does not call for operation in the absence of clinical indications. If the circle of Willis is patent, two vertebrals and a carotid may furnish sufficient circulation. In fact, angiography may strengthen contraindications to surgery; e.g., bilateral lesions or intracranial *and* cervical lesions on the same side almost always preclude operation on an extracranial artery. For a quick, less risky look for any difference in flow to the front half of the brain on one side or the other, a nuclear cerebral flow study is useful. Although not diagnostic, appropriate change on a flow study may be of help in deciding whether or not to proceed with arteriography.

Generally, I would not advise angiography or surgery for the apparently operable geriatric patient who has had a single TIA with only fleeting functional loss. As the clinical pattern grows more suspicious – that is, the patient experiences amaurosis fugax, there are retinal emboli, and limb weakness is severe and lasts for hours, or there have been several transient ischemic episodes – a recommendation for surgery becomes more justifiable.

The decision to do something or nothing for the TIA patient is delicate and complex. Besides the clinical profile, considerations include age, expected years of life remaining, collateral disease, the possibility of the patient's succumbing to something other than stroke, and the risks and benefits of surgery as such vs those of a possible alternative – medical therapy. It is when the patient seems *least* in need of help – that is, the patient is healthy despite a history of TIAs – that intervention may be most helpful and can be accomplished relatively safely. This is probably the best time for a neurologic or neurosurgical consultation. In completed stroke with notable residua, neither surgery nor anticoagulation can be recommended, even though these patients have the conditions that tempt us most to want to act.

What are the chances that TIAs are the forerun-

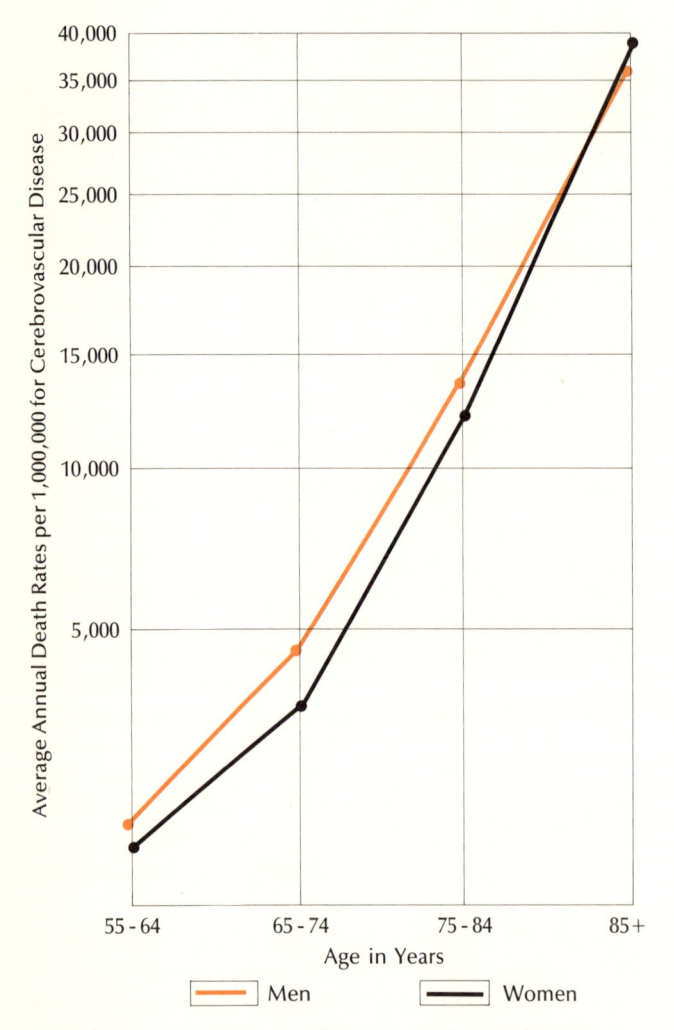

Graph shows steep rise with age in stroke incidence; note also absence after age 65 of any female advantage.

ners of completed stroke? As indicated before, the data vary considerably but suggest that many TIA patients experience no completed stroke or do not live long enough to have one. Some studies estimate that 50% to 70% of untreated TIA patients become asymptomatic. Others estimate that this occurs in only 25% or less. In one study, half of 82 untreated patients followed for an average of 39 months experienced a completed stroke. Another study found that 33% had a stroke one to eight years post-TIA.

If we put the question retrospectively – how many patients with completed stroke had had a previous TIA? – proportions of one half to four fifths appear in the literature. In one study, 81% of patients with angiographically proven carotid occlusion had one or more TIAs previously.

What are the risks and benefits of surgery? The risk varies in different hands. With appreciable operative experience, surgical mortality appears to be under 5% and is often only 1% to 3%. At the Mayo Clinic, endarterectomy carries a mortality or morbidity of 1% or 2% for neurologically stable patients having no medical risk, whether or not angiography discloses multiple lesions, malformations, or other arterial factors. The risk rises to 7% at Mayo for neurologically stable patients with significant medical illness, primarily cardiac disease, according to Thoralf M. Sundt Jr. and colleagues. They report that the risk is 10% for neurologically unstable patients, but this group experiences the most dramatic restoration of function. By and large, surgery is not indicated for progressing strokes.

Patients with unilateral carotid stenosis underlying a TIA apparently are the ones most likely to be helped by operation. Some 70% to 90% of TIA patients are asymptomatic or improved after carotid surgery, but 5% to 15% become worse or die as a result of surgery, the Joint Study of Extracranial Arterial Occlusion reported in 1969. However, *cumulative survival* at the end of 42 months was found virtually identical in surgical and nonsurgical management of TIA.

The balancing of risks and benefits of surgery for the TIA patient is a far different exercise from that involving the patient with breast cancer or another disease carrying a high probability of death without intervention. Even if a large proportion of TIAs proceed to completed stroke, the completed stroke often is not a total disaster. A decision against surgery is far from being a death warrant. Moreover, the incapacities sustained by the stroke patient may be subject to spontaneous improvement and may allow for a de-

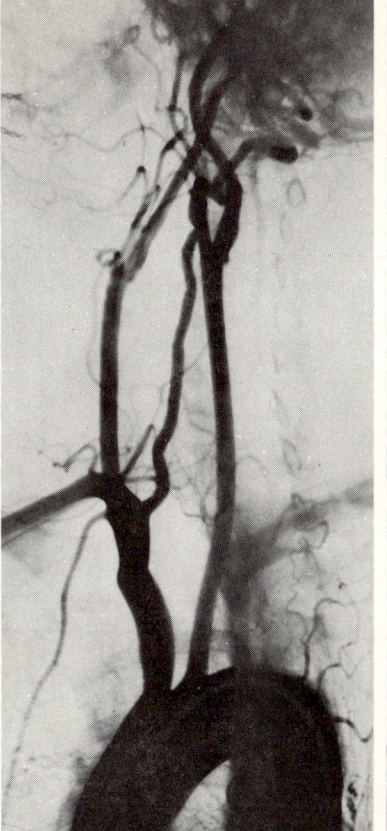

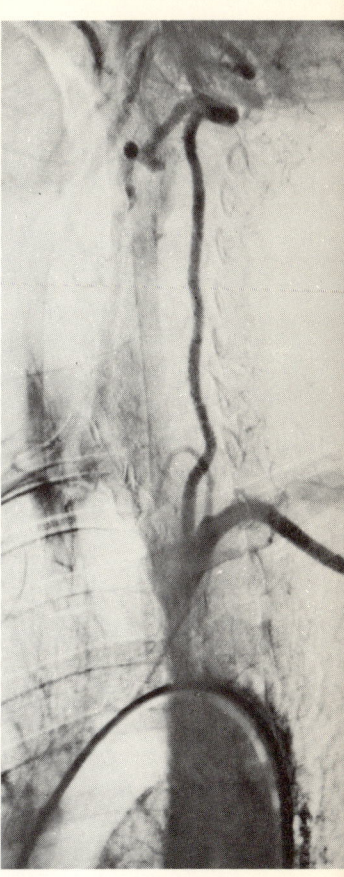

Angiograms provide unusually clear study of "subclavian steal." In view at left, carotid artery is filled but not vertebral or subclavian; in view at right, retrograde flow through vertebral now fills the subclavian.

cent quality of life. I would sum up the risk/benefit issues in a question: Is it worth taking a 1% to 5% risk of operative mortality to avoid, say, a 25% to 50% chance of stroke, which, if it did occur, might likely leave only a partial incapacity?

Is age per se an operability consideration? Generally, no. The appropriate concern is the patient's health status. I am far more eager to consider surgery for a 70-year-old patient who has no diffuse vascular disease than for the 55-year-old patient who does. Nonetheless, age does enter the picture. The older the patient, the less well is operation tolerated. There is much to be said for taking fewer risks in patients with fewer years of life expectancy. Age also enters the picture in another way: According to J. C. Goldner and colleagues at Mayo in 1971, if a first TIA occurs when patients are at least 65, the survival rate is similar to that of the general population. In their study, it made no difference to expected survival whether patients had primarily motor or sensory deficits. This picture confirms the view that collateral diseases weigh heavily in prognosis for any geriatric patient and dominate consideration of operability.

Are drugs an alternative to surgery? The extent to which TIA represents a thrombotic or embolic process amenable to drugs is not clear. Anticoagulants, vasodilators, aspirin, and other agents have all been tried. In recent studies, aspirin, which probably works by inhibiting platelet aggregation, has appeared to be the most successful. Fields et al, in the May-June, 1977 issue of *Stroke*, reported the results of a combined double-blind trial of aspirin for treatment of cerebral ischemia, in which a decreased frequency of TIAs was found with the use of aspirin, but no decrease in death or completed stroke. In the report of the Cooperative Study of Hospital Frequency and Character of Transient Ischemia Attacks, in *JAMA*, July 11, 1977, little difference in outcome was noted with various modes of treatment, including extracranial arterial surgery and antiplatelet aggregation drugs. However, the study did find a significant increase in mortality in patients treated with anticoagulants.

The most promising findings were reported by Barnett at the Third Joint Meeting on Stroke and Cerebral Circulation in 1977. (Abstracts of the meeting were published in the January-February, 1978 issue of *Stroke*.) The "Canadian Cooperative Platelet-Inhibiting Drug Trial in Threatened Stroke" evaluated aspirin and sulfinpyrazone, used individually or together and compared with placebo. Aspirin was found to confer significant benefit in normotensive males. Thus, the general trend is to use aspirin more and anticoagulants less. This is particularly true in the elderly, who fall more easily because of poor vision, joint dysfunction, and peripheral neurological and vascular disease as well as cerebrovascular disease.

For the elderly patient surviving a completed stroke, who cannot benefit by these interventions, the prognosis generally is often not dire. While there is a high frequency of occupational disability following stroke, most patients in the group we are considering are already retired. It is hard to say in the early postictal phase how much function will return. The longer the no-improvement interval, the worse the prognosis. A patient who has shown no improvement in two days may still do better. But the expectations are much less with no improvement after two weeks. At the end of a month, if improvement has not been made, none is likely. The patient who sustains both severe motor and sensory losses has a poor prognosis. Among other things, such a patient is deprived of the sensory inputs needed to support development of compensatory maneuvers. There are no sound bases for attempting to predict degree of recovery according to etiology of the stroke.

Early rehabilitation is of the utmost importance for patients with less severe losses. Fancy rehabilita-

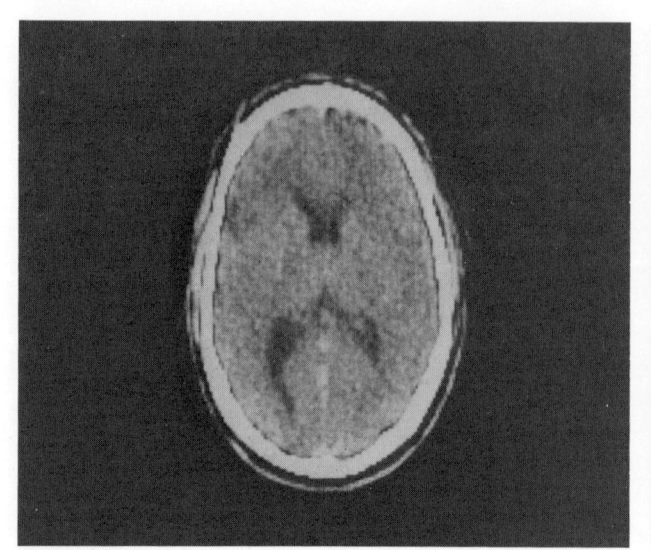

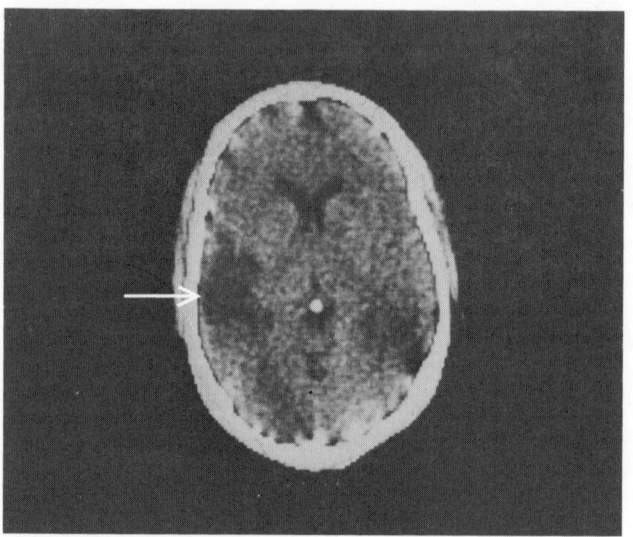

Computed axial tomography offers noninvasive approach to etiologic differentiation of stroke. Scan at left was made immediately after stroke occurred; it reveals a nontumorous lesion in the midcerebral distribution and minor edema of the tissues. Eleven days later (right) infarction in this area can be clearly seen (arrow).

tion units are not needed for the first and most important phase, mobilization. Early mobilization is necessary to preserve strength in unaffected muscle groups and for balance; unless this is done, when strength improves on the affected side the patient will be too weak to begin training for walking. The worst thing that can happen to an elderly patient with a small stroke is to be hospitalized and confined to bed for extensive, often unnecessary, workup.

It may help with ambulation to recommend weight reduction for the overweight patient with completed stroke. Any maneuver that will help the patient move about should be considered. It is not so much actual *recovery* of function but *ability to compensate for loss* that should be stressed in the rehabilitation phase. In the sense that patients find ways of compensating, they do "get better" even though they do not regain motor or sensory function.

All these considerations lay the foundation for what I tell the patient and family. Substance and tone are both important. For example, the TIA patient should be told frankly: We are uncertain whether another episode may or may not occur, but if one does, there are reasonable grounds to believe functional loss will be minimal if at all permanent. The patient should be urged to call the physician as soon as TIA symptoms appear. I tell the completed-stroke patient in the immediate postictal period that nobody can predict whether there will be improvement. I try to explain that most patients get better, but some do not improve and some worsen. I try to convey hope that the future is not necessarily bleak. I emphasize that medical, nursing, and rehabilitation assistance will be forthcoming to support patient and family.

Hope is justified not only because many patients improve physically but also because many patients do find ways to compensate for weakness. The patient with a paralyzed leg may find that he or she can move in and out of chairs. "I'm able to do it. I'm better," such a patient will say. And the patient is correct. Before a physician abandons hope, this dimension of patient potential – and means of encouraging it – should be carefully considered. On the other hand, given the uncertainties of surgery and chemotherapy, the patient must understand the futility of investing energies and resources in these directions, unless there are clear reasons for proceeding. My experience is that such reasons are not found in most geriatric patients with stroke. An example is the 72-year-old patient who presented with right-arm weakness. He had awakened with the condition three days before coming to see me, and there had been no

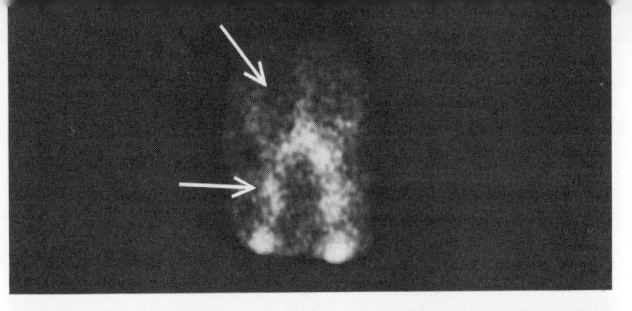

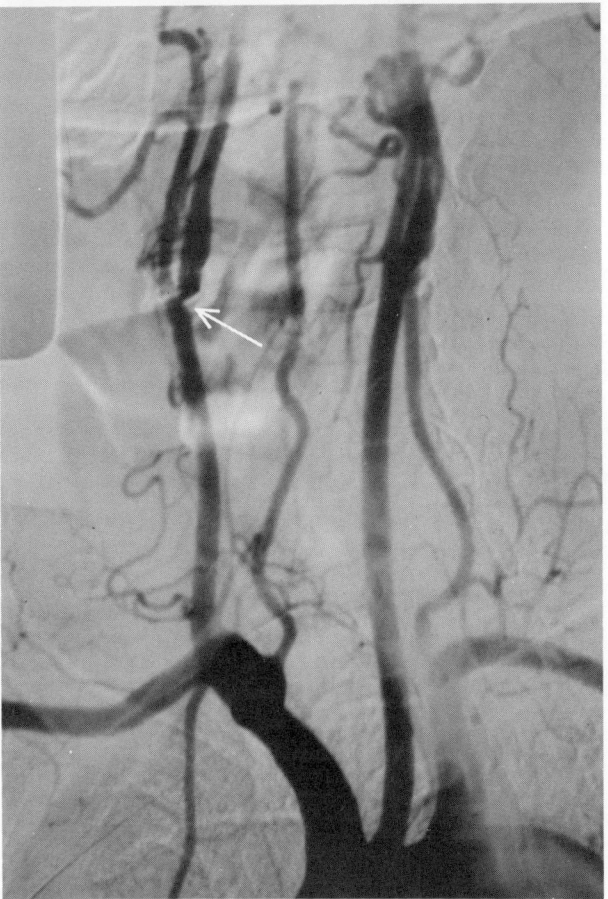

Case illustrated is one in which radionuclide scanning suggested advisability of angiography to evaluate operability of a lesion. Scan at top is 12-second image from anterior cerebral flow study (courtesy Dr. P. E. Dibos). Decreased activity is seen in region of right carotid and right cerebral hemisphere (arrows); angiogram confirms stenosis in right internal carotid (arrow).

change. Since the patient had no evidence of diabetes, syphilis, or other disease or condition requiring detailed studies, I did not recommend hospitalization. The patient had fair residual function, and the odds were that it would improve gradually.

If not hospitalization, would such a patient – or one more seriously impaired – need a nursing home? The answer varies, depending on the attitude of his family and the availability of home care services.

Many factors influence the decision to institutionalize; these are discussed fully by Dr. Jack Kleh in Chapter 23. The questions to pursue are: Is there someone at home who is physically and emotionally able to care for the patient? Is the cost of nursing home care beyond the family's means? Are home health services available or is there transportation for the patient to an institution for periodic medical, nursing, or rehabilitative care? If the answers are yes, then care at home is a reasonable consideration. When family members are reluctant, I find that the availability of home health services or close medical support produces a critical psychologic uplift; whether or not the service can be expected to improve the patient's condition, the family's recognition that outside support is available often makes the difference in willingness to accept the patient.

If care at home is inadvisable, the patient is entitled to an explanation of the reasons why. The patient should be informed what plans or options exist for care and what the long-term outlook is. One must guard against implying professional or family abandonment. Periodic appraisal of care at home or in the nursing home must be performed by the physician or a representative to protect the patient – as much against an excess as a lack of care. Sometimes a patient benefits from less rather than more attention; an overzealous family may produce an incapacitated individual by preventing the patient from trying to do something for himself or herself.

Stroke is a humbling disease to patient and physician. The temptation to try extreme measures is great. I am mindful of patients who have had such severe strokes that heroic measures resulted in protecting bodies without minds, while respirators became instruments of preserving non-lives. In caring for the stroke patient, one must develop a kind of watchful patience while hoping for spontaneous improvement. Some steps in fact may be counterproductive: The aged stroke patient who has a slight respiratory problem should not be placed on a respirator because one may not be able to wean him from it. If possible, more nursing should be offered in such a situation.

In summary, there are a few suggestions I might offer:

• Don't be didactic when making predictions about a patient with stroke, because anything is possible.

• Don't undertake complex, arduous diagnostic procedures routinely in all patients.

• Don't abandon the patient because you feel so little can be done medically for stroke as such.

9

Hematologic Problems

C. ROBERT BAISDEN
Johns Hopkins University

Some hematologic problems are essentially limited to older adults and respond to specific therapy. Yet a gradually developing anemia, for example, may also be a sign of serious disease affecting another organ system. The distinction is obviously important, but such signs and symptoms as may be present seldom help much in making it. Diagnosis in the elderly therefore begins with an appreciation that hematologic problems may – and commonly do – arise in several contexts. Hematologic evaluation is recommended on minimal indications, if not routinely, and only a complete hemogram will suffice.

This means more than the standard hemoglobin and hematocrit determinations and leukocyte and differential counts. The complete hemogram also includes several red cell indices – mean corpuscular volume, mean corpuscular hemoglobin, mean corpuscular hemoglobin concentration – as well as an absolute reticulocyte count, plus data as to observed form and structure of blood cells.

Any elderly patient with a suspected hematologic disorder should also be checked for occult blood loss, since the two often go together. And if the hematologic abnormality seems associated with chronic infection, the evaluation must include serum immunoglobulin determinations; immunoglobulin concentrations are decreased in several diseases found among the elderly, such as chronic lymphocytic leukemia, multiple myeloma, acquired immune deficiency syndromes, and others associated with an increased susceptibility to infection. An unexplained anemia is best studied by analysis of a bone marrow aspirate and, if necessary, marrow biopsy. This examination is also informative as to the cellularity of the marrow and the presence of specific cell lines; perhaps it may also reveal evidence of lymphoproliferative or myeloproliferative disease.

Before considering such possibilities, however, the primary physician needs to establish that a significant hematologic problem exists. He may be misled if he relies on standard adult values in interpreting the hemogram. Geriatric norms have only recently been worked out in any detail, as suitable populations have been studied; *among other things, they tell us that hemoglobin or hematocrit values unacceptable at younger ages may be quite compatible with health in the elderly.*

Consider the findings when Earney and Earney evaluated a group of 400 presumably healthy elderly subjects in a nursing home setting. The lowest hemoglobin value among the men was 10.11 gm/100 ml, the highest 19.75 gm/100 ml; hemoglobins in women ranged from 10.38 gm/100 ml to 18.30 gm/100 ml. Leukocyte and differential counts also ranged widely, from a low of 3.91 to a high of 11.07 (10^3/mm^3) for leukocytes, from 24.15% to 70.99% for the proportion of polymorphonuclear cells. Male and female values tended to overlap, indicating that the differences between the sexes observed in earlier decades become minimized with aging. Furthermore, age per se in the geriatric group was not a factor; similar values were recorded in ambulatory

Standard Adult vs Geriatric Hematologic Values

	Standard Adult	Geriatric
Erythrocytes (10⁶/mm³)	4.2 – 6.2	3.30 – 5.46
Hemoglobin (gm/100 ml)	11.5 – 18.0	10.24 – 19.04
Hematocrit (vol %)	37 – 54	31.01 – 53.29
Leukocytes (10³/mm³)	5 – 10	3.91 – 11.07
Polymorphonuclear cells (%)	50 – 65	24.15 – 70.99
Small lymphocytes (%)	25 – 40	18.64 – 64.20
Basophils (%)	0 – 1	0.00 – 2.34
Monocytes (%)	0 – 8	0.50 – 8.65
Eosinophils (%)	0 – 4	0.00 – 3.66

Data from Earney and Earney

subjects, whose ages ranged from 70 through 94.

I cite these details to stress that hematologic status in the elderly should be assessed only on the basis of appropriate geriatric reference values. Beyond that, each case must be evaluated individually, since the significance of any finding depends on the circumstances. A relatively low hemoglobin may be entirely appropriate in the presence of hypothyroidism because metabolic rate is also reduced. An elderly patient confined to bed in a nursing home will tolerate a lower hemoglobin than someone the same age who is ambulatory and relatively active. Specific questions must be asked as to activity level (How far can you walk without tiring? Can you climb stairs?) and the responses heeded. The individual slow to cerebrate may be manifesting signs of anemia rather than (or in addition to) cerebral arteriosclerosis.

As a practice we consider hemoglobin values in the 10 to 12 gm/100 ml range as the lower limits of normal in the elderly, but we always investigate if the hemoglobin goes below 10 gm/100 ml. In doing so, one must be wary of certain pitfalls. For one thing, red cell concentration may be reduced because of hemodilution, producing a spurious anemic state. The most obvious cause in the elderly is fluid retention due to congestive heart failure. Overhydration for any reason has a similar effect, creating a dilutional anemia that may then be overtreated. Unfortunately, treatment may take the form of blood transfusion, which is poorly tolerated in the elderly, especially in those with marginal compensation of cardiac function. The increase in blood volume may precipitate circulatory failure, not to mention possible exposure to transfusion hepatitis.

Transfusion, unless strictly indicated, is to be deplored. When it becomes a necessity, packed red cells rather than whole blood should be used to avoid excessive volume expansion.

One mistake is to assume that relatively low hemoglobin or hematocrit values in the elderly signify a reduced circulating blood volume. In fact, blood volume remains essentially unchanged with advancing age, nor is there any evidence for any age-related decline in two other indices, platelet count and a change in coagulation time. Put another way, an elderly patient manifesting thrombocytopenia, thrombocytosis, or a clotting abnormality requires careful diagnostic study. Most thrombocytopenia in this age group is associated with drug toxicity; the drugs in-

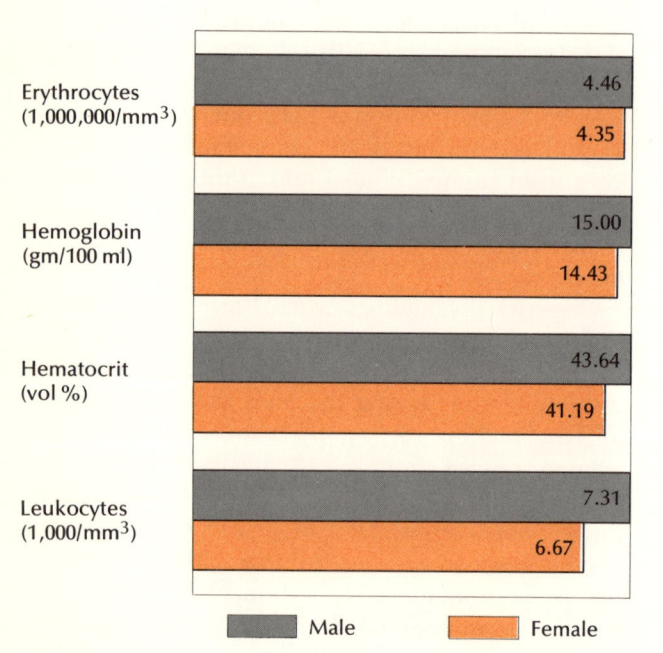

	Male	Female
Erythrocytes (1,000,000/mm³)	4.46	4.35
Hemoglobin (gm/100 ml)	15.00	14.43
Hematocrit (vol %)	43.64	41.19
Leukocytes (1,000/mm³)	7.31	6.67

Evaluating hematologic problems in the elderly requires reference to geriatric norms, exemplified by mean values recorded by Earney and Earney among presumably healthy nursing home residents 70 to 80 years old.

volved may either suppress platelet production or form platelet antibodies (see table on page 70). Bruising of the skin is often the first manifestation. If it appears in an elderly patient who is on chlorothiazide therapy, drug toxicity should be thought of immediately. A prolonged clotting time or a specific coagulation defect may occur with immunologic diseases such as systemic lupus erythematosus, rheumatoid arthritis, or pemphigus.

In general, problems that affect platelet count or coagulation time significantly are serious enough to warrant referral to a hematopathologist or an internist with a special interest in hematology. The same is true if anything about the blood picture suggests neoplastic disease of the blood-forming tissues. Other problems, certainly most anemias, can usually be successfully managed by the primary physician who knows the essentials of diagnosis and therapy.

An initial hemogram that reveals anemia may also suggest its type, provided that cell morphology and red cell indices are read correctly. As to the latter, the number of red cells as such is less meaningful than the relationship among cell number, quantity of hemoglobin, and volume of cells per unit of blood. A greater decrease in hemoglobin and red cell mass than in cell number signifies a reduction in the size of most red cells; the anemia thus produced is termed *microcytic*, or, if hemoglobin concentration within individual cells is also reduced, the result may be a *microcytic-hypochromic* anemia. Conversely, the number of red cells may be reduced more than hemoglobin or red cell mass, with cell size increased; the anemia is then termed *macrocytic*. This approach simplifies diagnosis, since it limits possible etiologies. On discovering a microcytic or macrocytic anemia, the physician knows what to test for or rule out.

Suppose that red cell indices are all reduced and the anemia is microcytic-hypochromic. One possible diagnosis is acquired sideroblastic anemia, a disease of the elderly associated with microcytic-hypochromic cells. The anemia might also be due to pyridoxine deficiency or a toxic drug reaction. However, most microcytic-hypochromic anemia in older adults is due to *iron deficiency*; therefore this diagnosis must always be considered first.

The initial workup includes determinations of plasma iron, total iron-binding capacity, and serum transferrin saturation to make certain an iron deficiency exists. A low transferrin saturation (below 10%) is virtually specific for iron deficiency anemia, whereas a high transferrin saturation is indicative of

Indications for Transfusions in Elderly Patients

Hemorrhage or severe blood loss associated with the following:
   Blood volume of less than 70% of normal
   Persistent pulse rate of 100/min or greater
   Central venous pressure of less than 50 mm saline

Hemolytic anemia in hypoplastic bone marrow crises

Aplastic anemia

Chronic anemias associated with:
   Cardiac failure
   Angina pectoris
   Cerebral insufficiency
   Infection
   Hematocrit below 25%
   Hemoglobin concentration below 8 gm/100 ml

iron overload, as in sideroblastic anemia. For a complete evaluation of body iron stores, one must examine a marrow aspirate that has been properly stained for iron particles. In anemia of chronic disease, especially infection, the marrow iron stores are generally abundant despite the characteristic lower serum iron and transferrin concentrations. The percent of transferrin saturation in chronic disease is usually greater

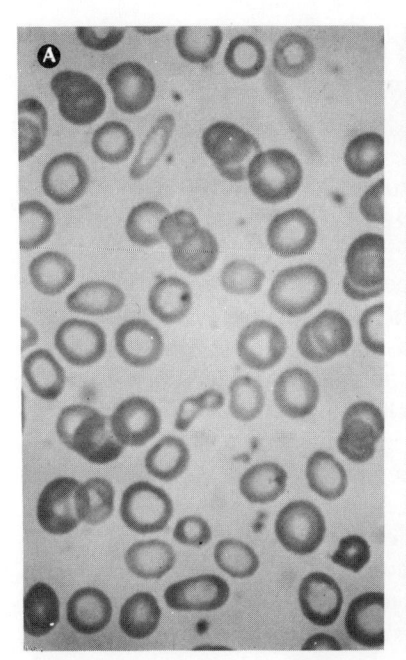

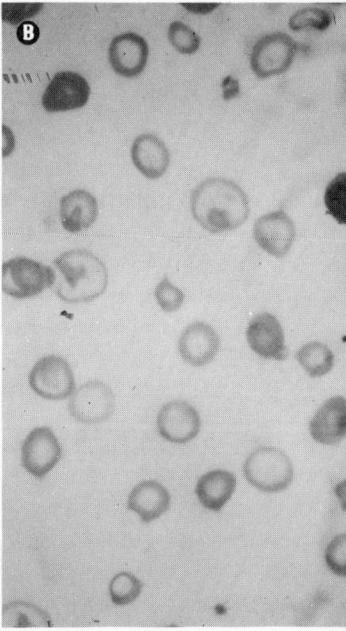

Blood smear shows microcytic-hypochromic anemia secondary to iron deficiency (A). Iron-vitamin B_{12} deficiency produces a macrocytic-hypochromic anemia (B).

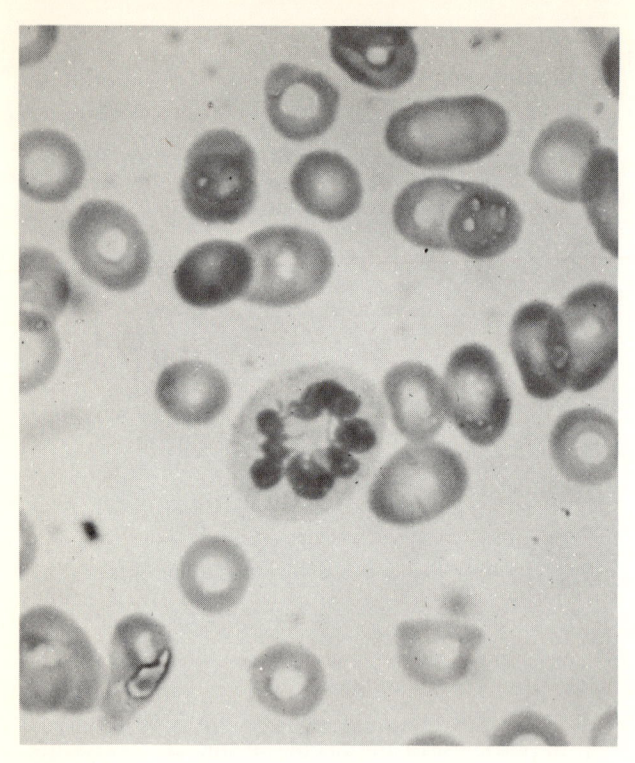

Treatment for vitamin B_{12} deficiency has produced hypochromic anemia secondary to unmasked iron deficiency. Hypersegmented neutrophil indicates recent B_{12} lack.

than that found in iron deficiency anemia.

Even a severe iron deficiency is correctable in most cases with oral replacement therapy. *But it is not enough to treat iron deficiency anemia and let it go at that.* The physician must also address the cause of the problem, since most iron deficiency anemia in the elderly is the result of a gastrointestinal disorder that is causing blood loss. Accordingly, the hematologic evaluation is incomplete without a check for occult GI bleeding, beginning with three stool guaiac tests for occult blood. Any positive finding calls for further investigation by means of fiberoptic endoscopy, x-ray studies, and sigmoidoscopy unless the patient's condition precludes it.

The cause of GI bleeding may be hiatus hernia, peptic ulcer, diverticular disease, or carcinoma of the colon; all have been associated with iron deficiency anemia in the elderly. Physical examination may reveal the presence of hemorrhoids; however, anemia may not be attributed solely to hemorrhoids until results of x-rays and endoscopy prove negative. One patient we studied was found to have an undiagnosed coagulation defect (Factor VIII deficiency) in addition to hereditary hemorrhagic telangiectasia.

A detailed history always helps. The fullest possible information should be elicited concerning surgery performed on the GI tract, and questions about use of geriatric vitamins should be included. Since these preparations are usually enriched with iron, the patient who faithfully takes his vitamins may effectively mask iron loss caused by occult GI bleeding. I know of several instances in which a large cancer of the colon was discovered only after belated diagnostic studies.

Of course iron deficiency anemia may also be secondary to disease or to a tumor that produces blood loss via the genitourinary tract. The dip-stick method of urine testing used in most hospitals does not rule out occult bleeding, I should add; the test is specific for hemoglobin, but the urine specimen must also be examined microscopically for the presence of red cells. Precise diagnosis and proper management of the bleeding lesion, whether in the GI or GU tract, are obviously of far greater importance than repletion of iron stores.

The anemia of iron deficiency is usually responsive to oral therapy, as noted earlier, and therefore any lack of response to such therapy must be checked out. Perhaps the patient is not taking the ferrous sulfate preparation because it is upsetting to the stomach. Perhaps the medication is being taken but not absorbed, as shown by serum iron values. On occasion the underlying problem proves to be sideropenic dysphagia related to development of an esophageal web or stricture (Patterson-Kelly syndrome, Plummer-Vinson syndrome); bougienage to overcome the stenosis and restore normal nutrition is usually required for therapy of the anemia. Iron supplementation is at best a temporary measure.

I referred earlier to sideroblastic anemia. It is uncommon in comparison with iron deficiency anemia but remains a possibility in any elderly patient who manifests a hypochromic anemia with high serum iron and transferrin. Given these findings, a bone marrow aspirate must be examined for the presence of "ringed" sideroblasts indicative of excessive iron deposition within mitochondria of normoblasts. What causes sideroblastic anemia? Disorders of heme or porphyrin synthesis have been implicated, but the etiology is really unknown. Nonetheless, this type of anemia often responds to pyridoxine therapy, which should be tried.

Let us turn to macrocytic anemia, which in older adults generally implies a *vitamin B_{12} deficiency*. This diagnosis should be thought of first in any elderly patient having macrocytic anemia associated with

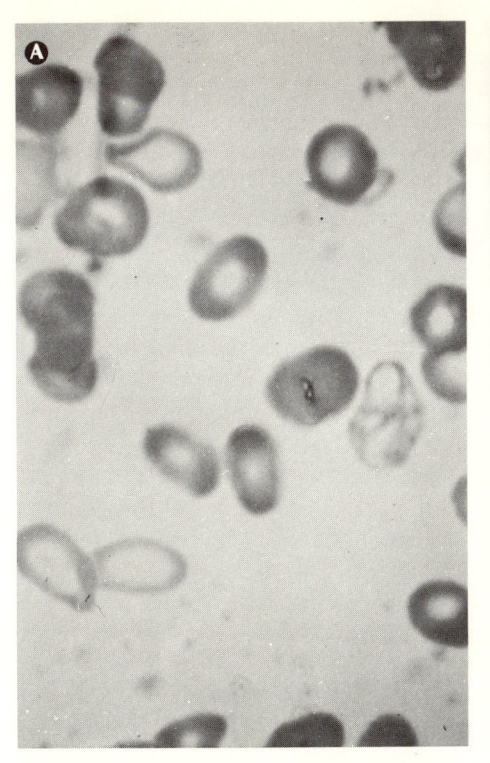

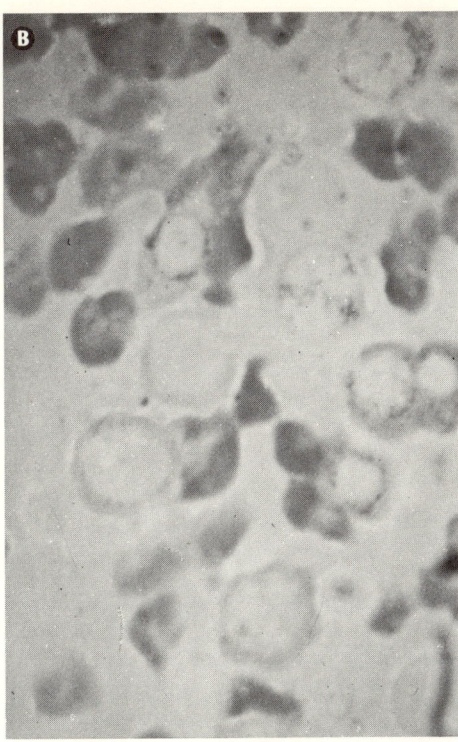

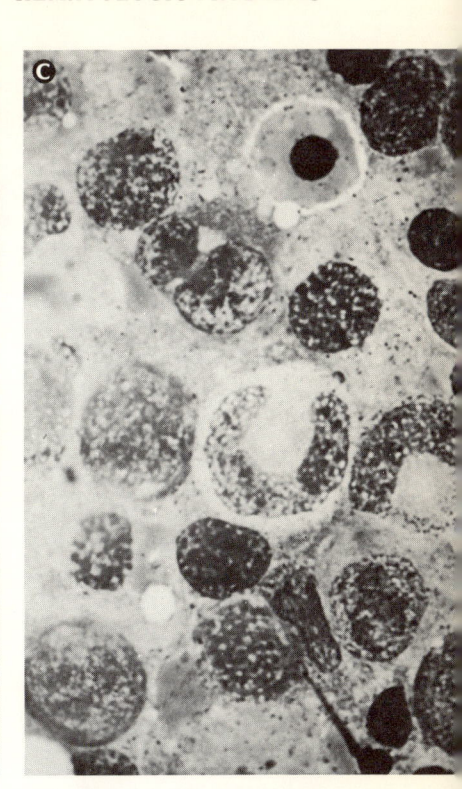

In blood smear of elderly patient, hypochromic red cells reflect an acquired sideroblastic anemia (A); confirmatory bone marrow study showed ringed sideroblasts due to excessive iron deposition within mitochondria (B). Marrow specimen with giant neutrophilic band is characteristic of early pernicious anemia (C).

increased mean corpuscular volume (MCV). False macrocytic indices may be produced by an underlying disease associated with cold agglutinins, or by prior administration of a hematinic evoking a marked reticulocyte response. In such cases the MCV is usually within normal limits.

Vitamin B_{12} deficiency is nearly always the result of defective absorption due to a lack of intrinsic factor. The fundamental defect may be gastric atrophy associated with loss of all gastric secretions, in other words, a classic pernicious anemia. Most victims of pernicious anemia are elderly. If the triad of weakness, glossitis, and paresthesia is present, the diagnosis is easily made. But initial symptoms vary and may suggest anything from a digestive disorder to cardiac or renal disease.

Intrinsic factor may be lacking in the elderly for a number of reasons. Carcinoma of the stomach may interfere with secretion of gastric juice. Depending on its extent, a surgical procedure may destroy most intrinsic factor secreting cells. Partial gastrectomy that removes a large portion of the stomach (70% or more) may do so. Surgery of the distal ileum may be even more damaging, since most vitamin B_{12} absorption takes place there. Macrocytic anemia has followed removal of the terminal 20 cm of small bowel.

The association is not always clear because there are extensive hepatic stores of the vitamin. *Two years may elapse after surgery or disease that affects secretion of intrinsic factor before vitamin B_{12} deficiency shows up.* For this reason it is unusual to encounter dietary B_{12} deficiency. By contrast, dietary folate deficiency develops more rapidly, since only two to four months' worth is stored. The elderly, whose intake of folate-containing foods is often low, are prime candidates for folate deficiency anemia. Macrocytic anemia in patients with alcoholic cirrhosis is almost always a consequence of folate deficiency.

With these considerations in mind, one evaluates a patient with macrocytic anemia for both vitamin B_{12} and folate deficiency. A Schilling urinary excretion test is ordered to measure B_{12} absorption. A marked reduction is indicative of pernicious anemia or another disorder in which intrinsic factor is lacking, whereas a more modest reduction suggests B_{12} deficiency resulting from intestinal malabsorption.

However, errors may be introduced if urine collection is incomplete or if renal disease is present. Uri-

> **Drugs Causing Untoward Hematologic Reactions in the Elderly**
>
> (ranked in decreasing order of frequency of side effect)
>
> **Associated with:**
>
> | ANEMIA | THROMBOCYTOPENIA |
> |---|---|
> | Chloramphenicol | Quinidine |
> | Methyldopa | Gold salts |
> | Penicillin | Ethanol |
> | Diphenylhydantoin | Chlorothiazides |
> | Phenacetin | Diphenylhydantoin |
> | Cephalosporin derivatives | Sulfathiazole |
> | Chlorpromazine | Rifampin |
> | Phenylbutazone | Quinine |
> | Ethanol | Acetazolamide |
> | Isoniazid | Digitoxin |
> | Sulfonamides | Acetaminophen |
> | Quinidine | Hydroxychloroquine |
> | Quinine | Chlorpromazine |
> | Para-aminosalicyclic acid | Cephalothin |
> | Aspirin | Phenacetin |
> | | Propylthiouracil |
> | **LEUKOPENIA** | Aspirin |
> | Phenothiazines | Reserpine |
> | Thiouracil and propyl- | Meprobamate |
> | thiouracil | Promethazine |
> | Methimazole | Sulfisoxazole |
> | Phenylbutazone | Sulfamethoxazole |
> | Sulfonamides | Mercurial diuretics |
> | Chloramphenicol | Spironolactone |
> | Meprobamate | Estrogenic hormones |
> | Penicillin | |
> | Aspirin | |
> | Procainamide | |

posed when an anemia is normocytic-normochromic. A broader variety of etiologies must be considered; moreover, this type of anemia is often a sign of serious disease. A normocytic-normochromic anemia frequently accompanies chronic infections, rheumatoid arthritis, or cancer.

When cell morphology and red cell indices are not very revealing, one looks first at red cell production, which is conveniently evaluated by means of a reticulocyte count. In normocytic-normochromic anemia related to renal failure, the reticulocyte count tends to be elevated; in the anemia of chronic infection, the count tends to be low.

Physiologically, bone marrow is capable of increasing red cell production six- to eightfold in order to compensate for anemia. This mechanism remains operative in the elderly, though it takes longer to achieve the maximal hematologic response. Therefore, whenever the reticulocyte count fails to increase proportionately to the degree of anemia present, it may be assumed that the bone marrow has been affected, either directly or indirectly, so that red cell production is impaired.

Marrow hypoplasia (or aplasia) must be presumed if the absolute reticulocyte count goes below 50,000 to 60,000/cu mm and is associated with leukopenia and thrombocytopenia. *The physician must be ever aware of the possibility that hypoplastic anemia in the elderly may be due to drug toxicity, since these reactions are unpredictable.* Bone marrow examination may show a large number of cells, primarily blasts, if it is performed during the regenerative phase. Unless the patient's history is known, these findings may be misinterpreted as leukemia.

On the other hand, leukemia may be present but unsuspected if it is asymptomatic or associated with nonspecific complaints only. This is especially true of *chronic lymphocytic leukemia*, the most common lymphoproliferative disorder of the elderly. This leukemia may be recognized in the course of evaluation for an unrelated disorder or when the patient presents for surgery. A presumptive diagnosis of chronic lymphocytic leukemia should be considered in any elderly patient who manifests persistent blood lymphocytosis accompanied by enlarged nodes or splenomegaly. Bone marrow examination that reveals an excessive number of lymphocytes provides confirmation of the diagnosis.

The important point about chronic lymphocytic leukemia is that its course is often quite benign in the elderly. Many patients remain relatively well for

nary excretion data should therefore be supplemented by serum B_{12} values or, preferably, a B_{12} radioimmunoassay should be performed in the first place. There is not only anemia as such to be concerned about but also the potential for neurologic damage associated with B_{12} deficiency. Serum folate levels are determined by radioimmunoassay.

Anemia due either to B_{12} or folate deficiency is reversible with vitamin replacement therapy. In treating any anemia in the elderly, however, one must anticipate that reticulocyte response may take several days longer than in younger individuals. A little patience prevents overtreatment of severe anemia (by transfusion), with its dangerous potential.

So far I have discussed chiefly the microcytic and macrocytic anemias. But there are other problems

some time and succumb eventually to an unrelated disease. In Wintrobe's series, median survival time following diagnosis was at least nine years, longer if the leukemia was diagnosed before symptoms appeared. The longest survivor died of pneumonia at 79 – 24 years after the diagnosis was made.

All of this usually dissuades us from employing antileukemic therapy, considering its known hazards and its questionable influence on survival. Once the diagnosis is made, the patient with chronic lymphocytic leukemia can usually be managed on an outpatient basis by the family physician, provided he is watchful for complications such as infection, development of hemolytic anemia, or impaired immune mechanisms. Adjunctive therapy is essential.

Another lymphoproliferative disorder, fairly rare, is Waldenström's macroglobulinemia. I mention it because it primarily affects the elderly. There may be vague symptoms, if any, before significant clinical manifestations appear. These relate mostly to the physicochemical properties of the macroglobulins, which give rise to the hyperviscosity syndrome. The diagnosis is established on the basis of the characteristic serum protein abnormality plus the presence of lymphoid cells in bone marrow.

This brings to mind *multiple myeloma*, a more common disorder also characterized by uncontrolled proliferation of cells normally involved in antibody production and synthesis of an abnormal globulin (M-component). The difference is that multiple

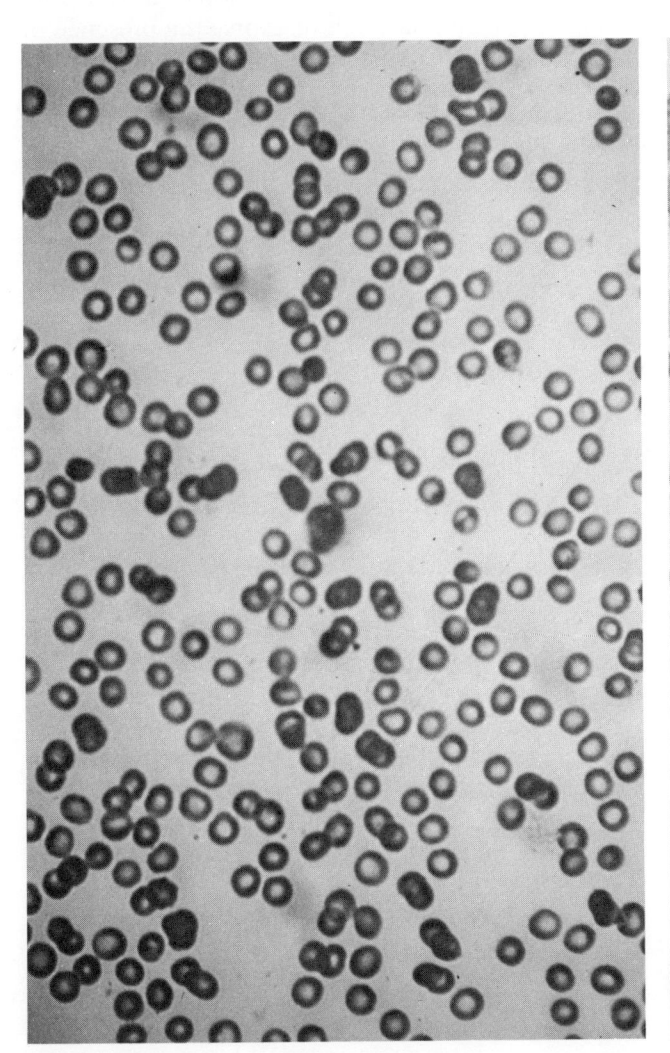

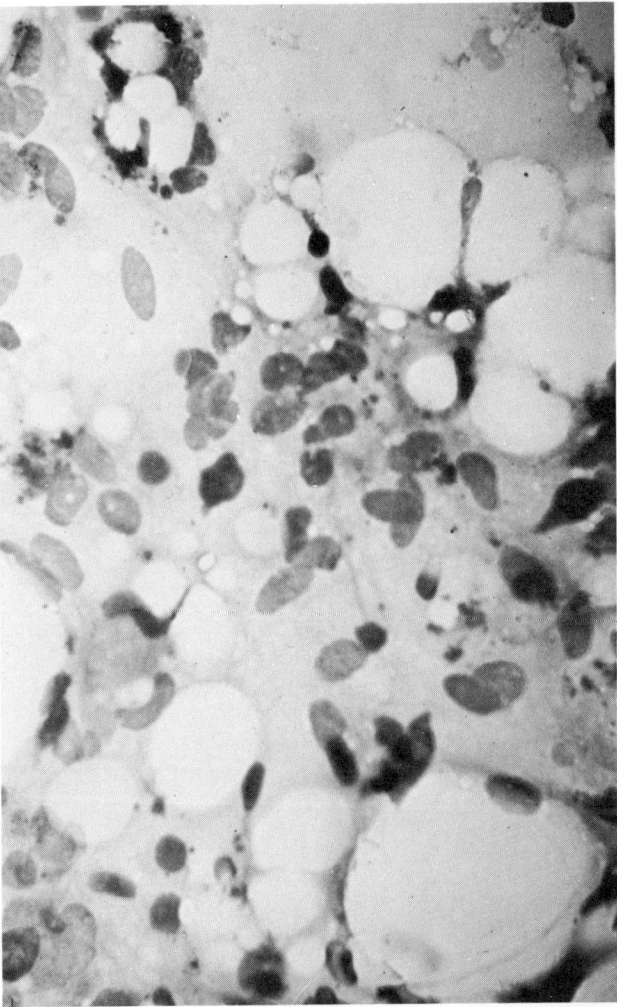

Untoward reactions to chloramphenicol include anemia combined with leukopenia and thrombocytopenia; note absence of platelets in blood smear (left). Another manifestation of chloramphenicol toxicity is bone marrow hypoplasia (right). Many drugs cause hematologic side effects in the elderly (cf table on page 70).

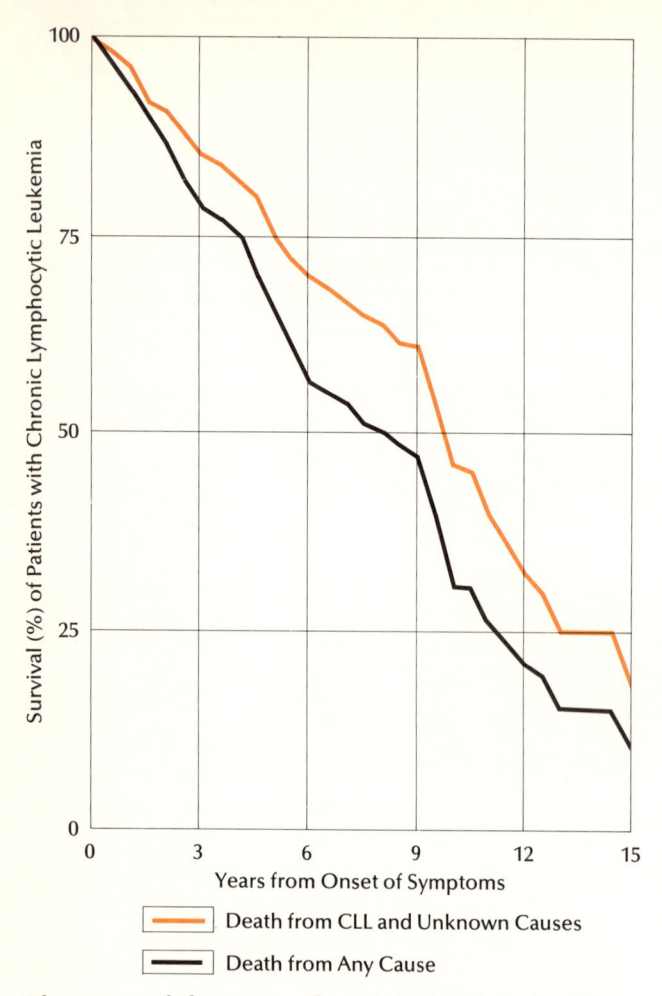

The course of chronic lymphocytic leukemia in the elderly is often quite benign, as indicated by Wintrobe's data on survival time after onset of symptoms in 130 cases.

myeloma is a plasma cell dyscrasia whereas a lymphocyte dyscrasia is responsible for Waldenström's macroglobulinemia. Physicians caring for the elderly should be aware of both disorders in the event diagnostic study seems warranted. Certainly it should be undertaken if plasma cells appear in the peripheral blood and there is a concomitant increase in total serum protein. If the cause is multiple myeloma, this should be detectable by serum and urine protein electrophoresis. The presence of 10% or more plasmoblasts in a marrow specimen confirms the diagnosis, though some increase of these cells in the elderly is not abnormal. Systemic chemotherapy is indicated, since multiple myeloma is a generalized disease, while painful bone lesions are treated by irradiation; both must be closely supervised by a hematologist.

Finally, *chronic myelocytic leukemia* must be mentioned along with two other myeloproliferative disorders, *idiopathic myelofibrosis* and *polycythemia vera*. All are usually associated with leukocytosis, thrombocytosis, and splenomegaly, and the first two with anemia.

Chronic myelocytic leukemia should be suspected if the peripheral blood smear shows an increased number of basophils, and of course the presence of Ph[1] chromosome in bone marrow strongly favors this diagnosis. In most cases of idiopathic myelofibrosis, the blood smear reveals poikilocytosis and nucleated erythrocytes. In polycythemia vera, individual red corpuscles appear quite normal; it is the striking increase in their number and in total red cell mass that is characteristic. In the classic case, the combination of polycythemia, ruddy cyanosis, and splenomegaly makes the diagnosis unambiguous. But presentation varies in the elderly and may suggest a cardiovascular or neurologic disease. If hematologic evaluation suggests any of the three myeloproliferative disorders a hematologist should be consulted.

A last word about *senile purpura* because it is so commonplace. The basic defect is a loss of dermal collagen, elastin, and subcutaneous fat, producing the familiar ecchymotic spots on extensor surfaces and radial borders of the forearms. When left alone the spots usually fade in a few weeks, leaving a residual brownish pigmentation. Though a minor annoyance to most patients, senile purpura exemplifies a useful principle: the hematologic problems of the elderly should neither be overlooked nor overtreated but must be managed according to their significance in the patient's total health picture and way of life.

Disorders of the Aging GI System

MARVIN M. SCHUSTER
Johns Hopkins University

Gastrointestinal disease in the elderly may differ in degree or in kind from GI disease in young adults. Differences occur in frequency of disease, clinical presentation, and the treatment required. The aged person is more subject to socioenvironmental stresses, has collateral diseases, and carries an accumulation of disabilities. Vulnerability to gastrointestinal difficulty, if not disaster, increases with the age of the patient. Malignancy appears more often, probably as a function of chronic exposure to carcinogens in the food supply and to atrophy of tissue in the stomach and elsewhere. In this age grouping, malignancy of the gastrointestinal tract rises to an incidence of 10%.

The aging gut is less resilient and if injured takes longer to heal. Motor and neurologic disturbances are more frequent, contributing notably to fecal incontinence. One of the few GI conditions found almost exclusively in patients over age 40 is diverticulosis; after age 50, perhaps 25% of the population has demonstrable diverticulosis, but by age 80 the proportion is 70%. As with many age-related changes in morphology, diverticulosis may carry no symptoms and require no treatment. Indeed, there are many gaps in our understanding of how – if at all – age-associated morphologic changes produce clinically significant functional consequences. One would like to link up tissue changes and malfunction, but we can do so only speculatively.

Functional Components

The psychosomatic factor in GI complaints is well recognized. True as this is of the young, it is all the more significant clinically in the elderly. Accordingly, any discussion of disorders of the alimentary tract in the elderly should begin outside the tract itself. When one reflects on the stresses that many elderly persons encounter – retirement, loss of income, death or impending death of spouse, self, and friends, and changes in health status – it should be no surprise that digestive complaints having no obvious organic basis are so common. Attempts to compensate for perceived physical and mental malfunction or weakness often lead to or intensify the use of drugs (including alcohol), often with adverse gastrointestinal effects. For example, excessive use of aspirin is very common. A thoroughgoing drug history thus is essential not only for geriatric assessment in general, as pointed out earlier (see Chapter 1, "Drug Prescribing for the Elderly," by P. P. Lamy and R. E. Vestal), but for evaluation of gastrointestinal symptoms in particular.

The degree to which GI complaints have an emotional basis was suggested by a study of 300 outpatients aged 65 or older at the University of Chicago clinics. As in the young, their GI disorders were preponderantly functional, and since they were followed for a year or more, their final diagnoses were fairly well established. These were: functional GI distress, 56%; GI tract malignancy, 10%; gallbladder disease, 8%; duodenal ulcer, 7%; gastric ulcer, 3%; colonic diverticulosis, 3%; and various other disorders, 14%. These figures seem consistent with the experience of most GI clinics, where perhaps 60% of the patients seen have some major emotional or psychologic problem.

Depression is more common in the elderly than in the young, in part because of the recognition of deterioration of internal processes, with increasing limitations on activity, such as loss of eyesight, ability to chew, to walk, to perform in athletics, etc. External deprivations occur, including loss of friends and relatives. These losses can gradually deplete the usual familial and supportive environment. Some of the cardinal manifestations of depression – anorexia, constipation, and somatic pains – can easily be mistaken for symptoms of primary gastrointestinal disease. In assigning appropriate weight to emotional components, one must be on guard not to "overreact." Symptoms of primary gastrointestinal disorders may be attributed mistakenly to a coexisting depression. In treating the depression, small doses of tricyclic antidepressant drugs can be very helpful in the elderly, especially when combined with a sympathetic ear and provision of support. Environmental manipulation may be more important in the psychiatric management of the elderly than in the younger group. This manipulation may include provision for adequate housing, appropriate social contacts, prostheses, food, and medication.

Nutritional disturbances exemplify the amalgam of organic and psychologic factors one sees in exaggerated fashion among the old. Decreased intake is more likely to be the cause of weight loss than malabsorption, provided malignancy is not involved. Depression, apathy, loss of status and income, and disorientation all prompt people to eat less. So, too, do loss of teeth or grinding ability; difficulty in swallowing; pain after eating; cerebrovascular changes that interfere with taste and smell, so that food no longer is as interesting or appetizing. Family problems may also interfere (for example, if a person accustomed to one style of ethnic cooking moves into a household run by a daughter-in-law who cooks in a different style).

The family physician often is in the best position to evaluate such multifaceted problems, offer counseling or medical management, or make referral to the appropriate specialist. By virtue of long association with the patient and family, he may also be best able to evaluate and treat ominous weight changes, taking into account the fact that women tend to lose weight after age 60, while men tend to gain (probably reflecting replacement of lean tissue with fat).

Some elderly patients resort to vitamin supplements in the belief they need more as they age. Actually, the only vitamin requirement that may increase with age is that of B_{12}, probably because there is less stomach acid available for its absorption. The most common deficiency seen in the elderly, of vitamin C, is due not to malabsorption but to curtailed intake of citrus fruits. This deficiency may be critical, since vitamin C is necessary for iron absorption and wound healing. In the person who has no natural teeth to brush, the bleeding gums characteristic of the deficiency will not be seen, which may make the diagnosis difficult.

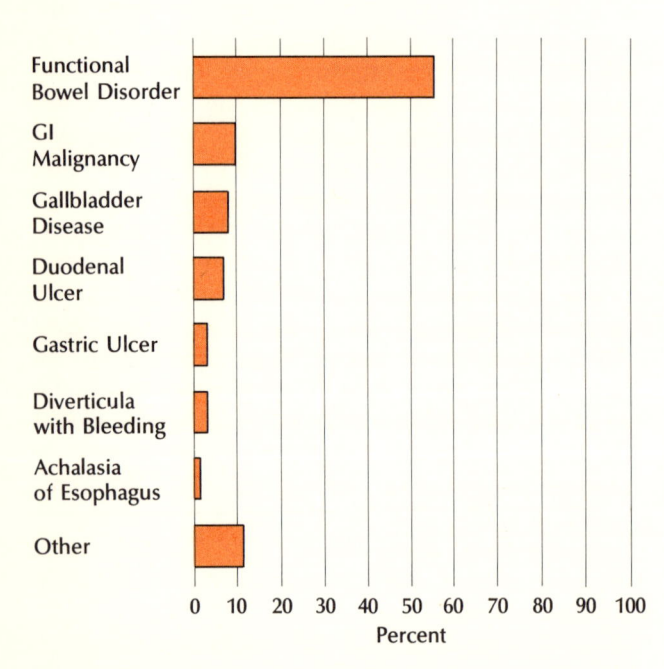

In patients who are over 65 years of age, as in younger people, more than half of all gastrointestinal disturbances are functional. The chart also demonstrates the incidence of other gastrointestinal disorders.

Esophagus

Having made these general comments I will turn now to specific organs of the alimentary canal, starting (as one would expect) with the esophagus. The normal elderly esophagus may perform differently from its younger counterpart; it may have decreased peristaltic response, increased nonperistaltic response, delayed transit time, and more frequent failure of the lower sphincter to relax upon swallowing. In addition, pathophysiologic states contribute to disturbances of esophageal motility.

In persons over age 80, and especially in nonagenarians, the peristaltic changes are strikingly apparent on cinefluoroscopy and manometry. There is an increase in contractions that are not peristaltic, a type found almost exclusively in the elderly. These are prolonged, spastic contractions of ringlike segments of the distal one to two thirds of the esophagus. The characteristic appearance on barium study gives rise to the term "corkscrew" esophagus. In the younger adult, the cause of such spasm more often is acid reflux; it may also be neurogenic or neuromuscular. The differentiation is made by the acid perfusion test, in which 0.1 N HCl is introduced by tubes into the esophagus (usually while recording pressure activity manometrically) or acid barium may be swallowed and the resultant spasm seen and recorded by cinefluoroscopy (neutral barium will have no such effect). A positive result calls for treatment with antacids.

Substernal pain may accompany esophageal as well as coronary spasm. It is commonly thought that these two entities can be differentiated with a trial of nitroglycerin. But since the drug dilates any smooth muscle, it reduces the pain of *either* type of spasm. It is thus not helpful for differential diagnosis but may be a highly useful treatment; in fact we frequently recommend that a nitroglycerin tablet be placed under the tongue before eating to decrease esophageal spasm in a susceptible patient. Eating often triggers spasm in such individuals.

The cause of reflux esophagitis – insufficient pressure of the lower esophageal sphincter – can be attacked experimentally through biofeedback, or operant conditioning. Healthy persons can learn to raise pressure from, say, 14 mm Hg to 28. Patients with insufficient pressure – 2 mm Hg, for example – can effect a doubling, but this magnitude is still not the normal resting level. Elderly persons have learned biofeedback techniques but it is not yet clear whether they, or any patients, can raise pressures to normal values and sustain them.

Urecholine, 25 mg *tid,* can be used to increase the tone of the lower sphincter; it may help some patients. The principal treatment for acid-induced esophagitis remains antacids and positional therapy plus diet; here I would like to emphasize that too often antacids and positional therapy are not given an adequate trial. The patient is then described as nonresponsive and is referred to a surgeon or gastro-

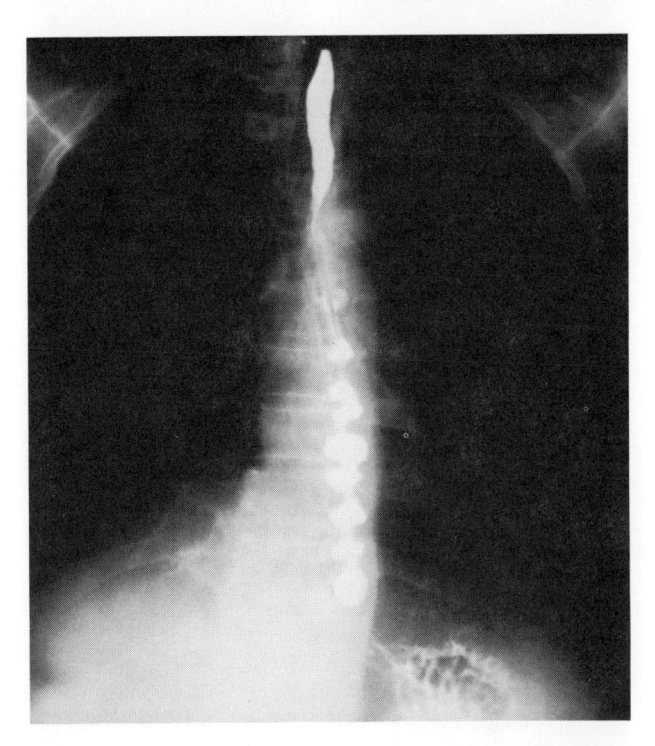

"Corkscrew" esophagus in the elderly results from prolonged, spastic contractions of the ringlike segments of the distal two thirds of the esophagus.

enterologist. The specialist often reverses these "failures" simply by careful instruction of the patient. Positional therapy is often not explained clearly enough. Most intelligent patients will cooperate and improve if they understand that their *shoulders* should be elevated 30 degrees, and why. Simply telling the patient to use two pillows may be taken to mean two pillows behind the neck, which only aggravates the reflux.

One pitfall with antacids is that patients are often told only to take a tablespoonful three or four times daily "before or after meals." This is wrong on two counts. First, taken right before or after meals, the antacid is useless because there is a natural buffer in the stomach during eating. Rather, patients need the antacid an hour or two *after* eating, when the stomach is empty. Since most elderly persons already have decreased stomach acid and impaired peptic digestion of food, taking antacids at mealtime can be counterproductive.

Another problem with the antacid prescription stems from the physician's assumption that patients eat three meals a day. But if one obtains a 24-hour log of patient activity, one may learn that the only meal eaten by an older person is supper. Though the

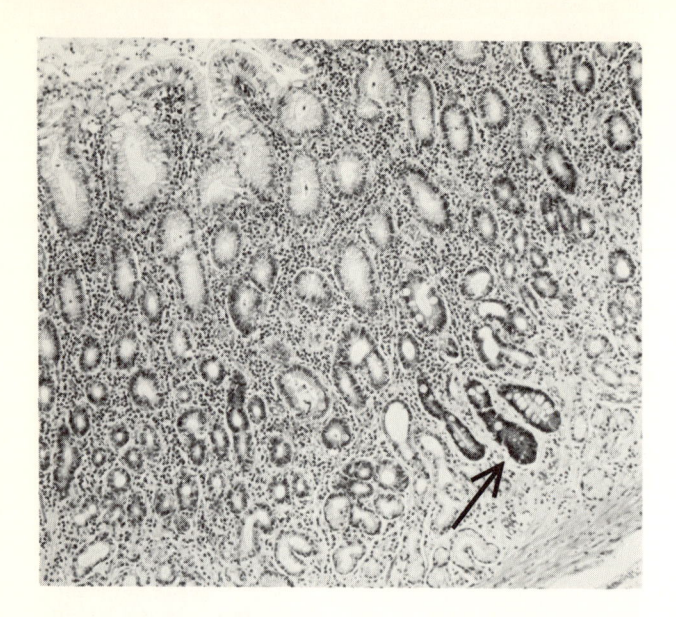

Gastric atrophic changes may be significant after age 50. Typical are lymphocytic infiltration and depletion of glands by about 25% as compared with young adulthood. Appearance of Paneth's cells (arrow) and absence of parietal cells signify degeneration to a more primitive state, or intestinalization (micrograph courtesy of Dr. R. Garcia Bunuel, Baltimore City Hospitals).

patient needs antacid most of the day because the stomach is empty, he construes the prescription to take antacids after meals as requiring him to take them only once a day. Or a log may show that a patient is skipping meals because he or she is dieting – and skipping the antacid too. Or if a patient has coffee and orange juice for breakfast, he may not count that rather acidic combination as a meal. Care must thus be taken in explaining how meals become the reference point for taking antacids. I do not recommend using anticholinergic drugs in treating reflux esophagitis because they decrease gastric emptying more effectively than they suppress secretion, which (especially in the elderly with impaired motility) is likely to leave a pool of acid available for reflux and worsening of the esophagitis.

The frequency of hiatal hernia increases with age; three fourths of all hiatal hernias are found in persons between the ages of 50 and 80. Most are of the sliding type, but perhaps only 1% are symptomatic. The high incidence in the elderly may result from an age-related relaxation of ligaments or muscle atrophy or may simply reflect prolonged intra-abdominal pressure. Occasionally, increased intra-abdominal pressure may be secondary to the weight gain accompanying aging, especially (as noted) in males.

Hiatal hernias, being so rarely symptomatic, infrequently require operative intervention. All too often symptoms of esophagitis are attributed to the hiatal hernia when the problem actually lies in an incompetent lower esophageal sphincter. Hiatal hernias may exist without esophagitis, and esophagitis can exist without hiatal hernia.

Stomach

Aging also is associated with secretory and morphologic changes within the stomach. Acid and pepsin secretion falls to about one third of that in younger adults. The efficacy of pepsin is compromised by the low-acid environment and absorption of iron and B$_{12}$ are diminished in this milieu. A combination of secretory factors thus tends to produce digestive impairment.

After age 50 or thereabouts, 80% of stomachs examined at surgery or autopsy show morphologic deviations from normal. Changes appear to occur through all layers of the stomach wall. While adipose tissue increases, smooth muscle thins out. Loss of parietal cells is reflected functionally in hyposecretion of acid. Muscular atrophy may be the morphologic correlate of age-related loss of stomach motility and may account for some nonspecific upper GI symptoms.

The thinning of the gastric mucosa, which seems to begin in the decade of the thirties, is sometimes accompanied by leukocytic infiltration and metaplasia of the glands of the fundus. The submucosa may become extensively infiltrated with monocytes and elastic fibers. These developments are thought to provide a background for neoplasia, either polypoid or cancerous. Since it is not the polyp as such that is precancerous, its removal does not by itself protect against malignancy. With diminishing acid protection both polyps and cancers become more frequent. Suspicious polyps often can be removed via the gastroscope, thus avoiding surgery.

Against this background it often becomes important to determine when a patient is at unusual risk of malignancy from chronic "atrophic gastritis" (which one study suggests carries a 20-fold increase in risk of gastric carcinoma). Recent technical advances, which have made it possible to perform polypectomy through the fiberoptic colonoscope, have transformed colonoscopy from a purely diagnostic to a therapeutic modality. It is hoped that early detection of polyps and cancer by this technique will result in decreased morbidity and mortality.

Unlike that of neoplasia, the risk of ulcer disease does not rise with age, but the secretory alterations produce age-related shifts in the epidemiology of ulcer types. The young and old share the same incidence of peptic ulcer, about 10%. But the ratio of duodenal to gastric ulcer, 10:1 in the young population, becomes 2:1 in the elderly. The duodenal ulcer's predominance fades with the age-related loss of acidity. There is also an age-related drop in mucin secretion, and it may be that the mucin-deficient stomach cannot protect itself as well against normal acidity, thus raising the incidence of gastric ulcer. Whether vascular changes contribute to ulcerogenesis in the elderly is not known.

Another epidemiologic change with age is in the sex ratio for duodenal ulcer. In middle age, male predominance is 11:1; in old age, 5:1. The recent increase in drinking, smoking, occupational, and other stresses in women may be the reasons why their risk has increased in modern times as women have assumed roles that in the past were traditionally reserved for men. The sexes have about the same incidence of gastric ulcer in old age. Ulcer treatment is empirical and paradoxical: antacids are recommended for both gastric and duodenal ulcer, even though normal secretion or hyposecretion characterizes the former and hypersecretion the latter. For most antacids, 2 tablespoons (or 2 tablets) should be taken one hour after meals and at bedtime (*qid* even if meals are missed).

Symptoms of ulcer in the elderly may vary from those in the young. Fever, leukocytosis, and other typical signs may be absent even when there is perforation. Although the incidence of bleeding does not increase with age, mortality from bleeding does, rising from 25% among people in their fifties with gastric ulcer to 65% in octogenarians. The corresponding rise in duodenal ulcer is from 12% to 50%. These statistics dictate earlier surgical intervention for the patient with bleeding gastric than with bleeding duodenal ulcer. The older the GI bleeder, the more likely he or she is to have sclerotic vessels, impaired hemostasis, and complicating collateral diseases. At the same time the elderly patient is less able to tolerate the hypotension, azotemia, and dehydration that accompany bleeding. These are among the factors that make the treatment of the elderly GI bleeder one of the most difficult problems in medical or surgical management.

Esophagogastroduodenoscopy, performed early while bleeding is still active, can be very helpful in saving time and lives by early localization of the bleeding site. Mortality from a massive bleed increases appreciably when diagnosis and treatment are delayed more than 24 hours, especially in the elderly. Modern fiberoptic instruments have overcome the problems imposed upon rigid instrumentation by arthritis, kyphosis, and vascular disease.

Small and Large Intestines

After age 40, the weight of the small intestine drops steadily, perhaps reflecting atrophy of the three layers of the intestinal wall. Fibrous tissue appears to replace parenchyma, there are fewer smooth muscle fibers (and these often are atrophic), and occasional cellular breakdown products are seen. In rats, net transport of essential amino acid constituents tends to fall off with age; if confirmed in man, such a reduction might explain some aspects of age-related mental decline. A gradual diminution of lipolytic activity starts at age 30, and eventually reaches a value 20% of that in young adults, but the clinical significance is unknown. As for information on enzymatic changes in the aging small intestine, it is either lacking or inconclusive.

Little is known about histologic, absorptive, and secretory changes in the colon with aging, but

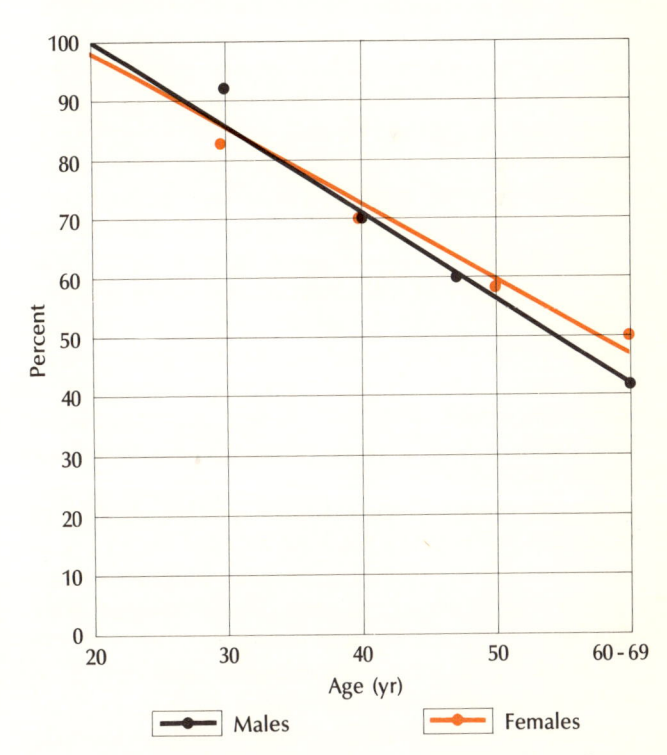

Secretion of acid (and of pepsin, not shown) falls with the increase in age, affecting the digestive processes.

chronic constipation is known to be a major GI problem of old people. The colon may be atonic, a state that predisposes to increased storage capacity, longer stool transit time, and greater stool dehydration. Other etiologic factors in constipation, such as the role of bacterial flora, are not well understood. In one study of geriatric patients in whom stool pH was alkaline, relief of constipation occurred after lactobacilli formation (stimulated by maltose) reduced the pH to less than 6.

Laxative abuse is of course very common; it is also the most common cause of diarrhea in this age group, especially among women. By the time the elderly patient seeks professional help for constipation, laxative dependency is likely to be well established. The vicious cycle is in full swing: the more the patient uses laxatives, the harder it becomes to induce a response to colonic distension. He or she then tries an even higher dose. Some patients ingest an amazing quantity and variety of drugs. One I can cite, habitually took 15 bisacodyl (Dulcolax) tablets, 30 senna concentration (Senokot) tablets, and 4 oz of castor oil *at the same time*.

The physician's first task is to try to reduce the laxative load and to transfer the patient to a high-fiber diet. This does not mean more roughage, or particulate matter, as obtained from corn or seeds. Rather, it means a diet rich in bran. If unprocessed bran is sprinkled over cereal or other food, its "sawdust" texture and taste will be disguised. The patient should be advised to expect bloating for a few weeks on a regimen of 4 tablespoons of bran, three or four times a day – a total of about 15 gm of unprocessed bran per day (the "all" or "100%" bran cereals contain about half as much bran as the same weight of unprocessed bran). For one in 10, the bloating or flatulence will be intolerable. Patients can be assured, however, that these symptoms will usually disappear in three weeks.

In conjunction with the high-fiber diet, the patient should be started on a bowel-training program, capitalizing on the gastroileocolic response. This is accomplished by having the patient regularly try to defecate after breakfast or supper, whichever is more agreeable, for five minutes. If no bowel improvement occurs, a hypertonic phosphate (Fleet) enema or suppository should be tried every other day. If followed faithfully, the regimen offers a good chance of establishing a response, but, as physicians well recognize, an established bowel pattern is hard to alter.

A mistaken idea of what is a normal frequency for bowel movements is often responsible for unnecessary drug taking. Fewer than three movements a week may be accepted as indicating constipation, but actually any figure is arbitrary. Constipation is not a disease but a symptom; if the patient does not complain, there is no cause for intervention, regardless of frequency of movements. My approach is to be skeptical about patient complaints of "constipation" until the picture is clarified by such questions as, "Are there fewer than three movements per week? Is there difficulty of passage? Is it painful? Are stools exceptionally hard? Are there complications (such as fissures and bleeding)?" If the answers are no, I advise the patient that no treatment is needed. Nonetheless, other possible causes may need investigation, and the patient may need counseling.

But if the physician ascertains that a particular patient does require a prescription, he should begin with stool softeners (such as a hydrophilic mucilloid, 1 tablespoon or dioctyl sodium sulfosuccinate, 50 mg *tid* orally), decreasing the dosage as soon as possible. Agents of this type should be taken soon after (or during) meals, so that they mix with the meal as stool is being formed. Two other drugs, senna and cascara, taken in high doses over a long period of time, may impair the ganglion cells that coordinate Auerbach's plexus, thus producing a condition akin to Hirschsprung's disease or esophageal achalasia. If colonic dilation suggests ganglion loss has occurred, biopsy may be undertaken for confirmation.

In persons whose severe constipation is related to ganglion loss, surgery may be indicated. A new approach, similar in principle to myotomy for esophageal achalasia, is to remove a longitudinal strip of muscle from the distal colon and internal sphincter. This overcomes sphincter resistance. Dr. Ghislain Devroede of Canada, who developed the technique, reports that two thirds of patients with severe constipation benefit from the operation. Other operative approaches have been much less successful.

Among the sequelae of severe constipation in the elderly is a paradoxical one, overflow incontinence occurring with fecal impaction. Bowel incontinence may also be caused by gradual neuromuscular deterioration and by the effects of intercurrent systemic diseases, such as diabetes with peripheral neuropathy. The paradoxical diarrhea and incontinence associated with fecal impaction are treated first by alleviating the impaction, then by treating the constipation. Disimpaction is best performed manually, since most attempts to relieve impactions by enemas are futile. Once the large impaction has been removed, appropriate medical management may prevent recurrence. Incontinence associated with neuromuscular pathology can respond even in elderly people to treatment by biofeedback techniques. In our experience, patients (including nonagenarians) can utilize operant conditioning to control impaired sphincters, even when this impairment has an organic etiology, such as surgical trauma, diabetes, and lesions of the spinal cord.

The appendix is the only part of the colon that shows definite histologic change with age. The lumen gradually begins to close, from the tip inward, and by age 50 has been obliterated in half the population. This may be part of an aging process or may be secondary to repeated inflammation. Of clinical importance is the fact that elderly patients with appendicitis may not display the classic symptoms of fever, leukocytosis, and rebound tenderness, even upon perforation.

Diverticula, uncommon below age 40, steadily increase thereafter, both with respect to people in a given population who develop diverticula and to the number likely to be found in a given individual. Those diverticula that are concentrated in a specific area (usually the sigmoid) are generally associated with increased pressures within the colon. High-fiber diets tend to increase the diameter of the colon and decrease the pressure. Antispasmodic medication may provide some relief of the pain associated with excessive spasms. Opiates, such as morphine and codeine, should generally be avoided because they increase spasm and aggravate constipation. Demerol is less likely to produce these undesirable effects. Antibiotic therapy may also be appropriate when associated fever and leukocytosis indicate inflammation, usually with microperforations.

Biliary Tract, Liver, and Pancreas

In general, biliary tract disease appears after the late thirties and the incidence of gallstones increases with age. However, if gallbladder disease is not present, there is no measurable change in gallbladder function with aging. Disease is not uncommon, however. In a series of 1,000 autopsies of patients aged 70 or older, 30% had gallstones and another 5% had previously undergone cholecystectomy. Among the 30%, gallbladder disease – inflammatory, obstructive, or neoplastic – was the immediate cause of death in one out of 12. Other factors affecting the recommendation for elective surgery in the geriatric patient will be discussed by Dr. Philip Ferris in a later chapter (see Chapter 20, "Surgical Management of the Elderly"), and therefore will be omitted here.

Surgery remains the treatment of choice for problematic gallbladder disease. Whenever possible, cholecystectomy should be performed, but occasionally a cholecystostomy is preferable, with drainage if necessary, as a primary procedure because of the elderly patient's poor condition. Chenodeoxycholic acid is presently undergoing investigation as a possible medical means of dissolving gallstones, but since this agent requires a long period to dissolve stones, it cannot as yet be recommended as a treatment for the acute manifestations or for the complications of gallbladder disease. Safety factors have also not yet been established.

A rare type of tumor that produces gallstonelike symptoms is noteworthy because it is deceptive and because its incidence may be on the increase. I refer to the Klatskin tumor, which until recently was seldom encountered. In the last year, however, four have come to my attention among elderly patients. These tumors at the bifurcation of the main hepatic duct are slow-growing and produce obstructive jaundice, with or without pain; occasionally, patients also have gallstones. In an elderly patient especially, it may be necessary to consider Klatskin tumor as the possible explanation of obstructive jaundice. The tumors require a special palliative approach: rather than a T tube in the biliary tree, a Rodney Smith

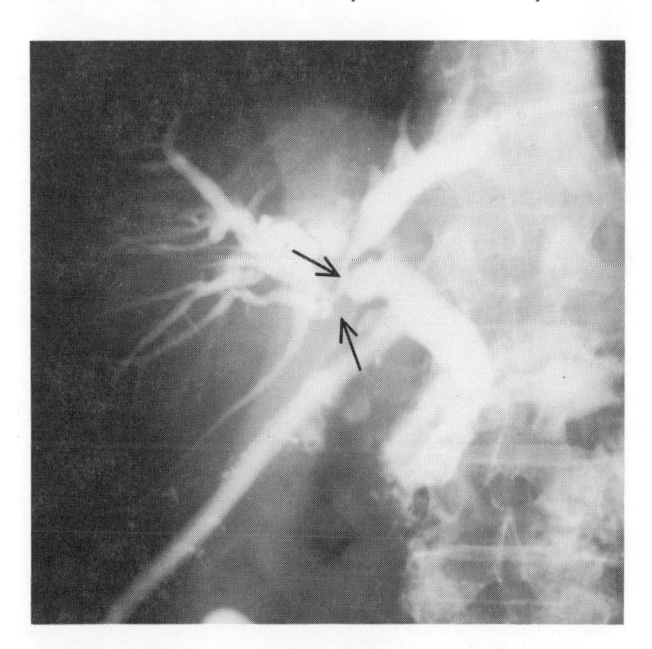

Klatskin tumor, an unusual condition, produces the constriction of the bifurcation of the left and right intrahepatic radicals seen in the above x-ray (courtesy Department of Radiology, Baltimore City Hospitals).

CHAPTER 10: SCHUSTER

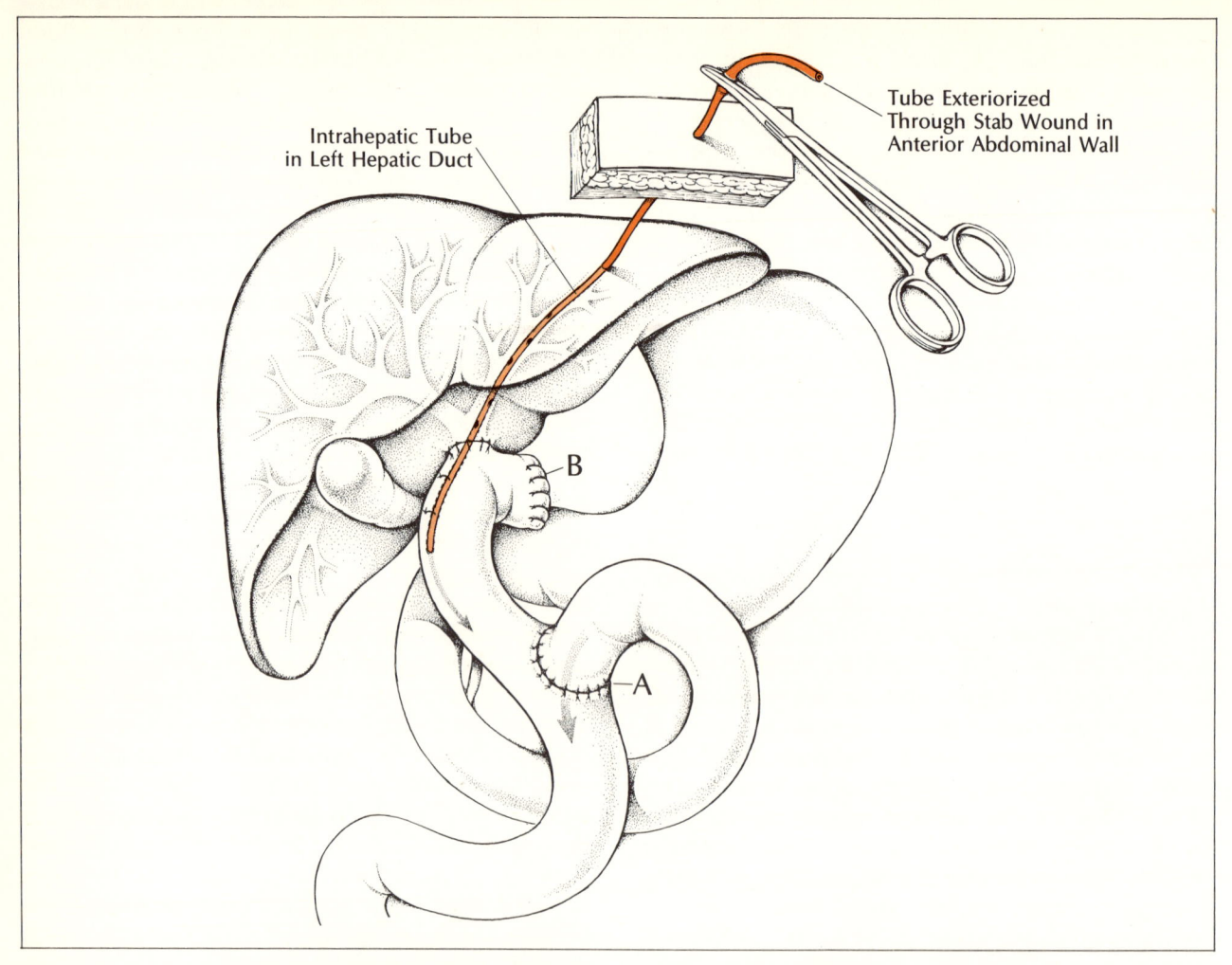

Rodney Smith tube for repair of high bile duct strictures permits drainage. A Roux-en-Y jejunostomy (A) is created with defunctionalized limb. Jejunal wall is anchored to liver capsule (B) around severed bile duct. Tube with side holes carries bile into the isolated loop of the jejunum. It can be left in place for many months.

tube is placed through the abdominal wall into the substance of liver to provide drainage from one of the major radicals. While not curative, the procedure may well palliate the effects of obstruction for the patient's remaining life-span.

The liver's weight diminishes with age by as much as 20% between ages 50 and 70, but because of its large reserve capacity, there seems to be little clinical effect. In a normal elderly population, liver function tests show little or no change; this statement includes BSP clearance and bilirubin tests. Morphologic changes do occur with aging but are unimportant in the absence of disease.

But while disease rather than aging appears to govern changes in the liver's chemical composition, there *are* suspected age-related reductions in hepatic enzymes, particularly the microsomal-induced enzymes involved in oxidation/reduction reactions significant to detoxification and drug metabolism. The evidence is far clearer in aged rats than in man. Impairments in these aspects of function may result from not only enzyme changes but diminished albumin synthesis (whether due to dietary deficiency or "aging") and reduced hepatic blood flow. (At age 65, liver blood flow has been estimated to be about 60% of the flow at age 25.)

Jaundice in the elderly is related to biliary obstruction in 80% of cases and to hepatocellular damage in only 16% of cases. Hepatitis, the principal cause of jaundice in the young, is thus a less important cause in the old, but its mortality is higher. Interestingly, at postmortem examination, the livers of elderly persons who had no frank liver disease often show a histologic picture like that of mild reactive hepatitis, but the clinical significance of this finding is not known. However, true hepatitis in the elderly is deceptive, tending to look clinically like intrahepatic obstruction. This makes it advisable to delay surgery for several weeks to see if the "obstruction" passes. The delay is warranted, since in any event surgery infrequently uncovers a remediable lesion.

In the pancreas, two histologic changes are seen with age: squamous metaplasia in the ducts and wide variations in size of parenchymal cells and their nuclei. We may speculate that the variation somehow relates to loss of endocrine reserve and reduced glucose tolerance with age, but we do not really know.

Malignancy of the GI Tract

The correlation of malignancy with age is of course well known, and the problem is statistically enormous. Among the 1.9 million deaths from all causes in the U.S. in 1975, there were 371,660 deaths from malignant neoplasms, among which those of the digestive organs and peritoneum numbered 101,880. The figure was slightly higher than in 1974 (98,913). Among the different neoplasms, the incidence of cancer of the colon appears on the rise in the U.S., that of cancer of the stomach on the decline, but the reasons for this are not clear.

What approach should one take to performing surgery for cancer in the elderly? The rate of five-year survival after surgery for cancer seems to be little affected by the age factor. The Lahey Clinic reports a 41% rate for patients over 70, and 44% for those under 70. I interpret this to mean that surgery should not be denied simply because a person is old. Early detection, of course, gives the optimal chance of success.

Concerning colon cancer, I would point out that changes have been occurring with respect to predominant sites. Ten years ago, 70% of colonic cancers were within reach of the proctoscope, now only 40% are. To reach the cancer sites higher in the colon, the flexible colonoscope must be employed. A good history, focusing on any change in bowel habits, and stool tests for guaiac positivity are vital in routine examination of the elderly. If there is a change in bowel habits or if one of three consecutive stools is positive, barium studies and proctoscopy are indicated. Sigmoid cancers are potentially curable if detected early.

This incomplete survey of the geriatric GI tract may exemplify a few major problems of managing the aged patient and describes some of the hard and soft evidence for age-associated changes in morphology and function. One might well wish for a way of ensuring that the intricate collaboration of GI organs continue untroubled well into old age. Whatever our shortcomings, our understanding has come a long way since the the nineteenth century surgeon Sir Arbuthnot Lane expounded the theory that toxic substances produced by putrefactive bacteria in the colon were largely responsible for senescence. Searching for a "fountain of youth," he inaugurated a fad for extensive colectomies – with what mortality history does not inform us, but one may assume that the operation was undoubtedly effective in preventing old age in a significant number of his patients. Remaining in the dark about any intrinsic aging process or processes, we can, while we wait for science to light the way, adopt a strategy not of attacking but rather of assisting and coaxing the aged GI tract to perform appropriately.

11

Endocrines and Aging

PAUL J. DAVIS
State University of New York at Buffalo

The possibility that waning endocrine function contributes to or dictates human aging has enjoyed waves of popularity and springs from the misconception that the menopause is a prototype of endocrine aging. In fact, the inevitable senescence in middle age of the human female reproductive tract is drastic and exceptional rather than typical of changes with advancing age in other endocrine glands. This false model has led reputable and disreputable scientists, alike, of other eras to graft young animal glands into old men in vain attempts to retard or reverse the aging process. Except for the ovary, changes with age in endocrine axes tend to be subtle and often are detectable only by challenging the responsiveness of the endocrine organs or feedback loops. The response of endocrine target organs, such as the human adrenal and thyroid glands, to their trophic hormones – ACTH and TSH (thyroid-stimulating hormone; thyrotropin) – is intact in the aged, but setpoints of neuroendocrine control of pituitary function may be altered in the old, sometimes on a sex-specific basis, as in the case of the hypothalamic-pituitary-thyroid axis. Excluding the menopause, none of the clinical features we associate with the normal aging process can be attributed to primary alterations in endocrine gland function. Nonetheless, a variety of changes in endocrine gland physiology accompany aging and, rather than directing it, appear to be secondary to changes in peripheral hormone degradation or target sensitivity. It is these changes that are the subject of the initial portion of this discussion.

Pituitary-thyroid axis: The serum thyroxine (T_4) concentration changes negligibly with age, although small declines in serum content of thyroxine-binding globulin (TBG), the major serum transport protein for thyroid hormone, do occur. A number of reports describe a decline in serum triiodothyronine (T_3) concentration, which may occur as a function of normal aging, owing, perhaps, to altered peripheral (i.e., extrathyroidal) conversion of T_4 to T_3. In other clinical circumstances in which serum T_4 concentration is stable but serum T_3 content falls, eumetabolism is preserved, and there is no reason to assume that any clinical consequences accrue in the aged because of small declines in serum T_3.

In elderly men there is a decrease in pituitary gland responsiveness to thyrotropin-releasing hormone (TRH) – that is, TSH release by the pituitary in response to TRH may be depressed or negligible in normal elderly men. TRH responsiveness in women is unaffected by age. It is unclear what, if any, physiologic meaning should be attached to these observations. Clinically, however, its importance is clear as we come to rely on TRH-testing in certain patients to confirm diagnoses of pituitary or thyroid disorders. The results of TRH-testing may be misleading in elderly men. Depressed TRH responses *in younger patients of both sexes and in elderly women* are consistent with pituitary gland failure, with hyperthyroidism (because excess thyroid hormone inhibits TSH release), or with exogenous thyroid hormone administration. Depressed TRH responsiveness cannot be viewed as indicating any pathologic process *in old men*. If a normal response – acceptable TSH output after TRH administration – occurs in men of advanced age, then we can conclude that the pituitary-thyroid gland axis is intact.

Pituitary-adrenocortical axis: Blood glucocorticoid concentrations are similar in healthy old and young persons. Levels are maintained in old persons because decreases in cortisol degradation rates are accompanied by appropriate declines in cortisol secretion by the adrenal cortex. The adrenal cortex in elderly persons is normally responsive to ACTH in terms of cortisol output. In contrast to glucocorticoids, the level of aldosterone in blood is decreased with advanced age. In intact young subjects, aldosterone secretion is sensitive to factors such as renin production and blood potassium content rather than primarily dependent upon pituitary ACTH production. There is a diminution with age in the responsiveness of the renin-aldosterone system to changes in posture and variations in salt intake, but it is unknown whether this diminished responsiveness has significant physiologic consequences. The *capacity* of the pituitary to release ACTH in response to controlled stresses (such as as hypoglycemia) or to reduction by pharmacologic means (metyrapone) of plasma cortisol levels is intact.

Antidiuretic hormone (ADH): Because the ability to concentrate urine decreases with age in man, it had been thought that ADH secretion might fall in the course of normal aging. It has been shown recently, however, that secretion of ADH may in fact be exaggerated in aged subjects as the distal renal tubule becomes less responsive to the presence of this hormone. Thus, exaggerated increases in serum ADH content in response to dehydration may be seen in aged subjects, but these increases are *secondary* to age-related changes in the kidney and are not a primary alteration of ADH secretion.

Other hormonal systems: Although age-specific data for serum immunoreactive parathyroid hormone (iPTH) levels in man are incomplete, there is a suggestion that iPTH levels may decline in normal individuals as a function of advancing age. Absolute insulin output in response to a glucose challenge is reduced in nonobese elderly normal subjects, and insulin release is delayed. Statistically significant declines in serum testosterone content with advancing age in men have also been documented; the variation among individuals in any decade of life in terms of testosterone secretory rates is so wide, however, as to discourage consideration of the thesis that failing androgen production is a clinically significant event in men. The ability of the pituitary gland to secrete growth hormone (GH) in response to certain stimuli is reduced in aged individuals, but at present no clinical significance is assigned to this finding. Although beyond the scope of this discussion, changes in peripheral tissue receptor sites for hormones are thought to explain certain changes in hormone responsiveness that occur with normal aging in animal models and in human fat cells. Whether there are clinical overtones to such observations is unknown.

This overview of alterations in endocrine physiology as a function of age leads to several conclusions. First, a substantive, primary limitation on endocrine organ secretion as a function of age is characteristic of the ovary, but not of other endocrine tissues. Second, physiologic changes with age in several endocrine axes are secondary to alterations in the peripheral degradation of hormones or to decreased target organ responsiveness. Third, aging of endocrine axes in certain instances involves sluggishness of response of neuroendocrine loops, such as TRH responsiveness in elderly men or the decreased output of GH in response to induced hypoglycemia. These changes are heterogeneous, and their significance is unclear.

The foregoing has dealt with *physiologic* alterations in endocrine function with *normal* aging. However, many patients with *pathologic* endocrine function are age 60 or older; accordingly, the second part of this chapter is concerned with the recognition and management of endocrinopathies in the elderly.

Relevant Clinical Features

Hyperthyroidism: It is estimated that 20% of the hyperthyroid population is elderly, although recently collected data suggest that as many as one third of thyrotoxic patients are older than 60 years. About 75% of elderly hyperthyroid patients have classic symptoms and signs of thyroid hyperfunction and pose little diagnostic difficulty. Severe ophthalmopathy is very infrequent in this age group.

In the remaining 25% of elderly thyrotoxic patients, however, the diagnosis is elusive. In contrast to younger hyperthyroid patients, elderly individuals with hyperthyroidism may present without goiter (one third of patients). Thyrotoxicosis disguised by phlegmatic or apathetic facies or obscured by the concomitant presence of severe nonthyroidal illness (such as congestive heart failure, stroke syndrome, or infection) mandates a low threshold for recognition of quite isolated findings consistent with thyroid disease. Examples of such findings are unexplained heart failure or tachyarrhythmia, recent-onset psychiatric disorder, or profound myopathy. A triad of

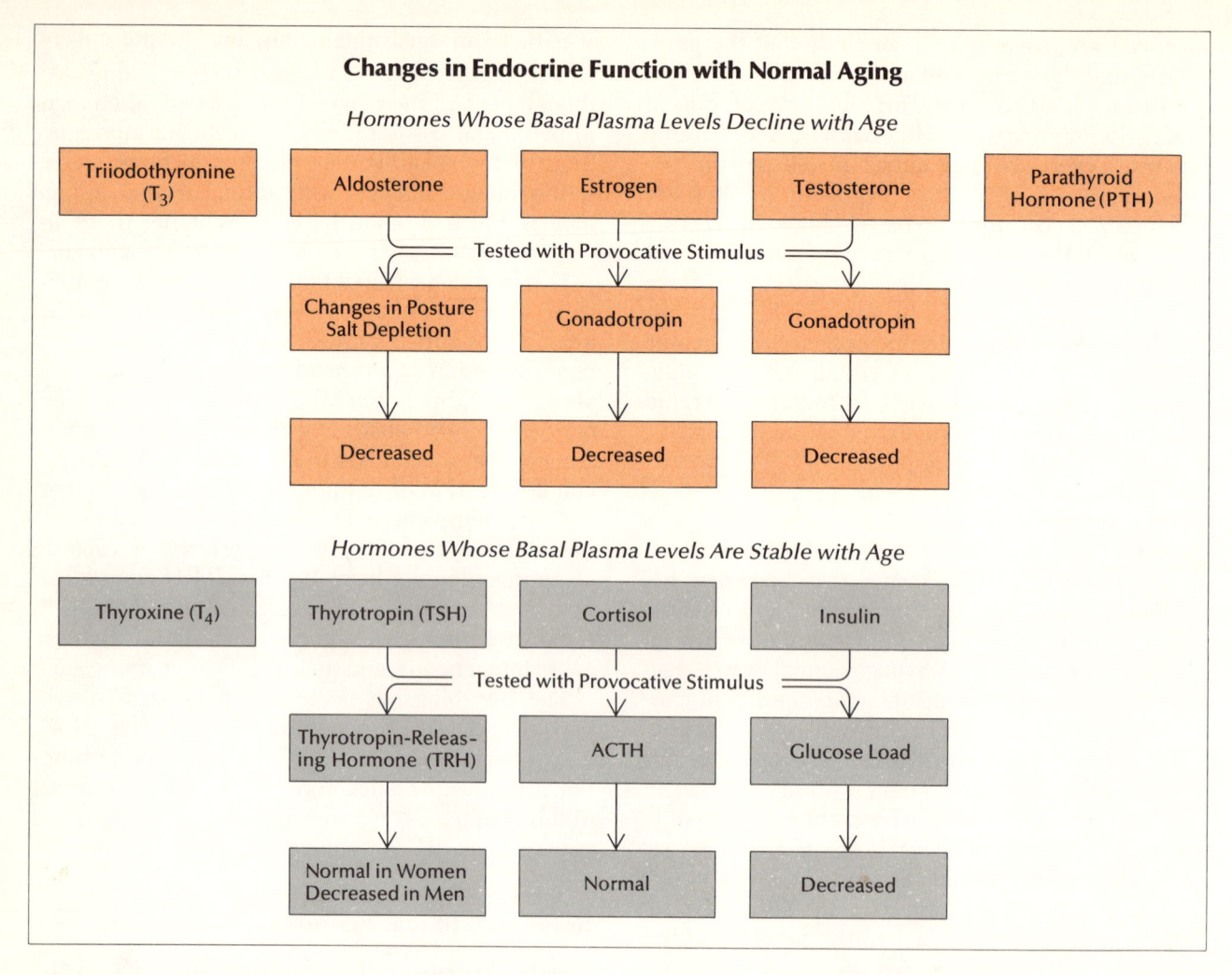

Changes in Endocrine Function with Normal Aging

Hormones Whose Basal Plasma Levels Decline with Age

Triiodothyronine (T$_3$)	Aldosterone	Estrogen	Testosterone	Parathyroid Hormone (PTH)

Tested with Provocative Stimulus

	Changes in Posture Salt Depletion	Gonadotropin	Gonadotropin	
	↓	↓	↓	
	Decreased	Decreased	Decreased	

Hormones Whose Basal Plasma Levels Are Stable with Age

Thyroxine (T$_4$)	Thyrotropin (TSH)	Cortisol	Insulin

Tested with Provocative Stimulus

	Thyrotropin-Releasing Hormone (TRH)	ACTH	Glucose Load
	↓	↓	↓
	Normal in Women Decreased in Men	Normal	Decreased

weight loss, anorexia, and constipation occurs in 15% of elderly thyrotoxic patients.

Of the two thirds of older thyrotoxic patients who do present with goiter, the incidences of diffuse gland enlargement and of nodular goiter are, in our experience, equal. There is a much higher incidence of atrial fibrillation in older hyperthyroid patients (35% vs approximately 5% in the younger patients). Ninety percent or more of young patients with atrial fibrillation revert spontaneously to normal sinus rhythm during antithyroid therapy, but only 50% of older hyperthyroid individuals with this arrhythmia convert spontaneously and maintain a sinus rhythm.

Laboratory findings in elderly thyrotoxic patients can be confounding. There is an appreciable incidence of normal serum T$_4$ concentrations in aged subjects who are shown to be thyrotoxic by two or more other independent laboratory parameters. The explanation for this is unclear, although some of the individuals with normal serum T$_4$ levels have been shown to have T$_3$ toxicosis. Measurements of serum free T$_4$ concentrations may be useful in confirming the presence of thyrotoxicosis when concomitant nonthyroidal illness is *absent*; the latter, of course, may result in misleading, usually modest, elevations of serum free T$_4$ levels in eumetabolic patients of any age. The vast majority of our own elderly hyperthyroid patient population have had diagnostically elevated thyroidal radioiodide uptakes. Attempts to confirm the autonomy of the thyroid gland in elderly subjects by use of suppression testing (i.e., determining the effect of thyroid hormone administration on thyroidal radioactive iodine uptake) is often troublesome; cardiovascular and other symptoms of thyroid disease may be exacerbated in already mildly hyperthyroid patients by the administration of exogenous T$_3$ as part of the suppression test. We have also occasionally induced thyrotoxic symptoms de novo in previously eumetabolic patients with autonomous thyroid nodules when we have carried out suppression testing with T_3 administration.

The treatment of choice for the mildly to moderately ill, elderly thyrotoxic patient is ablative radioiodide administration. I prefer to withhold treatment with ^{131}I until the patient is rendered euthyroid by thiourylene drugs (methimazole or propylthiouracil) or until symptoms of thyrotoxicosis are controlled with the cautious administration of propranolol. Certain older patients with hyperthyroidism may respond to as little as 40 to 80 mg total oral propranolol daily in divided doses (i.e., 10 to 20 mg *qid*), although the pharmacology of this drug would suggest that such low doses ought not to be effective. I recommend surgery for toxic goiter in this age group only when a large multinodular cervical or substernal thyroid gland is present, producing local, usually respiratory, symptoms.

Treatment of the severely thyrotoxic elderly patient is more problematic. The reason for this frequently is the concomitant presence of nonthyroidal disease that has its own morbidity and that may be exacerbated by thyrotoxicosis or by treatment of thyrotoxicosis. The management of congestive heart failure in the elderly hyperthyroid patient is not compromised by antithyroid agents such as thiourylene drugs and iodide, whereas the use of drugs such as propranolol or guanethidine to control thyrotoxicosis in individuals with mild heart failure can critically worsen the latter. However, if heart failure appears to be heart-rate related – that is, in those situations of hyperthyroidism in which the patient's heart rate is 140 beats per minute or higher – then *very* cautious titration of heart rate to the 100 to 120 beats per minute range may be attempted with small (0.5 mg) intravenous doses of propranolol. This measure is *rarely* indicated but can markedly improve heart failure when rapid heart rate due to thyrotoxicosis plays a substantive role in the genesis of failure. Conventional cardiotonic measures are, of course, indicated at the same time. In those instances in which heart rate is below 120 beats per minute and congestive heart failure is present, propranolol is *not* to be considered, and we rely on conventional diuretic and/or digitalis management of heart failure and handle thyrotoxicosis with oral or intravenous iodide administration and propylthiouracil or methimazole therapy orally. Parenteral reserpine may be employed in the "stormy" elderly hyperthyroid patient to control severe symptoms of thyroid disease without increasing the risk of heart failure; its unpredictable effects on the sensorium and blood pressure, however, drastically limit its usefulness in the elderly.

The dosages of methimazole, propylthiouracil, and iodide in older thyrotoxic patients are those prescribed in younger patients.

The preceding discussion has emphasized the effect of thyroid hyperfunction (and its treatment) on concomitant nonthyroidal illness. It is also well known that "stresses" of various types (nonthyroidal illness such as infection, surgery, and systemic drug reactions) may trigger a worsening of symptoms and signs of thyrotoxicosis, sometimes to a critical point ("thyroid storm"). Thus, in all thyrotoxic patients effective management includes attention to specific treatment of concomitant nonthyroidal illness and postponement of surgery until thyroid disease is adequately controlled.

Hypothyroidism: Primarily a disease of the fifth, sixth, and seventh decades of life, hypothyroidism has had its classic definition in the elderly age group. Younger patients with thyroidal hypothyroidism are not materially different in presentation from older subjects. Goitrous hypothyroidism occasionally occurs in younger patients whose thyroid failure reflects relatively recent Hashimoto's thyroiditis. Goiter is rarely found in elderly hypothyroid patients, unless hypothyroidism is iodide induced. The latter represents reversible thyroid hypofunction related to administration of agents such as saturated solution of potassium iodide for its "mucolytic" action in patients with chronic obstructive pulmonary disease. Very severe hypothyroidism – myxedema stupor and coma – is almost invariably limited to older hypothyroid patients.

The clinical recognition of hypothyroidism in elderly individuals is handicapped by the similarity of changes with normal aging in performance, attitude, and behavior to those that occur in hypothyroidism. Insidiousness of onset of hypothyroidism is a factor in patients' failure to appreciate that a process distinct from "getting older" is present.

The secure laboratory diagnosis of thyroidal hypothyroidism rests on the demonstration of an elevated serum TSH concentration. While the serum T_4 concentration is depressed in hypothyroid patients, it may also be low in both elderly and young patients with chronic, usually debilitating, nonthyroidal illnesses. Measurement of the serum T_3 concentration (T_3 radioimmunoassay) is not useful in the diagnosis of thyroid hypofunction. There is substantial overlap of the euthyroid and hypothyroid patient populations in terms of serum T_3 levels, just as there is in the case of serum free T_4 measurements. Basal thyroidal radioactive iodine uptake is now infrequently useful in confirming the presence of hypothyroidism, because the lower limit of the normal range for ^{131}I uptake is currently so low as to make impossible the distinctions between normal and pathologically low uptakes. Coupled with ^{131}I thyroidal uptake, the administration of exogenous (bovine) TSH can establish that there is no thyroid tissue to respond to thyrotropin with enhancement of radioiodide uptake ("TSH stimulation test").

We have already indicated that TRH testing is problematic in elderly men because of a depressed response that can occur in the eumetabolic state. Thus, use of the TRH test in elderly men, with subsequent failure to observe a significant rise in serum TSH concentration, could lead to the erroneous conclusion that pituitary hypothyroidism is present. In older eumetabolic women, on the other hand, TRH responsiveness is normal, and the test can be applied with the expectation that an exaggerated TSH response, consistent with the diagnosis of thyroid hypofunction, will be obtained in patients of any age with thyroidal hypothyroidism. Pituitary or hypothalamic hypothyroidism represents less than 5% of the hypothyroid patient population. Nonetheless, the possibility of pituitary or hypothalamic disease should be considered in any patient with thyroid hypofunction because of the therapeutic implications of pituitary failure: if thyroid hormone, alone, is administered as replacement to such patients, they may experience acute hypoadrenocorticism.

Elevations of serum concentrations of muscle-source enzymes such as creatine phosphokinase (CPK) are consistent with hypothyroidism as well as with acute myocardial infarction and skeletal muscle trauma. Persistence of CPK elevation until the administration of replacement thyroid hormone or measurement of serum CPK isoenzymes helps to distinguish hypothyroidism from CPK increases due to myocardial damage. Much or all of the serum CPK rise in hypothyroidism is of skeletal muscle origin (MB isoenzyme).

Although a good deal of attention has been paid recently to what constitutes full replacement thyroid hormone dosage, age-specific requirements for thyroid hormone have been studied only with regard to the pediatric population. In younger patients with hypothyroidism, full thyroid hormone replacement (0.15 to 0.20 mg L-thyroxine orally per day) can usually be instituted at the time of diagnosis without fear of cardiovascular consequences. In elderly hypothyroid patients such an approach carries risks because of the likely concomitant presence of arteriosclerotic heart disease, independent of thyroid disease. A starting dose in elderly thyroidally hypothyroid patients of 0.025 mg L-T$_4$ daily is instituted, and 0.025 mg is added to the dose every one to three weeks, until full replacement dosage of 0.10 to 0.15 mg daily is achieved. The end point is signaled by reduction of serum TSH levels into the normal range or by satisfactory remission of symptoms and signs of hypothyroidism. Sometimes the end point is the supervention of angina pectoris in the course of replacement therapy; 0.0125 mg increments in L-T$_4$ dosage, instituted at three- to four-week intervals, may permit gradual achievement of euthyroidism. Occasionally, we encounter patients whose angina limits any dosage increase and in whom the combination of propranolol and thyroid hormone is unsuccessful in permitting us to treat fully the hypothyroid state. Arrhythmias and worsened heart failure may also cause us to maintain patients on subreplacement amounts of T$_4$.

In the patient whose sensorium is impaired by hypothyroidism and in whom the latter has led to body temperature below 95° F, the administration of large quantities of thyroid hormone intravenously is justified as a lifesaving measure. The total body pool of thyroid hormone is replaced rapidly with 250 to 500 µg of L-T$_4$ administered IV, and a second comparable dose is given 12 to 24 hours later if substantial improvement in sensorium has not resulted. The value of corticosteroid administration simultaneously with thyroid hormone replacement is not clearly established, but use of steroids is certainly justified in those patients with hypotension or hyponatremia. As in the severely hyperthyroid patient, concomitant nonthyroidal illnesses – such as infection – may compromise outcome in the hypothyroid patient and must be treated specifically and early.

Thyroid nodules and cancer: Benign thyroid nodularity is a concomitant of apparently normal aging, and postmortem studies suggest that thyroid micronodularity is almost universal in patients older than 80 years. It is not clear that micronodule formation relates to the incidence of thyroid carcinoma in the elderly. Mortality from thyroid carcinoma increases with age, regardless of the histologic type of thyroid tumor. Even relatively benign-appearing, well-differentiated papillary carcinomas of the thyroid produce an importantly increased mortality in patients over 40. Nearly half of anaplastic thyroid carcinomas, which have the poorest prognosis of any thyroid neoplasia, occur in the older age groups.

It is not clear that surgical excision of thyroid carcinoma in the elderly has an effect on survival that is materially different from that of suppression of endogenous TSH with the administration of exogenous T_4. While many of us acknowledge this, we nonetheless recommend surgical excision of those thyroid nodules we believe to carry a high risk of containing thyroid carcinoma. It is possible with reasonable security to differentiate high risk and negligible risk of thyroid nodules in the elderly patients. Almost invariably benign are soft or spongy nodules that have been stable in size for some years or decrease in size on suppression therapy, are not "cold" on radionuclide scanning, and occur in the context of positive family history of goiter or in conjunction with elevated serum antibody titers to thyroid antigens.

Hyperparathyroidism: Nearly one third of patients with primary hyperparathyroidism are older than 60 years. Diagnosis of this disease in patients with equivocal serum calcium values has been facilitated in recent years by availability of assays of serum immunoreactive parathyroid hormone (iPTH). Many patients with borderline calcium elevations and inappropriately high iPTH values remain free for years of bone disease, urinary tract calculi, abdominal complaints, and myopathy. The symptoms and signs of hyperparathyroidism in the old and young are similar, but the diagnosis may be overlooked in the elderly because we accept demineralizing bone disease, asthenia, or joint complaints as concomitants of normal aging. The younger patient who is minimally hypercalcemic and asymptomatic is usually subjected to neck exploration for management of parathyroid adenoma or hyperplasia or both. In the elderly, the presence of minimal hypercalcemia in an asymptomatic individual with high iPTH levels does not mandate surgery. In these individuals, anesthetic and surgical risks and the concomitant presence of nonparathyroid disease (such as heart failure or pulmonary disease) represent greater threats than hyperparathyroidism. The development of significant hypercalcemia (>11.5 mg/dl) may force neck exploration if chronic medical management of hypercalcemia with oral phosphate or subcutaneous calcitonin is impractical or ineffective. Obviously, we should avoid the use of thiazide diuretics in such patients (e.g., for management of coincidental heart failure), since these agents may cause further elevation of serum calcium levels. The calciuretic effect of furosemide makes the latter an appropriate diuretic in these patients. While it is reasonable to recommend regular measurement of bone density by noninvasive techniques (such as photon absorptiometry)

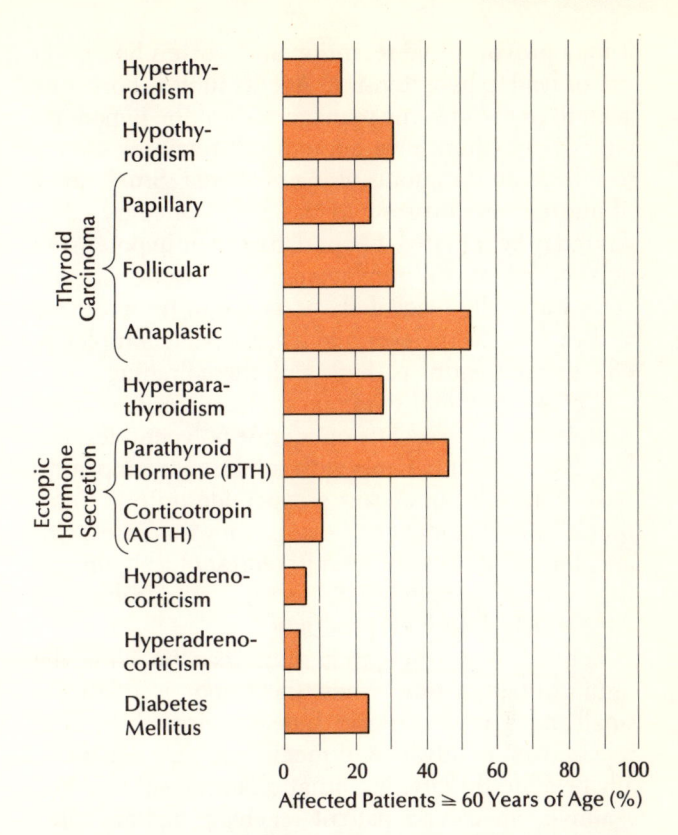

Substantial numbers of patients with endocrinopathies are aged 60 or above, though aging as such does not produce primary alterations in most endocrine glands.

in the asymptomatic elderly hyperparathyroid patient, it is not as yet clear what represents a pathologic rate of bone mineral loss in patients who are in the seventh or eighth decades of life. When normative data for such measurements are available, the decision regarding neck exploration in asymptomatic elderly hyperparathyroid patients may be made easier.

Adrenocortical diseases: The incidence of adrenal hyper- and hypofunction in the elderly is low, and the clinical features of both illnesses are not materially different in young and old affected patients. The hypovolemia and postural hypotension of hypoadrenocorticism do not prejudice survival in the young as they do in the elderly who have cerebrovascular or cardiac disease. Replacement glucocorticoid therapy is similar in old and young patients with Addison's disease. Overly liberal parenteral saline administration in elderly Addisonian patients may be complicated by the development of an overexpanded plasma volume and attendant problems. Similarly, the routine use of fluorohydrocortisone in elderly hypoadrenocortical patients is not recommended, since it may provoke fluid retention and worsen heart failure or lead to hypertension. Agents such as cortisone acetate in the chronic management of the hypoadrenal patient often have enough salt-retaining effects to relieve all symptoms of hypovolemia. Small doses of fluorohydrocortisone (0.05 mg/day or every other day) may be initiated if hyponatremia or hypotension persists when full replacement cortisone acetate (12.5 mg orally twice daily or 25 mg in the morning and 12.5 mg in the evening) has not been completely effective in treating patients with these findings.

Ectopic humoral syndromes: The majority of solid tumors appear to secrete endocrine polypeptides, but less than 10% of patients with solid tumors appear to have clinically significant polypeptide output. Inasmuch as the incidence of malignancy increases with age, older patients are seen to represent a significant fraction of patients with ectopic syndromes of ACTH, ADH, or PTH production.

Ectopic hormone production may be clinically significant at a time when the tumor is relatively small and is not metastatic. Indeed, ectopic hormone release well in advance of metastases may occasionally be a life-threatening situation in the elderly. For example, an elderly patient receiving digitalis who becomes hypokalemic as a result of ectopic ACTH production may develop digitalis toxicity and succumb before the tumoral source of ACTH and the hypokalemia is appreciated. Whether hypercalcemia of ectopic hormone origin potentiates digitalis intoxication, as do acute infusions of calcium, is not clear.

Diabetes mellitus: It is now apparent that criteria for distinguishing normal and abnormal glucose tolerance must be age-adjusted. In general, nonobese elderly persons show a decreased ability to release insulin following exposure to a glucose load. Insulin release is delayed, and the absolute quantity of insulin secreted in response to glucose challenge is reduced in apparently normal older subjects. More of the material released as "insulin" in the elderly may be inactive (e.g., proinsulin). Standards of glucose tolerance based on performance of young subjects may thus define many older persons as "diabetic" when their responses may be unremarkable for their age.

Even when age-adjusted criteria are used, however, it is clear that there is an appreciable incidence of diabetes in the older age group. It is widely recognized that the elderly diabetic appears particularly susceptible to hyperglycemic nonketotic stupor or coma and infrequently presents with ketoacidosis or diabetic lactic acidosis. An exception to the latter statement is, of course, the maturity-onset diabetic whose disease has been managed in part with phenformin. Approval by the Food and Drug Administration for phenformin distribution was recently withdrawn because of its tendency to provoke lactic acidosis in patients, usually the elderly, who are not prone to ketosis.

It is not known whether the risks of classic complications, such as retinopathy, renal disease, and neuropathy, differ in old and young diabetics. The classic complications of diabetes usually do not appear for at least a decade or more after onset of diabetes in younger patients, and obviously long-term follow-up data are harder to obtain in patients aged 65 at the time of diagnosis of diabetes. Elderly patients with mild diabetes mellitus do seem to be peculiarly susceptible to diabetic neuropathies involving the autonomic nervous system and large peripheral nerve trunks. Autonomic neuropathies include abnormalities of the cardiovascular system (postural hypotension and inappropriate heart rate changes in response to posture) and urinary bladder dysfunction. Disorders occurring with increased frequency in elderly diabetics, such as diabetic amyotrophy or "diabetic neuropathic cachexia," may represent large peripheral nerve trunk pathology (mononeuritis monoplex or multiplex). Amyotrophy is a usually asymmetric syndrome of hip muscle mass atrophy, weakness, and disabling pain. A practical aid in deciding which patients have abnormal glucose tolerance is shown in the illustration on this page. This is an age-adjusted nomogram of glucose tolerance constructed by Reubin Andres and his colleagues at the National Institute on Aging. One should also note that the values in the figure represent two-hour postprandial values, and that fasting blood sugar levels do not change as a consequence of normal aging. My policy is to treat asymptomatic diabetic patients with insulin when the fasting blood sugar value is greater than 200 mg/dl with the objective of maintaining fasting concentrations between 150 and 200 mg/dl. Symptomatic patients who usually have values above 300 mg/dl are always treated.

Results of the University Group Diabetes Program (UGDP) have influenced the philosophy and practice of diabetic management in several ways. The study is discussed here because its impact on oral sulfonylurea therapy affects primarily the maturity-onset diabetic population. First, the study indicated that oral sulfonylurea therapy fails to postpone the development of complications of diabetes mellitus in patients with mild-to-moderate carbohydrate intolerance. The original purpose of the study was in fact to deal with this particular issue of the effect of drug therapy on diabetic complications. The UGDP study also indicated that a group of patients treated with variable insulin dosage, with resultant rather good control of blood sugar, developed complications at a rate similar to that of the placebo-treated and sulfonylurea-treated groups. While these observations may foster a nihilistic approach to blood sugar control, insofar as prevention of diabetic retinopathy or nephropathy is concerned, data from other studies, usually involving animal models, have caused the American Diabetes Association to endorse renewed efforts by physicians to improve control of blood sugar in their diabetic patients in the hope of postponing complications.

Second, the UGDP study showed that while the incidence of cardiovascular "events" (myocardial infarction, stroke) was similar in placebo-treated, sulfonylurea- and insulin-managed patients, the risk of cataclysmic cardiovascular death was increased in the sulfonylurea cohort. This finding appears valid despite the dissimilar prevalence of certain cardiovascular risk factors in the treatment groups. It is this finding that stirred the greatest controversy, and led to the discontinuation by many physicians of oral agents in the management of many maturity-onset diabetics. The *return* of many elderly patients to insulin, as a consequence of the discontinuation of oral sulfonylurea therapy, has disclosed the existence of a small group who are at risk for substantive insulin allergy because of immunization with animal-source insulin prior to the oral agent era. In those affected, an anamnestic reaction occurs when insulin is restarted after a hiatus of many years, taking the form of serious cutaneous allergy or, rarely, anaphylaxis. The possibility that such reactions may occur in patients returned to insulin therapy after a course of oral agents should be kept in mind, although fortunately their incidence is quite small.

We encourage all of our diabetic patients to maintain themselves on insulin, and insulin therapy is mandatory in our patients under age 50 years. In older subjects, insulin use is strongly encouraged, but oral sulfonylureas are permitted where sociomedical circumstances discourage insulin use. Such circumstances include impaired vision or isolated living conditions that restrict patient travel. Carbohydrate restriction and weight control are of course recommended.

Iatrogenic endocrine disease: In the preceding sections I have already referred to several clinical situations in which the physician fosters endocrinopathy

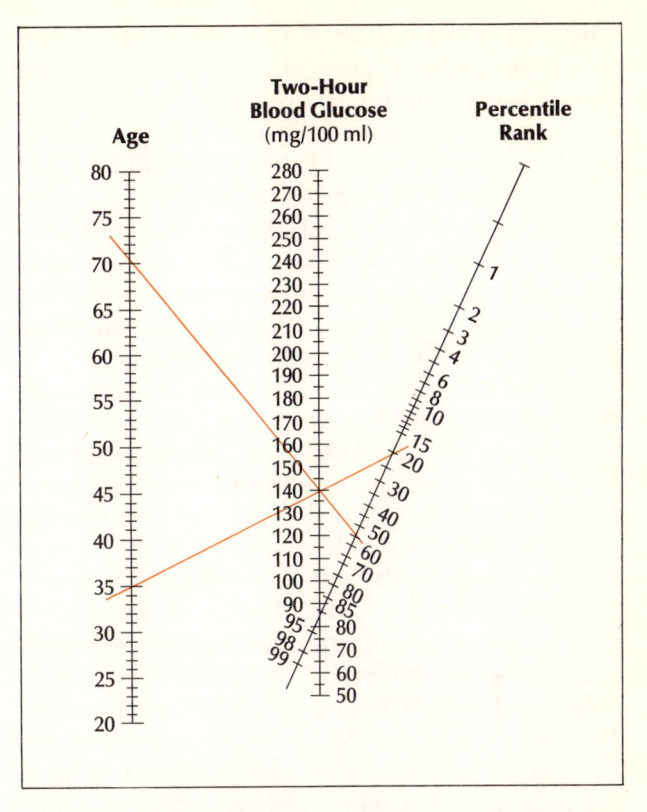

Nomogram for evaluating oral glucose-tolerance test (dose 1.75 gm/kg body weight) was developed by Andres et al. It is utilized by ruling line from age scale through test result and continuing it to percentile scale. At age 70 a subject with glucose concentration of 140 is about average; at age 35 same concentration ranks individual in 20th percentile, so 80% of age peers outperform him.

(e.g., the development of symptoms of thyrotoxicosis during T_3 suppression therapy and the unmasking of insulin allergy). Certain other iatrogenic endocrine problems particularly important in the elderly group include:

1) Induction of florid hyperglycemia with the use of thiazide diuretics or furosemide. While hardly restricted to the aged population, the use of diuretics is certainly more frequent in this group than in younger individuals. Profound hyperglycemia may be induced in the absence of antecedent abnormal glucose tolerance. In our experience, ethacrynic acid use has not eventuated in worsened carbohydrate tolerance and has been effectively substituted for furosemide or thiazides in patients who require diuretic therapy and have previously manifested hyperglycemia on thiazide. Directly, or via induction of potassium depletion, the thiazide diuretic effect on carbohydrate tolerance involves impairment of en-

dogenous insulin release by islet cells. Thus, the patient whose diabetes is being treated with 30 or more units of exogenous insulin a day will not have hyperglycemia provoked by thiazide use.

2) Induction of reversible hypoaldosteronism and hyperkalemia with heparin administration. This reaction is probably less likely to occur in a context of currently recommended low-dose heparin regimens. Occasionally, heparin or coumadin use may provoke hyperkalemia secondary to bilateral adrenal gland hemorrhage and acute hypoadrenocorticism.

3) Hyponatremia following chlorpropamide administration. This adverse effect is seen almost exclusively in elderly patients for several reasons. First, and most obvious, the agent is rarely used in younger diabetic patients. Second, hyponatremia during chlorpropamide therapy is particularly likely to occur in those individuals with previously established congestive heart failure or in those in whom oral diuretic treatment may also impair free water clearance.

Sex hormone production in the elderly: Estrogen depletion in elderly women and its management are discussed by Dr. Gerald Glowacki in Chapter 13. Changes in androgen production with aging have also been discussed above, and I indicated there are large variations in the androgen secretory capacity of individuals of any age. While there is statistical evidence to suggest in large series of individuals that androgen production declines as a function of age, longitudinal data are lacking to describe what happens to testosterone secretion in the same individuals over several decades. This statistical decrease with age in testosterone secretion cannot be viewed as a basis for espousing routine androgen replacement in elderly men. The loss of sexual potency that is coincident with advancing years is so complex a process that it is unjustified to attribute it primarily to decreased androgen production.

I will conclude this review by reiterating several themes: 1) The capacity of endocrine glands to secrete hormone is, with the exception of the ovary, generally intact throughout the life span; 2) there are changes that occur with normal aging in the responsiveness of neuroendocrine control circuits, particularly those involving the pituitary-thyroid axis, the pituitary-adrenal axis, and growth hormone secretion. The pathologic consequences, if any, of these changes remain obscure. Clinically, our treatment of older patients should be directed to the avoidance of iatrogenic endocrine disease and to the avoidance of treatment of physiologic changes expected with age, such as the fall in serum testosterone levels. We should, at the same time, lower our threshold for the diagnosis of endocrine disease in the elderly, since the presentations of such disease processes in this age group may be subtly or frankly altered by the presence of severe nonendocrine illness.

12

Bone and Joint Diseases

A. LEWIS KOLODNY *and* ANDREW R. KLIPPER
Franklin Square Hospital

By retirement age, 80% of the population has some rheumatic complaint; in fact, rheumatic diseases are so prevalent at this time of life they seem almost pathognomonic of human aging. The problem for the primary physician may then become one of sensing when symptoms are a signal for thorough investigation. The arithmetic of rheumatic disorders is that treatment is required in four of every 10 elderly persons. Moreover, arthritis in the elderly comprises many diseases including rheumatoid arthritis, degenerative joint diseases (osteoarthritis), gout, connective tissue diseases, polymyalgia rheumatica, osteoporosis, and others. The symptoms and signs of all may often overlap. Nevertheless, it must be understood that every ache and pain does not herald rheumatic disease.

In our experience as consulting rheumatologists, patients frequently are referred even though the primary physician had obtained all the information necessary for a correct diagnosis and could in fact have provided definitive treatment. In other patients, an incorrect diagnosis had been made because of incomplete workup, with the result that treatment was unavailing. Sometimes the result was that the patient had become depressed and desperate, resorting to – or ready to resort to – quack remedies.

Medicine is still a long way from comprehending the etiologic basis of the rheumatic diseases, although there have been notable "breakthroughs" with respect to therapy. But, by and large, physicians are still confounded as much by spontaneous remissions as by exacerbations. Even though specific cures do not exist for the "rheumatism" of old age, much can be done to make the patient comfortable and to minimize functional loss. The physician can relieve pain (in itself an enormous contribution to the quality of life), provide means to sustain if not improve the mobility of joints, suggest aids for the ordinary activities of daily living, and serve as a sympathetic protagonist of reality in helping the patient cope emotionally as well as physically with the disease. There is almost always something the physician can offer – even if it is nothing more than recommending inexpensive tools to help with buttons, zippers, eating, and grooming.

The rheumatic diseases cover so broad a front in medicine that it is often said to know them is to know almost all of internal medicine. For a relatively brief and practical look at this panorama, we recommend study of the *Primer on the Rheumatic Diseases,* prepared by a committee of the American Rheumatism Association and distributed to the profession by The Arthritis Foundation.

As it makes clear very quickly, the diagnosis of a rheumatic disease may require the piecing together of many signs and symptoms – in themselves often nonspecific – into a pattern that indicates pathology. Time often plays a part in revealing the diagnosis. In our own practice, to avoid the pitfall of premature labeling, we do not hesitate to describe a case nonspecifically, e.g., as "polyarthritis, symmetrical, additive, acute," while a meticulous examination is undertaken to see if the particular type of polyarthritis can be identified. Thus: Is this a small, benign fingertip lesion or the beginning of vasculitis? Is that elbow nodule rheumatoid? Possibly it, or a nodule along the ear, arm, finger, or toe actually represents tophaceous gout. Loss of the vermilion border of the lips and tightness of skin on face and hands may indicate scleroderma. Burning pain or tingling in the hands and difficulty in abducting the thumb may indicate carpal tunnel syndrome. In polyarteritis nodosa, finger pain often suggests rheumatoid arthritis. However, careful palpation reveals tenderness to be along the shaft of the finger between the joints. The location of tenderness coincides with the nerve and vessel bundles involved in the vasculitic process.

Pattern analysis will assist in differentiating the type of rheumatic disease present in the particular patient. This should cover such questions as whether the disease is or is not symmetrical, whether it affects small or large joints, whether the affected joints are proximal or distal, whether onset was gradual or violent. Such analysis may suggest rheumatoid arthritis if it is symmetrical (involvement of the proximal interphalangeal joints on one side is mirrored by similar if not identical involvement on the other). Or it will point to a form of psoriatic arthritis if it is asymmetrical (distal interphalangeal joints, proximal interphalangeal joints, and nails are involved on one hand only). Other small joints of the hand may also be involved. Although in many respects management of the two disorders is similar, use of antimalarial drugs for psoriatic arthritis could produce a lethal exfoliative dermatitis.

There are times when the problem in an elderly patient is not to determine which rheumatic disease is present but whether the signs and symptoms actually signify something else, such as an underlying malignancy. In a man who had "rheumatoid arthritis," the symptoms were found related to prostatic cancer. Polymyositis, with or without rash, may accompany malignancy of the lung. Pulmonary hypertrophic osteoarthropathy, which mimics osteoarthritis, may indicate malignancy of the lung or gastrointestinal tract. Systemic lupus erythematosus (SLE) can produce infiltrates that resemble pleural effusions produced by bacterial infection; nodules in the hilum of the lung may resemble lymphoma; and nodules of rheumatoid arthritis in the conducting system can cause heart block.

Osteoarthritis

Despite its name, osteoarthritis is not an inflammatory disease, but a degenerative one. More than a

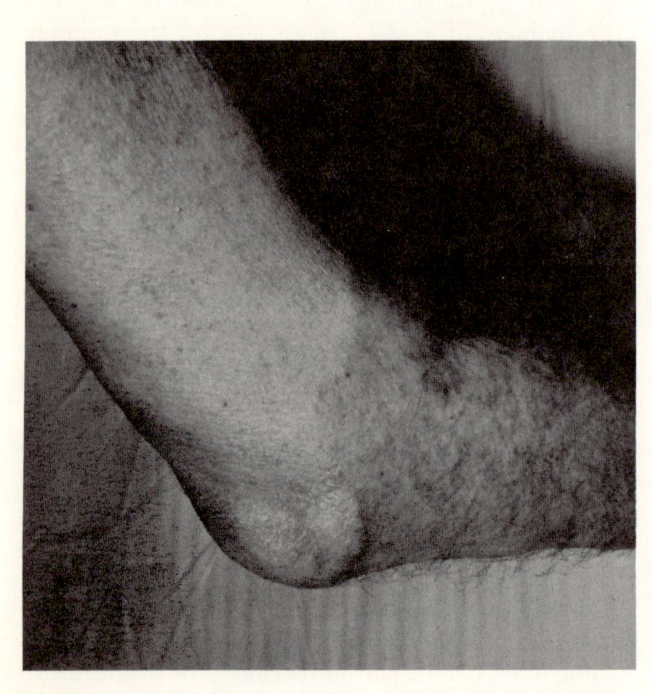

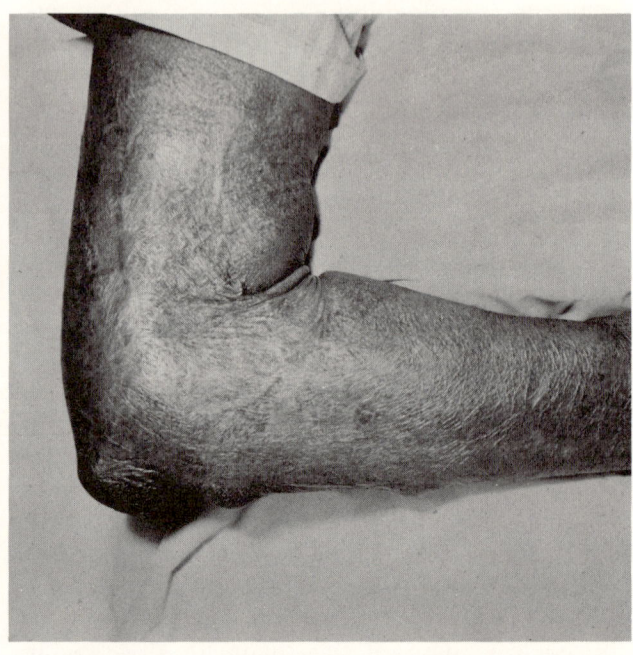

Diagnosis of rheumatic diseases is sometimes difficult because one condition resembles another. For example, tophus elbow (left) of gout patient appears to display the nodules of rheumatoid arthritis (right).

third of the population past middle age has this disease, but in a majority it is asymptomatic. All patients over 60 have roentgenographic or physical evidence of osteoarthritis, but symptoms occur in only 25% of women and 15% of men. Clinical strategy in this disease is directed at alleviating and at arresting or even reversing functional losses. Patients need to be reminded that osteoarthritis does not produce the widespread symptoms of rheumatoid arthritis. The disorder may involve the central and peripheral diarthrodial joints, producing Heberden's nodes of the distal interphalangeal joints and, less commonly, Bouchard's nodes of the proximal interphalangeal joints, the carpometacarpal joint of the thumb, and the major weight-bearing joints – hips, knees, cervical, thoracic, and lumbar.

The disorder may occur alone or be secondary to rheumatoid diseases, trauma, congenital defects, diabetes, and other conditions. Hence, it is important for proper management to determine whether the patient has primary or secondary degenerative disease. Primary osteoarthritis can be differentiated from rheumatoid arthritis by history of onset and symptoms, as mentioned above, and at times roentgenographically. For example, degenerative disease involves one compartment of the knee at a time. Usually, with rheumatoid disease, all three compartments are involved simultaneously. Synovial fluid will show no inflammatory features, though debris from degenerative cartilage may be present and account for a low-grade synovitis.

A treatment program should be directed at normalizing weight and decreasing stress on weight-bearing joints. Conservative management would employ rest, physical medicine modalities, and analgesic anti-inflammatory agents for relief of pain. Local arthrocentesis and injection of corticosteroids may be helpful (but not systemic use of corticosteroids).

Some patients may require surgery. The orthopedic measures comprise such varied interventions as laminectomy, spinal fusion, hip, knee, and small-joint replacements, and arthrodesis. If the patient is reasonably well, age per se is no contraindication to surgery. Our experience with total hip and knee replacements and hand reconstruction has been good. More recently, experimental prostheses for shoulder, wrist, elbow, and ankle have been developed.

Rheumatoid Arthritis

Turning now directly to rheumatoid arthritis, to which the larger part of this chapter will be devoted, we would point out that at least half of the 3.6 million Americans who have this disease are in the older age groups (50 and above). The course in the elderly differs from that in younger patients, often progressing relentlessly despite all measures to counter inflammation. The explanation may be related in part to the diminished immunocompetence seen with aging. The classic rheumatoid patient is easily recognized, but if a patient presents with ambiguous, minor signs and symptoms, the rule is to watch and wait. Aches and pains may indicate a cold, viral syndrome, mononucleosis, or vaccine reaction. However, if symptoms have persisted for six weeks, such transient entities are ruled out.

The American Rheumatism Association has systematized the criteria for diagnosis of rheumatoid arthritis. Eleven observational elements are given, in-

---

Drugs for Osteoarthritis

Nonanti-inflammatory analgesics
 Propoxyphene hydrochloride 32-65 mg *q4h*
 Propoxyphene napsylate 100 mg *qid*
 Acetaminophen 500-1,000 mg *qid*
 Ethoheptazine citrate 75 mg *qid*
 Pentazocine hydrochloride 25-50 mg *qid*

Skeletal muscle relaxant analgesics (*often given in combination*)
 Carisoprodol 250-300 mg *qid*
 Methocarbamol 6 gm/day may be given in four divided doses, with dosage as small as 2 gm/day
 Chlorphenesin carbamate 400 mg *qid*
 Orphenadrine citrate 200 mg/day in divided doses
 Metaxalone 800 mg *qid*
 Chlorozoxazone 250-750 mg *qid*

Anti-inflammatory analgesics
 Salicylates (aspirin) 325-1,300 mg *qid*
 Salicylates (choline salicylate) 5-10 cc *qid*
 Phenylbutazone 100 mg *qid* (short-term therapy only)
 Indomethacin 100-200 mg/day
 Ibuprofen 400-600 mg *qid*

Other anti-inflammatory agents listed for treatment of rheumatoid arthritis are still only experimentally used

Corticosteroids – these are not acceptable for systemic use in osteoarthritis; intra-articular steroids may be used cautiously

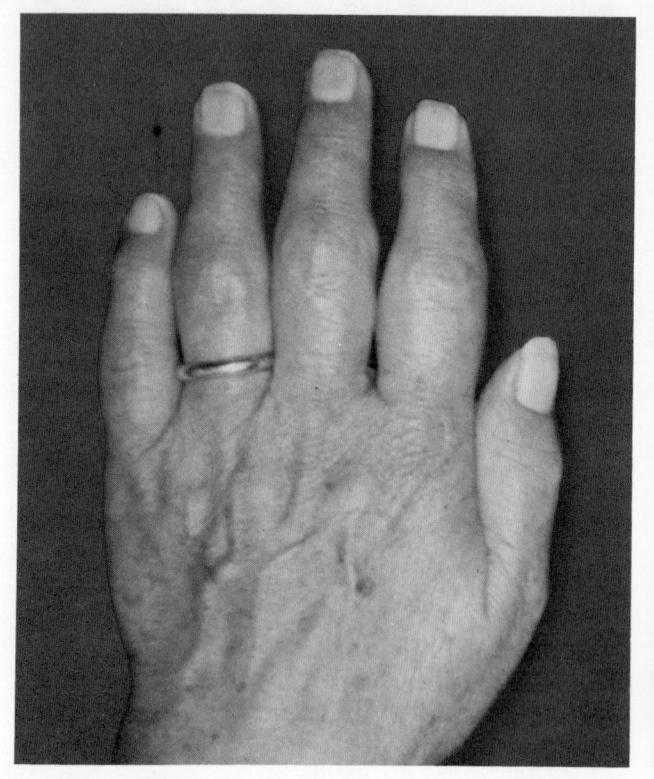

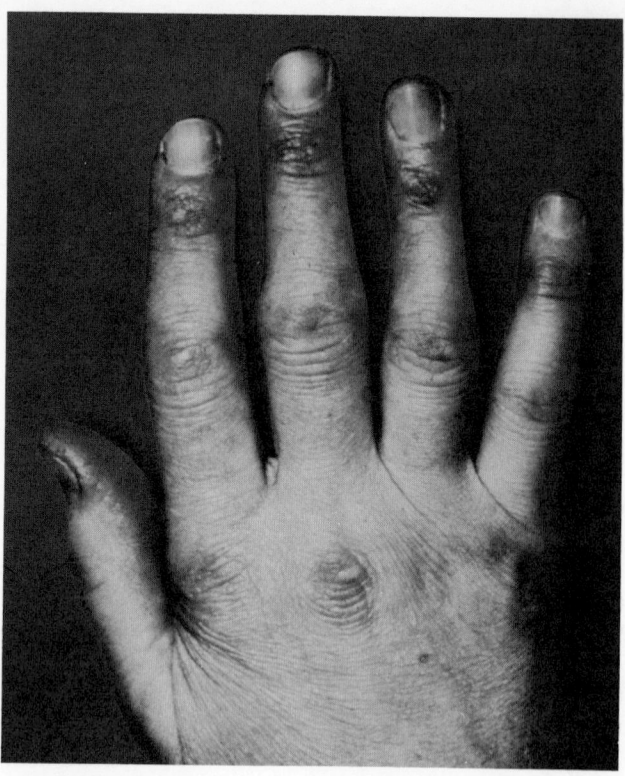

Hand of patient with osteoarthritis (left) displays Heberden's and Bouchard's nodes, produced by hypertrophic spurs. There is a resemblance to swelling seen in hand of a patient with rheumatoid arthritis (right).

cluding morning stiffness, pain on motion or tenderness as observed in at least one joint, swelling in one or more joints, and symmetrical joint swelling. If these elements have been present continuously for six weeks or more, they are considered indicative of the disease. Other criteria include subcutaneous nodules, roentgenographic changes, a positive test for rheumatoid factor, poor mucin clot from synovial fluid, and histologic changes in synovium and in nodules (demonstrating granulomatous foci). The presence of seven of these 11 findings warrants the diagnosis of the classic disease; of five, that of definite disease; and of three, that of probable disease. There is a list of 20 conditions, the presence of any one of which excludes the diagnosis of primary rheumatoid arthritis. This highly varied list, which points up the need for meticulous examination, includes the typical rash of systemic lupus erythematosus, histologic evidence of polyarteritis nodosa, persistent muscle swelling or weakness of dermatomyositis, definite scleroderma, tophi, and histologic evidence of joint tuberculosis.

Since rheumatoid arthritis tends to be bilaterally symmetrical and polyarticular, the finding of only one affected joint raises suspicion of prior trauma to that joint, infectious arthritis, gout, or pseudogout. If a single large joint, such as the knee, is inflamed, the possibility of infection must be excluded by examination of synovial fluid. If monoarticular disease persists, synovial biopsy may be necessary to rule rheumatoid arthritis in or out. In such a questionable case, further close observation over a prolonged period of time is required to establish diagnosis. Synovial fluid examination, culture, and biopsy may eliminate some diagnostic possibilities, such as mycobacterial arthritis, while leaving the door open to others. A search should be made for crystals of monosodium urate monohydrate, which would indicate gout, and for calcium pyrophosphate dihydrate, which would indicate pseudogout. A low complement level in synovial fluid, the presence of rheumatoid factor (RF) in the fluid, and of RA cells tend to confirm the diagnosis of rheumatoid arthritis. Low viscosity, poor mucin clot, low glucose, a polymorphonuclear leukocyte count >50,000/cu mm point at septic arthritis. One in five or six patients with rheumatoid disease may experience complete remission, suggesting caution in interpreting the claims for therapeutic effectiveness of any drugs or nostrums. If the symptoms persist, recur, or worsen in the course of a year or more, the chances of complete remission diminish. The appearance of subcutaneous nodules at the extensor aspect of the elbow in the patient with chronic disease is virtually pathognomonic, provided the nodules are differentiated from tophi. Eventually the nodules appear in 25% of RA patients. Where the diagnosis is in doubt, nodular biopsy may demonstrate a characteristic histologic pattern.

Rheumatoid arthritis and osteoarthritis also can be confused, especially when the (rheumatoid) arthritis occurs atypically in only one or two joints, and when osteoarthritis or gout is polyarticular. The pain of osteoarthritis differs from that of rheumatoid arthritis; in the former, stiffness is brief, is relieved by activity, and recurs upon rest, while in the latter, morning stiffness is prolonged. With advanced arthritis, pain in the weight-bearing joints can be disabling.

The treatment of uncomplicated rheumatoid arthritis in the elderly, as suggested earlier, is often best handled by the primary or family physician. The same holds true for uncomplicated osteoporosis and osteoarthritis. Generally, these conditions represent problems in managment of pain and emotional and environmental factors that condition the perception of pain or obstruct the patient's mobility. These factors are far more readily apparent to the primary physician who has known the patient for years than to the specialist. Heat, exercise, rest, gait training, splinting, corrective shoes, and other supports form the basis of managing rheumatoid arthritis, along with chemotherapy for pain and inflammation.

However, if the primary physician is unsure of the diagnosis or finds intractable pain, systemic manifestations indicative of any connective tissue disease (such as SLE, dermatomyositis, and vasculitis), and nonimprovement or worsening of the disease, referral or consultation is appropriate with a rheumatologist, orthopedist, or other specialist. The orthopedist is especially helpful in considering the need to reconstruct a joint that has become unstable or intractably painful, despite medical management.

Any primary physican undertaking chemotherapy for arthritides must know the drugs intimately and feel comfortably in employing them. As with drug therapy of hypertension, there is a drug "pyramid" for rheumatoid arthritis. At the base of the pyramid is aspirin. If efforts with aspirin to control pain and permit mobilization of joints fail, other drugs are added to to the regimen. Aspirin must be given at relatively high doses, with attention to hemorrhage, ulcer, and other potentially adverse gastrointestinal effects. Aspirin is most effective when given in doses sufficient to achieve serum values of 20-30 mg/100 ml. Serum values need to be monitored because salicylate absorption may be erratic, especially in the enteric-coated form. Most clinical laboratories perform serum salicylate determinations; if the laboratory capacity is not locally available, therapeutic dosage is established by finding the ototoxic dose and reducing it to the point where tinnitus disappears. If aspirin is not tolerated, choline salicylate may be substituted.

Alternatives to salicylates are indomethacin at 100 to 200 mg daily. Indomethacin must be watched for gastric irritation. A new group of nonsteroidal anti-inflammatory agents, such as ibuprofen, tolmetin, naproxen, and fenoprofen have analgesic properties useful in rheumatoid arthritis patients who develop gastrointestinal intolerance to aspirin. However, these agents carry their own risk of this adverse reaction. Ibuprofen should be given at 400 to 600 mg *qid* for adequate effect. Tolmetin is given at 1,200 to 2,000 mg daily, naproxen at 500 to 750 mg daily, and the dose of fenoprofen is 2,400 to 3,200 mg daily.

If these drugs are ineffective in controlling morning stiffness and pain, antimalarial drugs such as hydroxychloroquine may be added to the basic regimen with aspirin because they have moderate anti-inflammatory effects. For hydroxychloroquine, 200 mg is given daily at bedtime. It may take a month or two before the therapeutic effect is appreciable. Because of potential adverse effects on the eye, the patient

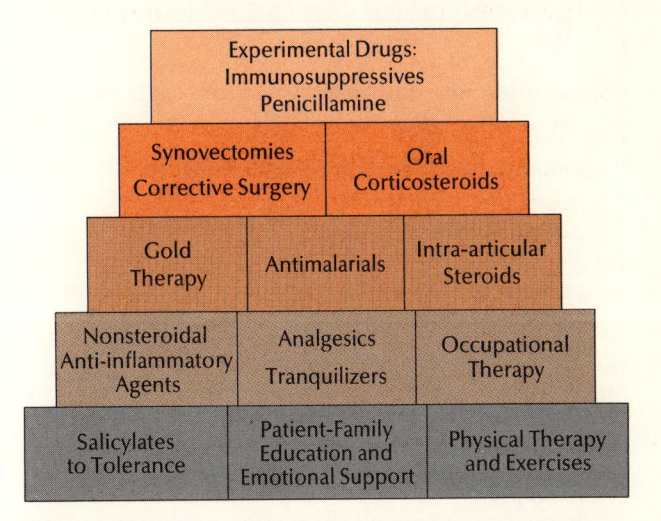

Drug "pyramid" for treatment of rheumatoid arthritis has aspirin at base. If base modalities are inadequate, the next level is tried, and so on to the top, where extreme caution in drug use is essential.

> **Drugs for Rheumatoid Arthritis**
>
> **Nonanti-inflammatory analgesics** (*only of limited value*)
>   Propoxyphene hydrochloride 32-65 mg *q4h*
>   Propoxyphene napsylate 100 mg *qid*
>   Acetaminophen 500-1,000 mg *qid*
>   Ethoheptazine citrate 75 mg *qid*
>   Pentazocine hydrochloride 25-50 mg *qid*
>
> **Anti-inflammatory analgesics**
>   Salicylates (aspirin) 975-1,300 mg *qid*
>   Salicylates (choline salicylate) 10 cc *qid* sufficient to have blood salicylate level of 25-30 mg/100 ml)
>   Phenylbutazone 100 mg *qid* (short-term therapy only)
>   Indomethacin 100-200 mg/day
>   Ibuprofen 400-600 mg *qid*
>   Tolmetin 1,200-2,000 mg/day in three or four divided doses
>   Naproxen 500-750 mg/day in two divided doses
>   Fenoprofen 2,400-3,200 mg/day in four divided doses
>
> **Gold salts**
>   Gold sodium thiomalate 10 mg/week IM starting dose; second week 25 mg; thereafter, 50 mg/week until 1,000 mg given; maintenance dose of 50 mg thereafter
>   Aurothioglucose – dose same as above
>
> **Antimalarial**
>   Hydroxychloroquine sulfate 200 mg/day in one dose
>
> **Corticosteroids** – dosage individualized cautiously according to indication
>
> **Immunosuppressives and penicillamine** – these agents should only be used experimentally by experienced investigators

should be examined by an ophthalmologist before chloroquine therapy is begun and then be seen at least quarterly. If drug deposits in the eye are noted, the drug should be withdrawn; usually the deposits will disappear and there will be no effect on vision.

Chrysotherapy is an alternative to antimalarials. Gold salts, preferably gold sodium thiomalate, may produce remission in some patients after several months or a year. However, chrysotherapy is relatively costly, requires periodic IM injections indefinitely, and has major side effects. Leukopenia or severe proteinuria are absolute contraindications to continuing or restarting gold therapy. Albumin or blood in urine, skin rash, or oral ulcers warrant suspending chrysotherapy but then restarting it when these conditions clear, utilizing small doses and raising them by small increments to test tolerance.

The next level of the drug pyramid is occupied by the corticosteroids. Their potency and toxicity require that they be used carefully in the lowest possible doses. At 5 to 7.5 mg daily for the short term, prednisone may tide over patients with intense rheumatoid arthritis until other drugs, such as antimalarials or gold, have a chance to take effect. Steroids can mask or reduce inflammation but probably do not stop progression of the RA. Some patients get into trouble because the steroids produce a sense of well-being, virtually eliminating morning stiffness. They take excessive amounts and thus risk hyperadrenal side effects and osteoporosis. They should be warned against taking the drugs without physician approval.

At the apex of the pyramid are two groups of drugs that have no place in primary care: immunosuppressants and penicillamine. These should be reserved for patients in whom the disease is uncontrolled and life-threatening. Especially in the elderly, in whom immune processes appear to be less effective than in younger people, these agents may aggravate susceptibility to infection and malignancy.

Acute flareups of rheumatoid arthritis may be benefited by phenylbutazone 100 mg *qid*. If not effective in a week, phenylbutazone should be withdrawn because of the risk of hematologic side effects.

Concerning pain, we would point out that its perception is influenced by the patient's personal level of anxiety, by attitudes toward suffering instilled at an early age, and by his or her past experience with pain. Some patients tend to magnify and some to minimize or ignore pain. Living alone or with a friend or relative and conscious of physical and economic vulnerability, many elderly persons perceive as a calamity the actual or impending loss of function from rheumatoid arthritis. The family physician, with extended knowledge of the patient's life, often is in the best spot to help the patient maintain self-respect and confidence. We find it critically important to allay fears with a sympathetic attitude and, if necessary, judicious prescription of psychotropic drugs. By eliciting and responding to questions about treatment and prognosis and by taking the patient's wishes into consideration in choosing alternative

BONE AND JOINT DISEASES

modalities of care, the psychologic trauma of the disease – and the patient's pain – often can be modified.

The patient's hopes must not be raised unduly. We emphasize that seven in 10 patients can be significantly helped by timely care of various kinds of polyarthritis. At least some degree of benefit is achieved by an additional patient or two. The possibility of remissions is explained to the patient. We try to make clear our objective of restoring joint function to the level the patient had before symptoms began, helping the patient protect himself against risk of falls and other trauma, and finding ways of compensating for functional loss. We review the patient's daily activities to see what potentially dangerous situations can be eliminated and what activities can be facilitated.

Perhaps nothing buoys up the patient better than providing him with practical aids to activities of daily living. For the patient with deformed hands and limb limitations, there are inexpensively made or bought implements for combing hair, turning water taps, holding playing cards, pulling zippers and buttoning, putting on trousers, and manipulating keys for doors and automobile ignitions. Such devices or plans for making them are available from a nonprofit volunteer organization, The Independence Factory, P.O. Box 597, Middletown, Ohio 45042.

Counseling of the family is important. The household may need to be rearranged to promote the patient's ability to do things for himself. Provision may be necessary in a working family for outsiders to come in during the day, to do something for or with the patient – such as preparing a meal or just to talk. Where the patient wants to continue at paid or volunteer employment, the physician may need to make suggestions to his or her work associates. The primary physician may also need to organize and coordinate the services of other professionals, such as physiatrists, orthopedists, physiotherapists, nurses, social workers, and occupational therapists. In short, the patient with rheumatoid disease often needs more than purely medical help.

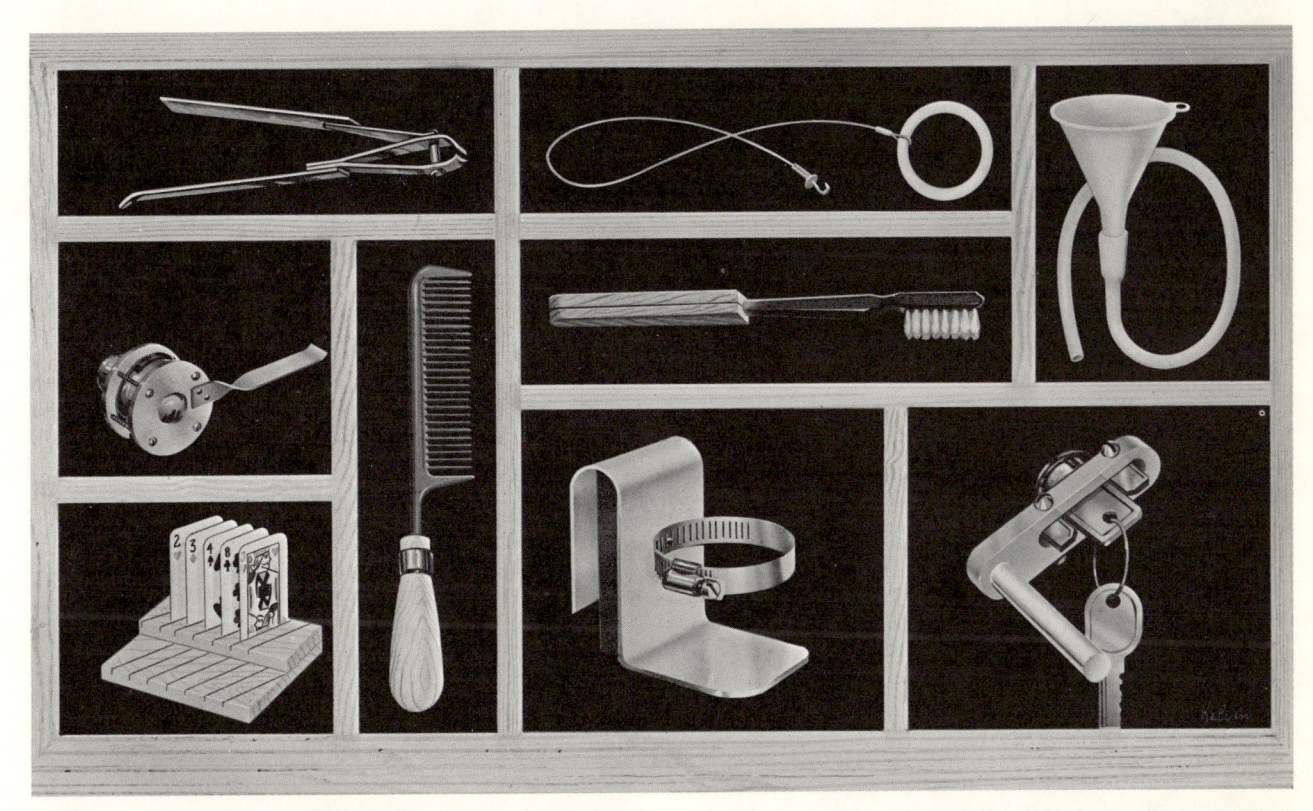

Some practical aids for the arthritis patient (illustrated above) include, in the left segment, nail clippers with metal strips welded on, lever on doorknob, playing-card holder, and rattail comb with file handle. Middle segment shows a zipper pull, enlarged-handle toothbrush, and drink holder for wheelchair. At right are a funnel and tube for urination, and a lever device to slip over auto-ignition switch. Such aids can be made at home or obtained from the Independence Factory, Middletown, Ohio. Factory will also provide plans.

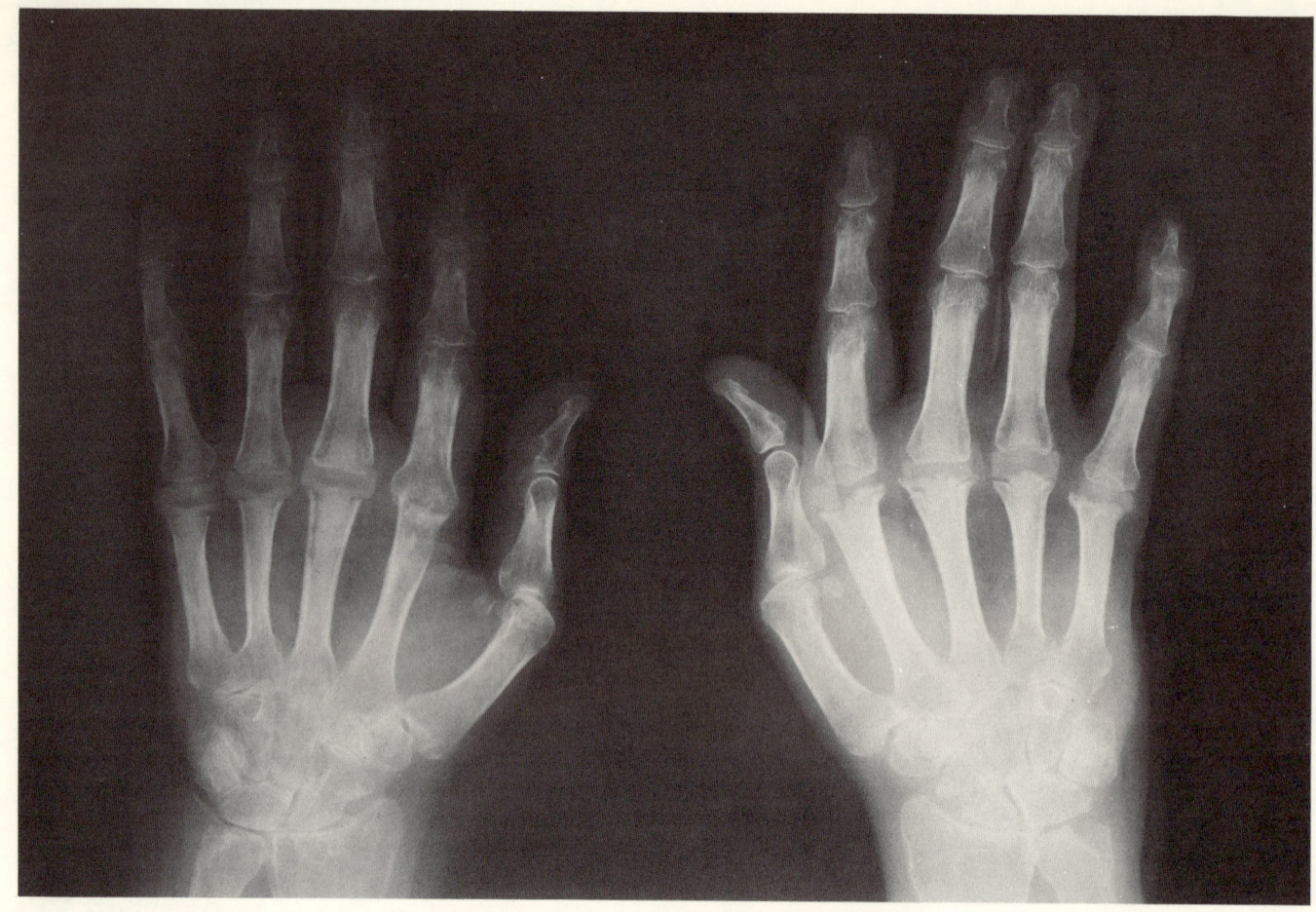

Hands of 45-year-old female RA patient reveal prostheses at metacarpophalangeal (MCP) joints. Severe osteoporosis can be seen in proximal interphalangeal (PIP) joints and MCPs. Carpal bones are also involved.

Osteoporosis

Osteoporosis increases in incidence from the fifth decade onward, is more prominent in women, and is thought to result from the postmenopausal imbalance between the anabolic sex hormones and the glucocorticosteroids that catabolize collagen. The effects are most marked in the spine, pelvis, sternum, and ribs. Vertebral collapse may cause patients to lose several inches in height and display marked kyphosis. Such collapse may occur spontaneously as well as from trauma. Intertrochanteric fractures may occur in the osteoporotic hip with slight trauma or none at all. If the patient then experiences a fall, the true cause of the fracture may become impossible to determine. When signs of osteoporosis appear on the x-ray film (bone structure appears to be lighter and the vertebral margins have greater density than the shaft), then at least 50% of bone mass is lost.

Particularly significant in diagnosis and management is the fact that pain from collapsed thoracic and lumbar vertebrae may radiate to the chest. The neuritic intercostal pain may resemble coronary pain superficially, but there is no sweating or radiation to the neck, shoulder, and to one or both arms. The pain of thoracic vertebral collapse may resemble that of hiatal hernia, but it is aggravated by activity.

The basic approach is to alleviate the pain with analgesics and to safeguard the patient against falls and other trauma by providing braces and other supports and by safeguarding the home environment in consultation with the family. Treatment aimed at strengthening bone is available, but its efficacy is by no means assured. Such therapy stresses the use of estrogen or testosterone as anabolic agents, together with supplementary calcium and vitamin D to facilitate its absorption. Some clinicians add fluoride to the diet with the goal of hardening bone, but this is

BONE AND JOINT DISEASES

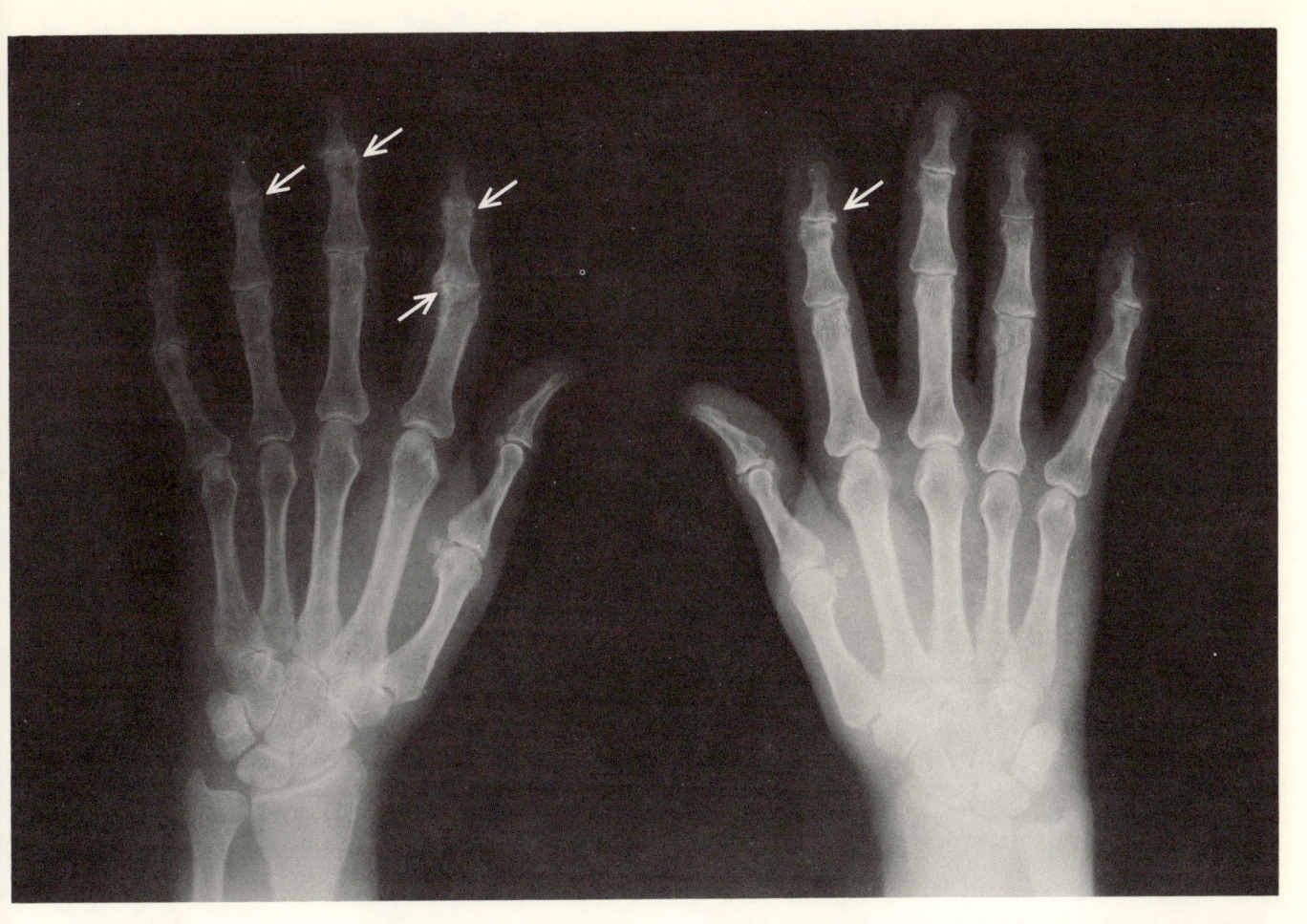

Osteoarthritis in 59-year-old female is seen on x-ray. Arrows indicate Heberden's and Bouchard's nodes and marginal erosions of the PIP joints, but MCP joints have been spared and there is no osteoporosis.

an experimental maneuver, and many months or years may need to elapse before one can detect improvement roentgenographically. In general, one evaluates the success of clinical maneuvers by symptomatic relief rather than by objective findings.

If the weakened bones fracture, orthopedic measures are undertaken. Hip replacements and prostheses are increasingly used in the elderly instead of pinning, provided the patient's physical condition permits the more complex operative procedure. The first sign of hip fracture – pain and decreased range of motion – may be mistaken for rheumatoid arthritis, osteoarthritis, or bursitis of the hip. In any elderly person who has had even a minor hip injury, complaint of hip pain should prompt immediate x-ray. The method of repairing a fracture should be left to the judgment of the orthopedist. It may be preferable to choose a lesser procedure if the goal is to mobilize the patient as promptly as possible, which is an important consideration in the elderly. In general, because of the risks of pneumonia, thrombophlebitis, muscle atrophy, and of the secondary osteoporosis in a joint left idle too long, it is preferable to avoid keeping the patient in a cast or in traction for extended periods of time.

Polymyalgia Rheumatica

A most important nonarticular rheumatic disorder of the older groups, polymyalgia rheumatica affects mostly middle-aged or older females. It is a disorder often misdiagnosed. Its presentation is frequently acute, with shoulder girdle or pectoralis pain and proximal muscle pain of the lower extremity, with considerable stiffness. Polymyalgia rheumatica is often mistaken for osteoarthritis, fibrositis, or psychogenic pain. Until recently, muscle pathology was never demonstrated by either biopsy or electromyog-

Rheumatic Diseases of the Elderly

Disease	Age	Sex Ratio	Clinical Features
Rheumatoid Arthritis	20-60 years, peaks at 35 and 45 years	2.5F:1M	Polyarthritis plus systemic manifestations
Osteoarthritis	After 55-64 years, 85% of persons involved	F greater after 55 years M greater under 45 years	Noninflammatory polyarthritis No systemic manifestations
Gout	Peak age onset, fifth decade	1F:20M F after menopause	Monoarticular or polyarticular, extra-articular manifestations: renal tophi
Chondrocalcinosis	36-92 years	1F:1.4M	Monoarticular or polyarticular, accompanying diseases such as hyperparathyroidism, hemochromatosis, gout, osteoarthritis
Systemic Lupus Erythematosus	20-60 years, peaks at 35 and 40 years	2.5F:1M	Systemic manifestations plus polyarthritis
Progressive Systemic Sclerosis	Increases third to fifth decade	1.5F:1M	Systemic manifestations plus polyarthritis
Polymyositis and Dermatomyositis	Peaks 45-64 years, fifth-sixth decades highest	2F:1M	Systemic manifestations plus polyarthritis; occult malignancy may be present
Polyarteritis Nodosa	20-50 years up to eighth decade	1F:3M	Systemic manifestations plus polyarthritis
Polymyalgia Rheumatica	Over 50 years, most over 65 years	1F:1M	Nonarticular systemic manifestations
Osteoporosis	Increases with age after 50 years	Greater in females, same after 70 years	Generalized bone involvement; no arthritis

raphy studies. However, recently, Dr. M. Brook and Dr. H. Kaplan demonstrated, with special histochemical staining, abnormalities of type 1 muscle fibers and atrophy of type 2 muscle fibers. Other laboratory tests are not significant with the exception of elevated erythrocyte sedimentation rates (ESR) ranging from 50 to 100 mm per hour. Nonspecific hypochromic anemia and α-2-globulin elevation may be noted.

Because giant cell arteritis may accompany this disease, early diagnosis is most important to prevent sudden blindness. The carotid artery and its branches, particularly the temporal artery, can be involved so that tenderness or pulsation over the temporal artery should be investigated. Such symptoms as temporal headache, diplopia, blurring of vision, and abnormal visual fields may also signify temporal arteritis. Temporal artery biopsy is confirmatory. In differentiating for polymyalgia rheumatica, one must take into account a disease described by Takayasu. It involves vasculitis of a number of large arteries including the common carotid, subclavian, innominate, and ilials. The disease, sometimes called aortic arch syndrome, pulseless disease, or giant cell arteritis of the aorta, is usually found in women under fifty. The ESR is greatly elevated. Differentiation from polymyalgia rheumatica is facilitated by leukocytosis, sometimes with eosinophilia, and elevated IgG, IgA, and IgM levels. In addition rheumatoid factor, antinuclear antibodies, and lupus erythematosus cells may be found.

Ordinarily, we treat polymyalgia rheumatica with 40 to 50 mg of prednisone daily, gradually reducing the dose as the ESR decreases. If there is any evidence of temporal arteritis, the dosage of prednisone is again increased. Maintenance of 5 to 7.5 mg of prednisone may be necessary for two or more years.

Gout and Pseudogout

Although the incidence of primary gout peaks in the 40s and 50s, postmenopausal women may develop it. Nevertheless, primary gout is much less common in older people than secondary gout associated with renal disease. Although recurrent acute gout episodes eventuate in tophaceous gout in only a minority of cases, early recognition is important to prevent the damage of chronic gout.

Acute gout may be confused with chondrocalcinosis, which may occur in a pseudogout pattern as well as pseudorheumatoid arthritis, pseudo-osteoarthritis, or asymptomatic groups. Indeed a pseudoneurotrophic joint pattern has been described.

Diagnosis of gout is dependent, not just on simple hyperuricemia but upon the discovery of urate crystals in synovial fluid, synovia, or tophi. Similarly, diagnosis of pseudogout requires finding calcium pyrophosphate crystals in either synovial fluid or synovia. Examination of synovial fluid under polarized light differentiates urate crystals from pyrophosphate crystals.

Classically, acute gout may involve the great toe, ankle, knee, wrist, hip, and elbow. Pseudogout more commonly starts with acute arthritis involving larger joints such as the knees, but all other joints may be involved. X-rays of involved joints during early stages reveal no bony abnormality. Characteristic changes occur during the tophaceous stage of gout and the chronic stage of pseudogout.

Management of acute gouty attacks is multifaceted. If synovial effusion occurs, arthrocentesis with removal of fluid and injection of corticosteroid affords effective relief. Oral colchicine therapy affords excellent relief if 0.6 mg is given every half hour until nausea, vomiting, or diarrhea supervenes. However, we prefer – when possible – to administer phenylbutazone, 200 mg every four hours for four doses, to be followed by 100 mg *qid*. Pseudogout acute synovitis may sometimes respond to colchicine, but in a less predictable manner. The use of phenylbutazone, joint aspiration, corticosteroids, and salicylates may also offer relief.

In our practice we use uricosuric agents in gouty patients demonstrating underexcretion of urates, using the following criteria for initiating therapy: 1) hyperuricemia persistently over 10 mg/100 ml, accompanied by frequent acute attacks of gout; 2) the presence of tophi in skin or bone; 3) evidence of renal damage.

A xanthine oxidase blocking agent, allopurinol, is also frequently employed in the presence of the following indications: 1) hyperuricemia brought about by overproduction of uric acid; 2) urolithiasis and/or renal pathology severe enough to interfere with the action of uricosuric agents; 3) failure to respond or sensitivity to uricosuric agents.

Our choices of uricosuric drugs include probenecid, given orally from 0.5 to 3.0 gm daily, or sulfinpyrazone in an oral dose of 400 mg daily. Concomitant use of salicylates will reverse the uricosuric effect of these drugs. Allopurinol is given orally in a dose of 100 to 300 mg daily. Aspirin does not interfere with its pharmacologic action. Colchicine should be prescribed with all of these drugs in a dosage of 0.6 mg once or twice daily. Diet restriction is also advised in the form of avoidance of foods high in purines, such as sweetbreads, liver, kidney, brain, anchovies, and rich gravies.

In summing up, we would stress that clinical strategy begins with alertness to any reports of joint pain. The primary physician, often possessing an extensive patient and family history, may be able to interpret the pain and in many cases rule out major disease. When the diagnostic picture is clouded, meticulous examination – a review of body systems – may furnish missing elements of a pattern of evidence implicating rheumatic disease. When the diagnosis remains doubtful, the condition worsens, or the pain is intractable, consultation is advisable. Systematization of rheumatoid arthritis with suggestion of vasculitis such as fever, vasculitic rash, neuropathy, and eye complications also warrants immediate consultation. Generally, the primary physican can manage the uncomplicated disorder. The patient's need for emotional support to face chronic disease may be best met by the sympathetic primary physician – all of which is to emphasize that the care of the geriatric patient with bone and joint disease belongs, as much as possible, within a familiar professional orbit.

13

Postmenopausal Gyn Problems

GERALD GLOWACKI
Johns Hopkins University

The presenting complaint of the postmenopausal, geriatric woman is rarely the vasomotor or psychologic symptoms of the menopause as such but rather some problems related to osteoporosis, neoplasia, or atrophy of the generative tract. Perhaps a decade has passed since her ovaries stopped producing estrogens, and her body has been adjusting to an estrogen-deficient environment. Calcium has been dissipating from the bony matrix, setting the stage for compression fractures of the spine and "wear-and-tear" osteoarthritis. There has been a loss of tone in skin and mucosa. She may at one time have been placed on estrogen replacement therapy to counter her menopausal symptoms, but it is highly probable that, as these waned, and studies began to be published indicating a higher risk of endometrial cancer in patients receiving such therapy, she has been taken off this regime.

My concern in this chapter will be with the specific gynecologic problems encountered in the aging or aged woman and the therapy that can be offered to her, including an assessment of the role of estrogens in her management. The broader subject of the management of the menopause itself is best left to another discussion, though some overlap is inevitable – as in the first aspect to be discussed: the history.

The physician seeing either the perimenopausal or the postmenopausal woman for the first time needs to obtain as accurate a historical record of her reproductive career as possible, beginning with maturation and including menstruation, childbearing, changes during the climacteric and menopause, and concluding with her current gynecologic complaints. Often, pelvic abnormalities may be explained by high parity, or by unattended, midwife-attended, or difficult childbirth. A history of markedly irregular menstrual periods suggests a premenopausal imbalance in secretion of estrogen and progesterone; some investigators have correlated such a history with a significant increase in risk of endometrial and breast cancer, though it has not been conclusively shown whether this higher risk continues past the reproductive period. Age at onset of menopause is relevant: late onset (past 50 years) has been associated statistically with a higher incidence of endometrial carcinoma. Since the prolonged influence of estrogen on the uterus may indeed be an etiologic factor in some individuals, it is necessary to ascertain whether any hormonal therapy was used during the climacteric, and if possible what it was.

In reviewing gynecologic symptomatology, a line of questioning that parallels that of a normal pelvic examination should be followed. One begins with vulvar symptomatology, proceeding then to vaginal, cervical, uterine, tubal, ovarian, and general pelvic symptomatology. Any investigation of vulvar or vaginal problems also calls for evaluation of the urinary system. Let us follow the same sequence in this review. In the pelvic examination itself, the emphasis is on the discovery of any generative tract prolapse or growths or both.

POSTMENOPAUSAL GYN PROBLEMS

Vulva

With the decrease in endogenous hormonal support, the patient becomes susceptible to inflammatory and traumatic disorders in this area; at the same time, if urinary incontinence is present, the vulvar environment is constantly moist, a situation that favors skin maceration and infection.

Candidiasis is probably the most common inflammatory process and may in fact suggest a basis for the diagnosis of diabetes, which has a high correlation with monilial infection. If diabetes is confirmed as an underlying etiologic factor, proper diabetic management can often reduce the tendency of candida infections to recur. The inflammation itself can usually be eliminated by the use of either nystatin vaginal tablets twice a day for two weeks or a miconazole nitrate cream nightly for the same period. Application of a 0.01% cortisone cream, either with or without supplemental nystatin, will usually provide immediate relief to the affected vulvar area.

Vulvar inflammation caused by trichomonal vaginitis is treatable with povidone-iodine vaginal gel twice daily for two weeks. Metronidazole is more effective but is being studied for possible oncogenic activity. In chronic vulvar dermatitis with pruritus, systemic antibiotics may be necessary to reduce the hazard of infection secondary to scratching. If possible the etiologic agent should be identified. Unless a viral infection is responsible, an acute flare-up usually is amenable to 0.1% cortisone cream. For refractory cases, local applications of estrogens, or androgens, or both, may be helpful. If pruritus persists, local alcohol injection or denervating surgery may be indicated to help resolve this very difficult problem.

In general, prompt biopsy for unexplained vulvar lesions is advisable, because vulvar carcinoma has a peak incidence in the geriatric years. No time should be lost in investigating lesions that are unresponsive to therapy, appear ulcerative, or otherwise look sus-

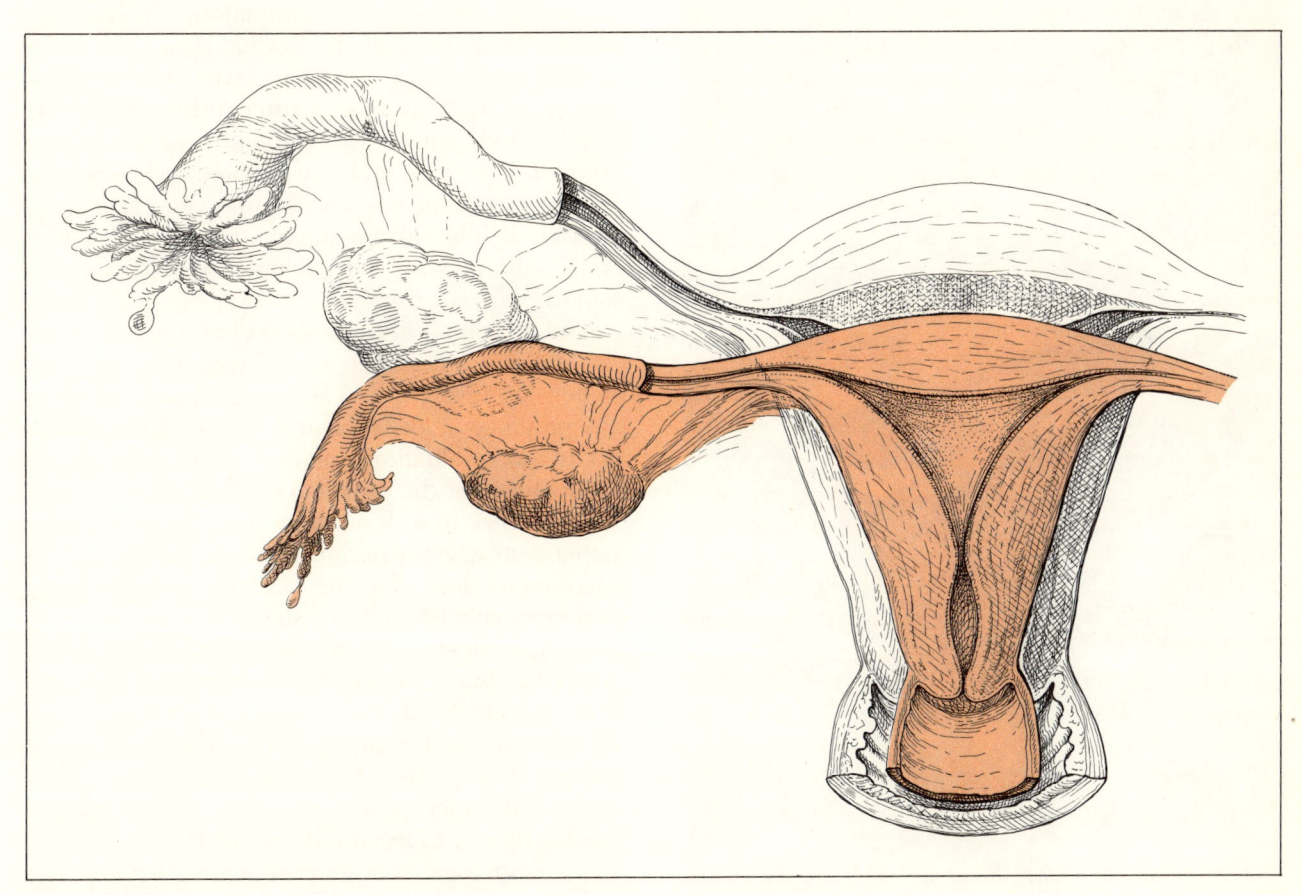

Atrophied postmenopausal generative tract is superimposed on premenopausal tract. Shrinkage of cervix makes endocervical lesions hard to detect. Any enlargement of uterus or ovaries requires investigation. Even such vague symptoms as persistent abdominal bloating or pelvic pain may be associated with ovarian Ca.

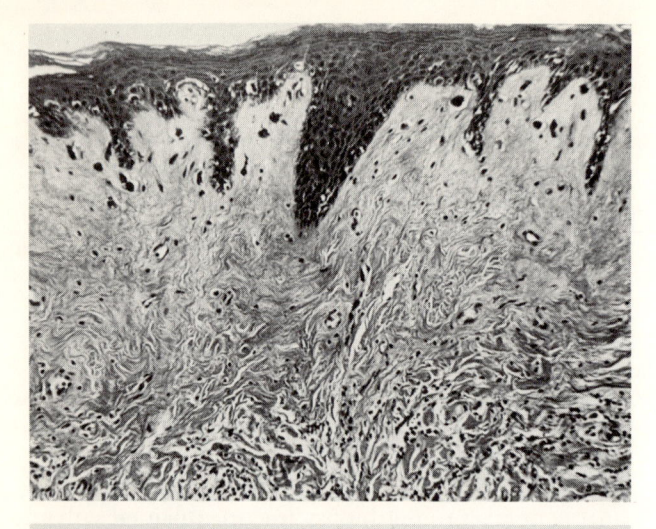

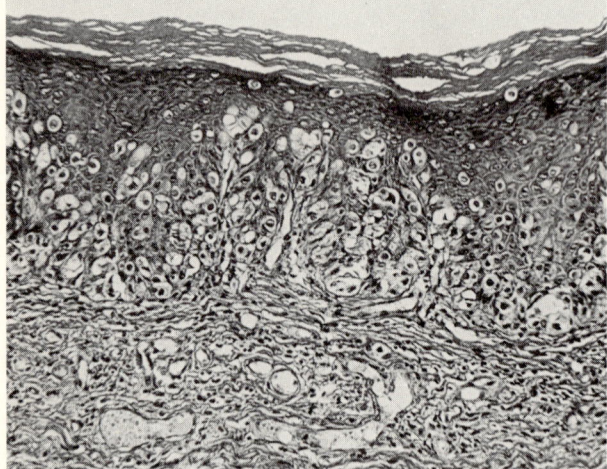

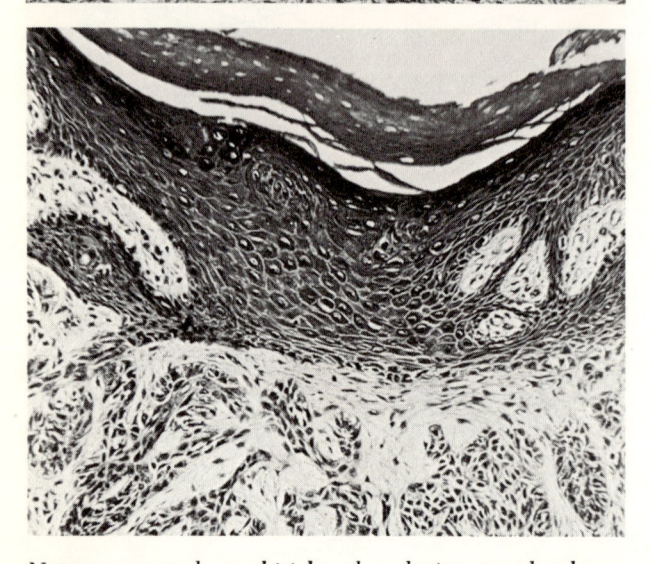

Not uncommonly a whitish vulvar lesion may be shown on biopsy to be lichen sclerosus (top). Paget's disease (middle) may present as reddish lesion, while blue or ulcerative lesions may be basal cell carcinoma (bottom).

picious, though a whitish lesion is not necessarily precancerous. It may be revealed by biopsy to be lichen sclerosus, a very common vulvar dystrophy that has a thin parchment-type appearance. About 5% of these lesions do show varying degrees of atypia. Treatment is with topical testosterone or one of its analogues, plus corticosteroids to reduce inflammation. Reddish lesions may indicate Paget's disease, while blue or ulcerative lesions may herald basal cell carcinoma. Such lesions also require immediate, liberal tissue sampling.

Vagina

Much of what has been said above applies also to inflammatory processes in the vagina, where vulvar infections often originate. With or without intercurrent infection, the senile vagina bleeds easily from spontaneous rupture of the now fragile vasculature, or, most commonly, following douching and/or coitus. This postmenopausal senile vaginitis is readily revealed by the physical examination, which demonstrates the absence of the normal rugal folds of the vaginal epithelium. Topical estrogens – nightly creams or suppositories for three or four weeks – are highly effective in providing the necessary hormonal support. The rugal folds are restored and the elasticity and compliance of the vaginal vault greatly improved. If intercurrent infection is present, adding triple sulfa creams to the regimen speeds estrogenization and recovery.

The relaxation of the vagina consequent to estrogen deficiency is also associated with development of cystoceles, urethroceles, enteroceles, and rectoceles, the presence of any of which must be taken into account in evaluating vaginal symptoms. As the competence of the proximal urethra declines, stress incontinence may develop, even to the point where patients must wear perineal pads at all times. If the involuntary loss of urine becomes incapacitating, and especially when it is associated with chronic infection, evaluation by cystoscopy and cystometry is indicated. Such investigation is mandatory if surgery is being considered.

Other modalities are available if surgery is contraindicated, perhaps by intercurrent illness. These include use of vaginal pessaries, a trial of antispasmodic agents, especially if the bladder dysfunction has a neurologic component, or microvoltage vaginal pessaries that provide constant bladder neck stimulation.

Moreover, as with bleeding, better hormonal sup-

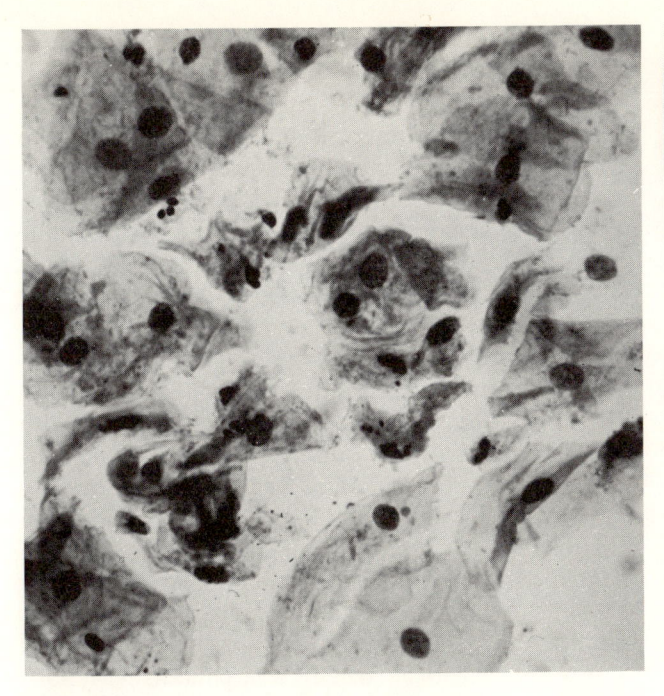

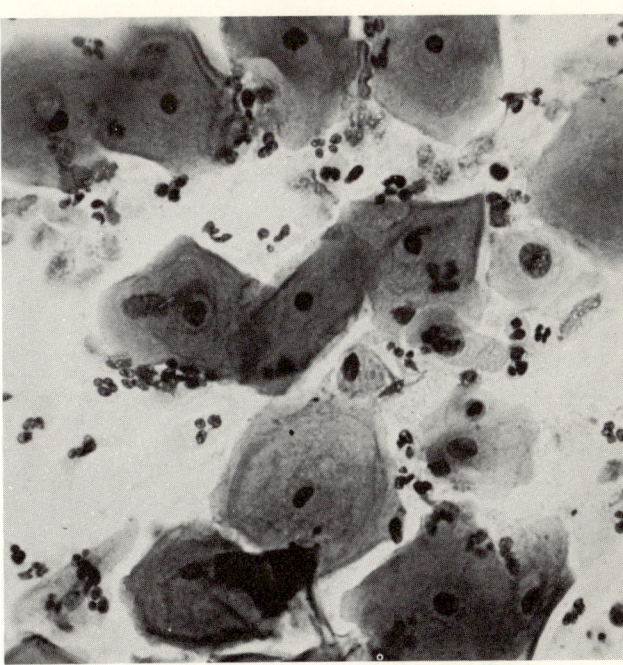

Typical atrophic changes of vaginal mucosa are seen in Pap smear specimen (left); a marked improvement in the cellular architecture occurs following therapy with topical estrogen (right).

port of the vaginal tissues may greatly relieve the incontinence problem and should be tried first, utilizing topical estrogens, creams, or suppositories. In up to 70% of patients in several series, topical estrogen applied to the vaginal mucosa achieved considerable, if not complete, restoration of urinary continence to a level esthetically acceptable to the patient. Even if surgery is contemplated for long-term correction, prior estrogenization is indicated to strengthen the fascia underlying the vaginal mucosa. Topical estrogen should also be continued postoperatively, since, without its supportive effects, relaxation may recur.

A problem in this age group related to enterocele and rectocele, which is seldom perceived as having a gynecologic basis, is tenesmus. Usually its presence is elicited only on direct questioning. Surgery is generally not indicated unless the symptom becomes a major hindrance to normal bowel function.

Vaginal vault prolapse is another common problem, especially so in the 50% or so of women who have had a hysterectomy by the time they reach the menopausal years; the incidence among women who no longer have a uterus has been put at 10%. Once again, the patient's general condition must be fully assessed before surgery is considered. Resuspension of the vault is the preferred procedure for women who are still sexually active; a combined abdominal and vaginal approach is utilized. In those who do not seek preservation of the vagina, obliteration of the vault by colpocleisis is a highly effective alternative. If uterine and vaginal prolapse coexist, vaginal hysterectomy together with vaginal support or obliteration provides total correction.

Primary vaginal carcinoma is a relatively rare lesion (accounting for less than 1% of female cancers) but must be ruled out if bleeding is present. Adequate visualization of the vaginal epithelium at the time of pelvic examination is vital, with cytologic sampling undertaken in the symptomatic patient to provide information on areas not visualized. Ulcerated or exfoliated lesions should be biopsied. If cytologic studies are suspicious but there are no gross vaginal lesions, colposcopy may identify the source of abnormal cells. Persons who have had cervical or vulvar dysplasias tend to have a relatively high incidence of vaginal dysplasias and should be tested by Pap smear annually.

Cervix, Uterus, Tubes, Ovaries

The postmenopausal shrinkage of the cervix makes endocervical lesions hard to detect. If smears suggest a squamous lesion of either the cervix or vagina, colposcopy, endocervical curettage, and/or

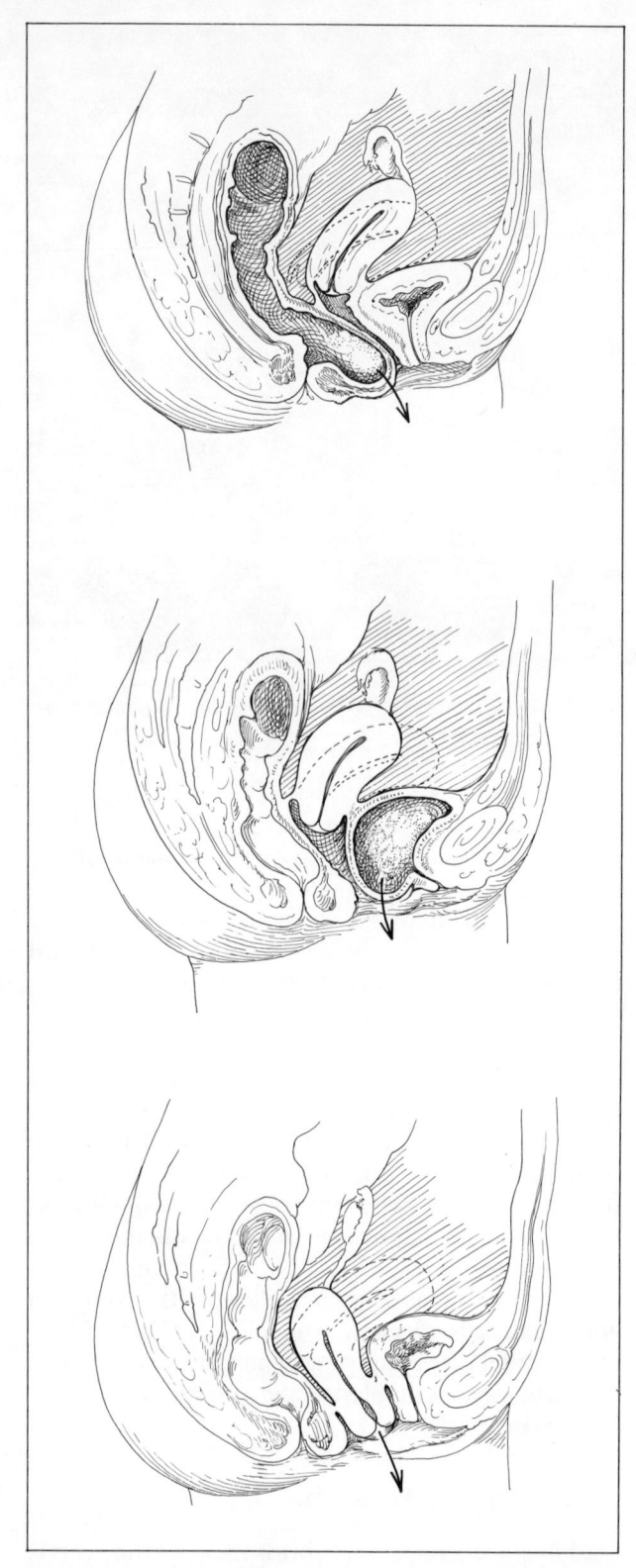

Relaxation of the vagina as a consequence of estrogen deficiency is associated with rectocele (top), cystocele (middle), and prolapse of the uterus (bottom).

cone biopsy may be required. Cervical polyps are a common cause of postmenopausal bleeding. If asymptomatic they can be excised as an office procedure, but the specimen should always be submitted for pathologic sectioning and review. When there is undetermined postmenopausal bleeding and the cervical canal is patent, it becomes necessary to sample the uterine cavity to rule out an endometrial lesion.

Several new methods have been developed for this purpose. Endometrial washing (as with the Gravely Jet apparatus), the endometrial brush, and endometrial biopsy (with or without aspiration) are usable in the office; their accuracy, in combined studies with D&C in patients with confirmed endometrial cancer, has been about 90%. Whether such techniques can detect early lesions such as hyperplasia of the endometrium has not yet been sufficiently studied. If outpatient procedures are unable to explain the etiology of postmenopausal bleeding, fractional D&C (fundus and endocervical canal) should be carried out. On a statistical basis 10% of patients with postmenopausal bleeding will prove to have endometrial cancer; the others will have bled for reasons such as atrophy of the endometrium, estrogen-related therapy, or benign factors, including endometrial polyps.

It is probably not necessary to dwell on the fact that any enlargement of the uterus in an elderly woman calls for investigation; it is likely to indicate that a pathologic process is under way. The postmenopausal uterus should be smaller in size than the premenopausal, and the same is true of the ovaries. The consensus with respect to the ovaries is that in the majority of patients they should no longer be palpable at, perhaps, five years postmenopause. In one small study, 60% of women with postmenopausally palpable ovaries proved to have ovarian cancer. At present, only one in four patients who undergo laparotomy for ovarian carcinoma survives for longer than five years; the other three are already beyond cure by surgery, radiotherapy, or chemotherapy. Given the lethality of this disease, there is no point in preserving the ovaries in a postmenopausal patient who is being treated for abnormalities, either benign or malignant, of the uterus or cervix.

Meticulous bimanual pelvic examination, at yearly intervals, is still the main approach to diagnosis of ovarian enlargement. Culdocentesis, which is helpful in suspicious cases, is not a feasible screening procedure, but the noninvasive technique of ultrasonography may well prove invaluable in detecting ovarian masses if it can be carried out on an annual schedule. Vague abdominal symptoms, i.e., persistent abdominal bloating or mild but persistent pelvic pain, should all be viewed in the postmenopausal woman with suspicion that there may be ovarian pathology.

Little need be said about the fallopian tubes in concluding this part of the discussion. Carcinoma of the tubes as a primary lesion is extremely rare. Nonetheless, when vaginal pool cytology is positive and investigation of vagina, cervix, and uterus proves negative, the tubes must be considered a possible source for the observed malignant epithelial cells and investigated by direct visualization – laparoscopy or laparotomy.

Estrogens and Osteoporosis

Although, as noted earlier, this chapter is not primarily concerned with the menopausal woman or the controversial question of the role of systemic estrogen replacement in managing her symptoms, the subject cannot be avoided when we turn to prophylaxis against osteoporosis. In the decade before menopause, women begin to lose cortical bone calcium. Initially gradual and minor, this loss accelerates after menopause. In the absence of ovarian estrogen and without treatment, it takes perhaps five to 15 years for calcium to leave the bony matrix. Disability associated with osteoporosis is both cosmetic and functional; vertebral compression can cause not only "dowager's hump" but severe pain. Secondary osteoarthritis can further exaggerate the condition, and diminished cortical bone integrity is, of course, a significant factor in the high incidence of fractures among elderly women.

Considerable evidence suggests that physiologic doses of estrogen can reduce the rate of calcium loss sufficiently to avert the osteoporotic pathologic consequences. While topical therapy often suffices to minimize or abolish tissue or vascular changes in the vulva and vagina, by definition it is hardly relevant in the context of prophylaxis against osteoporosis. By the time the patient presents with osteoporotic symptoms, estrogen replacement may stem further calcium loss and provide significant relief of pain, but it will not restore the status quo ante. In fact, after three years of estrogen deficiency, the existing bone changes may be considered irreversible.

In discussing the value of estrogen therapy for prophylaxis of osteoporosis, one therefore cannot help stepping into an area of debate, given the findings concerning a higher risk of endometrial cancer (five to 14 times higher according to different studies) in treated populations vs untreated controls. Moreover, while short-term estrogen therapy on a symptomatic basis induces a stable calcium balance and reduction in bone resorption as measured by microradiography and radiocalcium, no macroscopic radiographic evidence of estrogen-induced increase in bone mineral content has been published. Recently an ad hoc task force of an FDA advisory committee was assigned to produce guidelines for long-term clinical studies of estrogen therapy for osteoporosis.

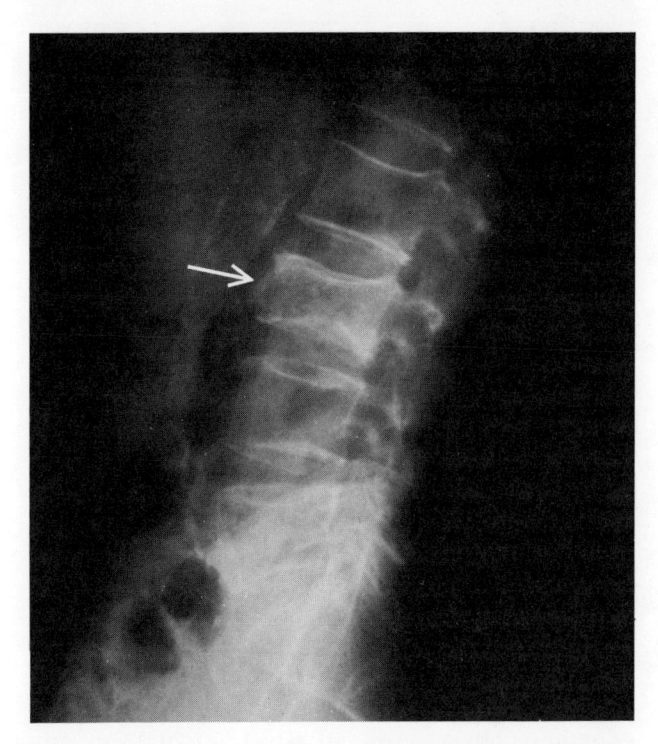

Common osteoporotic lesions shown are compression fractures (arrow) of the T-12 level of the thoracic spine. Estrogen will ease pain but not reverse bone changes.

Pending results of such studies, it is my own view that low-dose estrogen therapy begun within three years of onset of menopause appears effective in prevention and early treatment of postmenopausal osteoporosis. If six or more years have elapsed since ovarian function ceased, prophylactic measures do not seem justified; rather, one would then employ estrogens for their effect on symptoms.

Is it possible to define a low-dose regimen that may have a diminished carcinogenic potential? Preliminary evidence suggests that some products may carry a lesser risk: estradiol products appear retrospectively to be preferable in this respect to those containing a large proportion of estrone, the latter being the case with most conjugated esterified products. Products

> **Recommended Estrogen Therapy for Osteoporosis (Intact Uterus)**
>
> 1. Use lowest effective estrogen dosage
> 2. Use estrogenic compounds predominantly containing estradiol
>   - Ethinyl estradiol 0.02 mg
>   - 17-beta estradiol 1 mg
>   - Other estrogenic compounds in use
>   - Diethylstilbestrol 0.1 mg
>   - Conjugated estrogen 0.625 mg
>   - Estrone sulfate 0.625 mg
>   - All drugs to be used in cyclic fashion
> 3. Periodic challenge with a progestational agent
>   - Provera 10 mg x 5 days/month. Repeat in successive months until no withdrawal bleeding. Challenge then at three-month intervals as above.
> 4. Sample endometrial contents on a yearly basis with one of the presently available screening methods.

containing ethinyl estradiol, which is partly converted to estrone, appear to rank with the estradiol agents. The dosage that stems calcium loss, which is followed by monitoring urinary calcium and phosphorus excretion, is generally 0.01 to 0.02 mg/day of ethinyl estradiol, 0.6 to 1 mg/day of estradiol, 0.3 to 0.625 mg/day of conjugated estrogens, or perhaps 0.1 mg/day of diethylstilbestrol (which has not been studied for its oncogenicity in women whose childbearing days are past).

Patients receiving such therapy who still have their uterus (as noted earlier, at least half *do not,* some 600,000 hysterectomies being performed annually in the U.S.) should be monitored for endometrial changes by washing, biopsy, or aspiration biopsy at yearly intervals.

If these invasive methods are unacceptable or infeasible, an alternative is to give a progestogen for five days after the termination of the initial 25-day cycle of estrogen treatment. Agents that may be used for this purpose are Provera, progesterone in oil (IM), or Delalutin. If the estrogen dosage has caused endometrial proliferation, spotting or bleeding will occur, and it then becomes mandatory to ascertain and study the tissue from which the bleeding arose. If no contraindications to continuing the therapy are identified, one should reduce the estrogen dosage for the next cycle and repeat the challenge. In *all* cases, progesterone challenge should be instituted at three-month intervals as long as systemic estrogens are administered.

How long should replacement therapy be continued? Again, no satisfactorily scientific answer can be offered at the present time. With close supervision such as that described above, one may opt for indefinite maintenance since, on the one hand, symptoms will probably emerge whenever it is terminated, and, on the other, the physician has every likelihood of keeping ahead or abreast of any untoward consequence of the therapy per se.

The question of follow-up brings me to my concluding point. Which physician should have primary responsibility for the gynecologic problems of the postmenopausal woman? Since the cancer risk applies only to those patients in whom the uterus is still intact, probably only they need to be seen regularly by the gynecologist, while others can generally be managed by the family physician. In the hysterectomized patient, problems related to senile atrophy of the generative tract or osteoporosis do not require the same concern for carcinogenesis in assessing the risk/benefit ratio of estrogen therapy, though consultation may, of course, be indicated in individual circumstances. But it is probably unwise to initiate or continue estrogen therapy except under gynecologic supervision in patients with intact uterus. The gynecologist in turn should be advised on any problems, such as hypertension, blood clotting, or myocardial infarction, that may affect his evaluation of the appropriateness of estrogen therapy. Such sharing of information is indispensable to optimal management of gynecologic problems of the geriatric years.

14

Cancer in the Elderly

ARTHUR A. SERPICK
University of Maryland

Since cancer is preeminently a disease whose incidence rises with age, it could be argued that the manifestations of cancer in the elderly are the "norm," whereas cancers seen in younger individuals might be looked upon as "abnormal." Be that as it may, from the epidemiologic and other viewpoints, there are some significant differences among different age groups with respect to cancer. I would like to emphasize at the outset, however, that from the standpoint of therapy, cancer should be regarded similarly in all age groups. No patient should be denied the full employment of all appropriate therapeutic modalities on the grounds of old age alone. To put it as simply as possible, cancer treatment should be the same for young and old.

Although tumors and leukemias of course occur in childhood, in terms of actual numbers these are rare diseases. In general, cancer incidence and cancer deaths both rise continuously with age and are highest among the oldest. Thus the longer a person lives, the more likely he or she is to develop cancer. This applies regardless of whether the overall death rate for a particular cancer or site is increasing, decreasing, or remaining unchanged. For example, the death rate in the United States for cancer of the stomach has been declining steadily and strikingly since at least 1930. It was 308 per 100,000 white males aged 75 to 84 in 1930 and only 86 per 100,000 in 1975. Nonetheless, in 1975 as in 1930, its death rate increased steadily with age in both men and women (see graphs, pages 110, 111). The incidence of cancer of the uterus started to decline even before the Papanicolaou smear was introduced in the 1940s and has continued to do so, but it remains higher in older than in younger women. Breast cancer death rates in women have not changed significantly over the years, and they have always shown the same pattern of steady increase with age. For reasons unknown, pancreatic cancer, which is quickly fatal and largely untreatable, has been increasing alarmingly since 1930, and it, too, has always shown the same correlation between rising death rates and advancing age. Lung cancer, which has grown to epidemic proportions among men, is an exception in that death rates for U.S. males in 1975 were 195 per 100,000 in the 55 to 64 age group, 366 for those 65 to 74, 427 for ages 75 to 84, but 274 for ages 85 and over. (The death rates among women aged 65 and over are in the range of 65 per 100,000.)

The greater frequency of cancer with advancing age is thought to be at least in part a result of the accumulation of or repeated contact with chemical, physical, or biologic carcinogens. The relation between bone cancer and exposure to radioactive paint became apparent in the 1930s, when after a latent period of 10 to 25 years, many workers who had used such paint developed cancer. There may be a delay of 10 to 20 years between first asbestos exposure and the development of bronchogenic carcinoma and

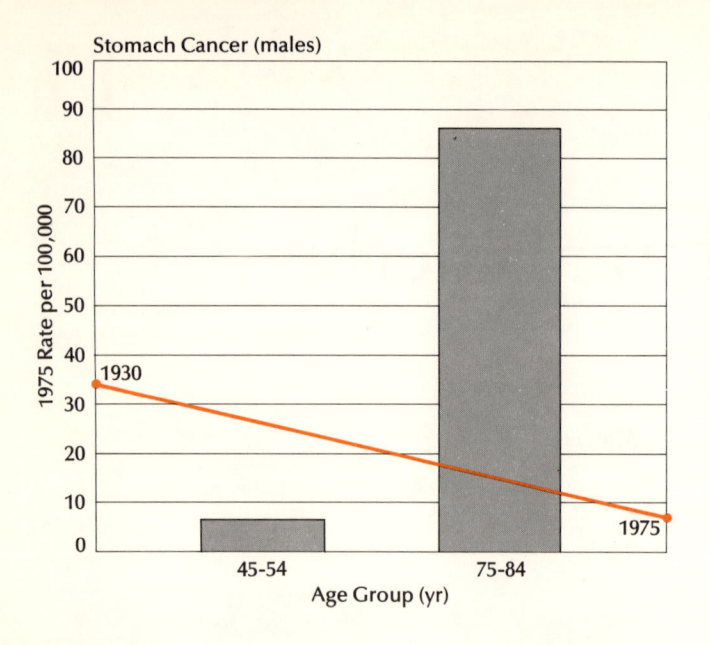

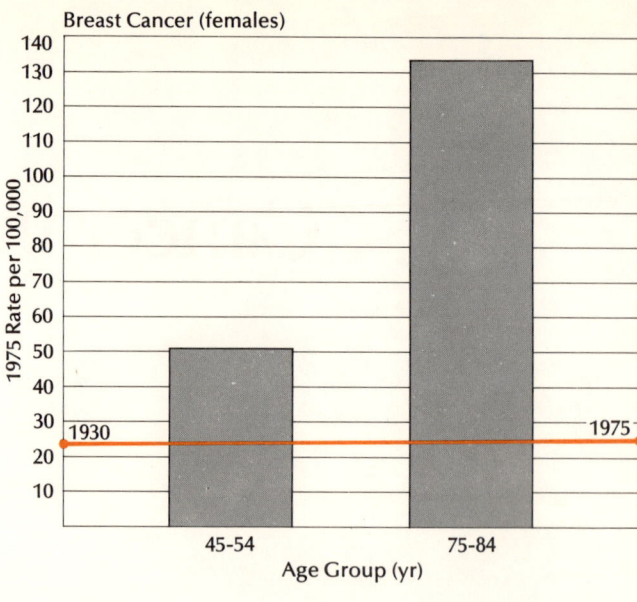

Incidence of cancer generally rises with age, as indicated in graphs above (1975 data from American Cancer Society). This pattern holds whether case rate of the particular cancer has been decreasing (stomach in men), remaining

mesothelioma. Lung cancer may be associated with nickel compounds, chromate compounds, and radioactive ores in trace quantities, and again there is a long period of latency.

Reduction of host resistance with age also probably helps explain the increase in cancer in the elderly. It is thought that many cancers arise and are destroyed early by the immune system in younger persons, but that in the elderly the immune system is less effective. Possibly this results in part from an accumulation in older people of exposure to many antigenic stimuli, possibly also from a decline in the production of certain hormones. This antigenic stimulation in the elderly results in the high incidence of positive latex fixation tests and of monoclonal peaks on serum electrophoresis.

A very few sites account for the majority of cancers in the elderly. Skin cancer is almost exclusively a disease of older persons, and since nonmelanoma skin cancer is by far the most common of all cancers – an estimated 300,000 new cases in all age groups in 1977 (but only 1,500 deaths) as compared with some 690,000 new cancers in all other sites – one can be grateful that it is easily detected and easily cured, usually with surgery or irradiation. Omitting skin cancer, data compiled by the End Results Group of the National Cancer Institute showed that the prostate accounted for one fourth of all cancers in men 75 years and older (another study showed that 80% of men over 85 had prostate cancer). Cancers of the stomach, large intestine, and rectum accounted for an additional 25%. Among women in the same age bracket, the breasts accounted for 21% of all cancers, and the stomach, large intestine, and rectum for 28%. Thus, half of all cancers in the elderly originate in only four organs: the prostate, the breast, the stomach, and the bowel. The lung, too, is the site of many cancers in elderly men, and although the rate in women is much lower, it is rising.

As these statistics imply, in older patients one must be particularly alert for symptoms of cancer at the high-risk sites. For example, the older patient especially should be asked if there has been a change in bowel habits, and any change must be taken seriously. If the patient has to bear down on evacuation or has alternating diarrhea and constipation, carcinoma of the bowel must be given primary consideration. Many older patients do not verbalize their complaints as well as younger people do, perhaps accepting the symptoms as normal concomitants of old age, and the physician must more actively seek information. As with treatment, so with diagnosis: the older patient should be given as much diagnostic attention as, and in fact may need even more than, the younger patient.

Aside from the annual Papanicolaou smear and

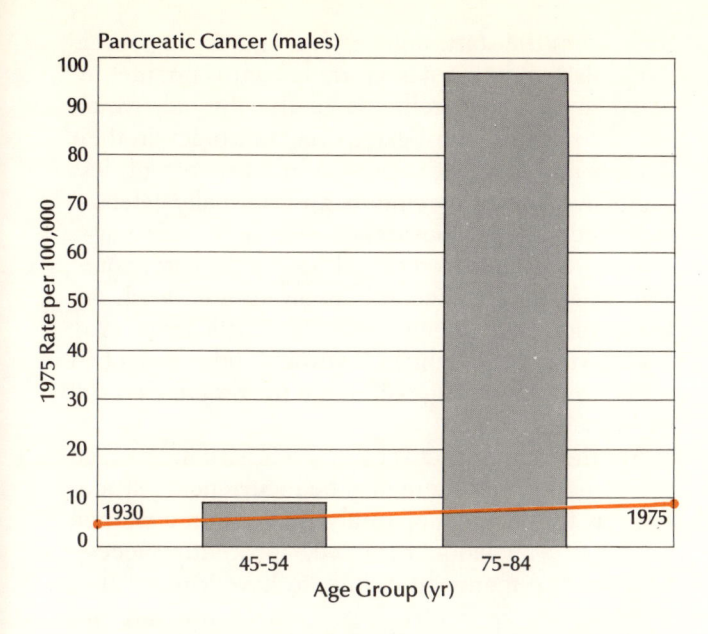

the same (breast in women), or increasing (pancreatic in men), as shown by age-adjusted rates for 1930 and 1975.

monthly breast self-examination for women, and an annual rectal examination in both sexes, there is no general agreement on what should be done routinely to detect cancer. With what frequency should individuals have a chest x-ray? Or a physical examination including proctoscopy? Many physicians would say annually for the chest x-ray, especially in cigarette smokers, but so far as the second question is concerned, I do not think the results justify routine annual proctoscopic examinations even in older people. Seldom is anything serious found in asymptomatic individuals. The person with a complaint, however, should be vigorously investigated. The cure rate of bowel cancer has not been shown to be higher when cancer is found in asymptomatic individuals than in patients who were thoroughly worked up after the first complaint, such as blood in the stool or a change in bowel habits.

Another example of a common complaint of the elderly that should be taken quite seriously is the backache, particularly in a patient who has or has had a carcinoma. The backache may result from metastases to the vertebrae, and occasionally is the first sign of an unsuspected primary tumor. Likely primary sites are prostate, breast, lung, and kidney.

From the perspective of this chapter, malignant tumors can be divided into three main groups: 1) those whose prognosis is the same in young and old; 2) those that have a better prognosis in the aged; and 3) those with a worse prognosis in older persons. The first group, which includes cancers of the gastrointestinal tract, oral cavity, larynx, and lung, will not be discussed here, since my principal concern is with cancers that are different in one way or another in the elderly or that are seen primarily only in older people. The major cancer with a better prognosis in the elderly is breast cancer. In the third group are such cancers as malignant melanoma and those of the thyroid. To begin with the cancers confined to or more prevalent in women, I would point out that breast cancer is particularly aggressive in women who are pregnant or still menstruating. Although the older a woman is, the more likely she is to develop breast cancer, the more years since the menopause the less aggressive the disease will be. This applies also to breast cancer that first occurred prior to menopause and recurs afterward. If the first tumor occurs postmenopausally, it often grows slowly and causes no symptoms or alarm for a long period. Recurrences in younger women are more likely to involve the liver and the lungs, producing disability and death. In older women recurrences tend to metastasize to bone and soft tissue, which is a less life-threatening situation. The difference is apparently related to hormonal factors that are not fully understood. Often painful bone lesions and soft tissue masses respond dramatically to radiation therapy,

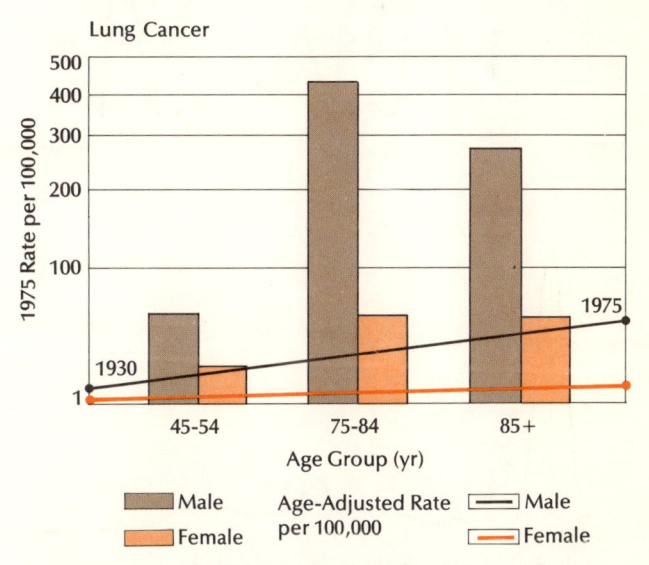

Lung cancer, which has of course become vastly more prevalent since 1930, displays slightly different pattern of rise in incidence with aging. In men, rate peaks in 75- to 84-year age group but drops after age 85.

and more general bone involvement may be treated with estrogens, or the newer, relatively non-masculinizing androgens, or with antiestrogens. Thus, therapy for the older woman can be less aggressive and debilitating than the the systemic drug therapy often necessary in younger women, and the older patient can be given the assurance that she is less likely than the younger to be disabled or killed by the disease.

Two types of gynecologic tumors occur predominantly after the start of the 60s. One is carcinoma of the vulva and vagina, the other carcinoma of the endometrium. The latter particularly affects obese, diabetic women and generally presents as postmenopausal bleeding. Extirpative surgery is the treatment of choice in both situations, with a trend toward additive radiation treatment in endometrial carcinoma.

As mentioned, thyroid gland carcinomas usually behave differently in the young and the old. Papillary carcinoma of the thyroid is relatively benign and easily treatable in a 30-year-old woman, whereas in those over 60 it is more aggressive, is very often metastatic from the start, and survival figures are poorer. Particularly fulminant is a form known as undifferentiated anaplastic carcinoma of the thyroid, which seems to occur almost exclusively in women in their late 60s and older. It may arise in a preexistent, less aggressive type of carcinoma and is usually detected from the sudden appearance of a large neck mass. Over several months regional nodes, the liver, bone, and lungs tend to become involved, and death occurs quickly. In recent years, the anticancer drug Adriamycin (doxorubicin hydrochloride) has been found to produce regression, but the prognosis is still early death.

Another tumor that is more aggressive in the aged is melanoma, and there may be recurrences particularly in the postmenopausal female. Some women have had a melanoma excised, apparently successfully, before menopause, only to have it recur after menopause. Evidently hormonal factors are involved; unfortunately hormone therapy for malignant melanoma has a dismal record. Early adjunctive cytotoxic drug therapy and immunotherapy are being explored as therapeutic approaches in those

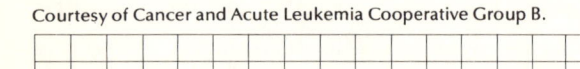

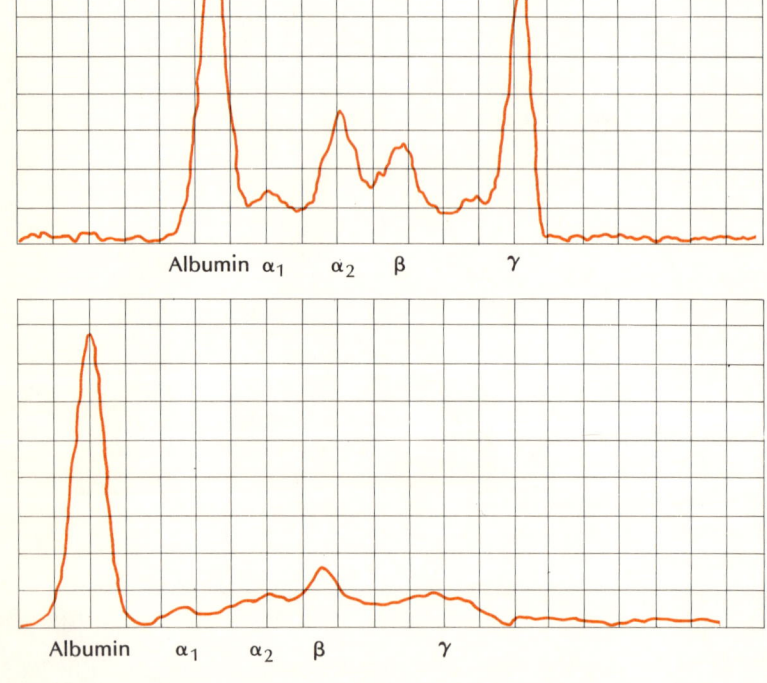

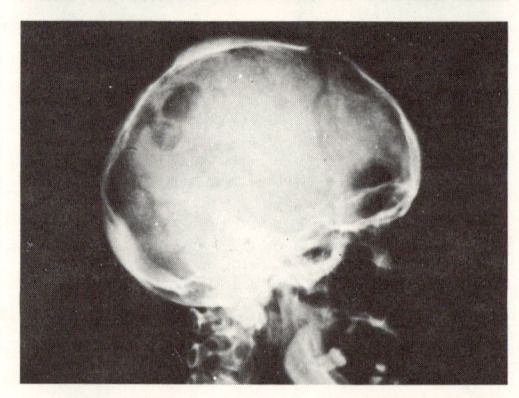

Courtesy of Cancer and Acute Leukemia Cooperative Group B.

Before treatment (top), male patient with multiple myeloma had "punched-out" lesions of skull and extensive abnormalities of serum zone electrophoretic pattern.

Combination chemotherapy led to disappearance of abnormal immunoglobulins and apparent recovery from skull damage, seen two and a half years later (bottom).

patients with recurrent melanomas or with deep levels of invasion at the time of primary diagnosis.

Turning to men, the most common cancer among those past age 50 is carcinoma of the prostate. It is exceeded only by lung cancer as the most frequent cause of cancer deaths in adult males (estimates for 1977 are 68,000 lung cancer deaths in males vs 20,000 prostate cancer deaths). Nine out of 10 cases are discovered in men 60 and older, the frequency increasing greatly with advancing age. The prevalence of prostate carcinoma at autopsy or on pathologic examination following prostatectomy for bladder obstruction far exceeds its clinical recognition, and this has led to the concept of the disease as the "pathologist's cancer." An illusion exists that prostatic cancer is not a lethal disease and that much can be done to alter its course at any stage of its progression. That this is not so is indicated by the figure of 20,000 deaths cited above. Hence cancer of the prostate should be diagnosed and treated in the early stages, when it is highly curable, although treatment is not necessarily started when it is first discovered, since it does usually progress slowly. Because the prevalence is so great, an annual rectal examination is recommended for older men.

When it is decided not to treat immediately, the patient must be followed with semiannual rectal examinations, x-rays of the pelvis, and a blood test for prostatic acid phosphatase. This enzyme is released by the cancer once it spreads beyond the prostatic capsule. The invasive carcinoma, of course, is a different story and may require prostatectomy, orchiectomy, drugs, and irradiation.

Carcinoma of the bladder is uncommon, but again is a disease seen almost exclusively in older people. The death rate in 1975 for men aged 45 to 54 was 2.6 per 100,000, jumping to 11.6 for those 55 to 64, to 38.2 at ages 65 to 74, 88.1 for 75 to 84, and 137.9 at 85 and over. (For women in the 75 to 84 age group the rate was 23.5, and for those 85 or over, 44.3.) The rate in the three oldest groups of men has been increasing since 1930 but has dropped in younger men, and in women it has gone up only in the very oldest group.

Bladder cancer is positively correlated with smoking, although it is not clear why. This association may help explain its increase in older men, which resembles that seen in lung cancer. Workers in the aniline dye industry also have a disproportionate rate of bladder cancer. The earliest symptoms may be blood in the urine, prolonged cystitis, and a feeling of a bladder load. Diagnosis involves cystoscopy and bi-

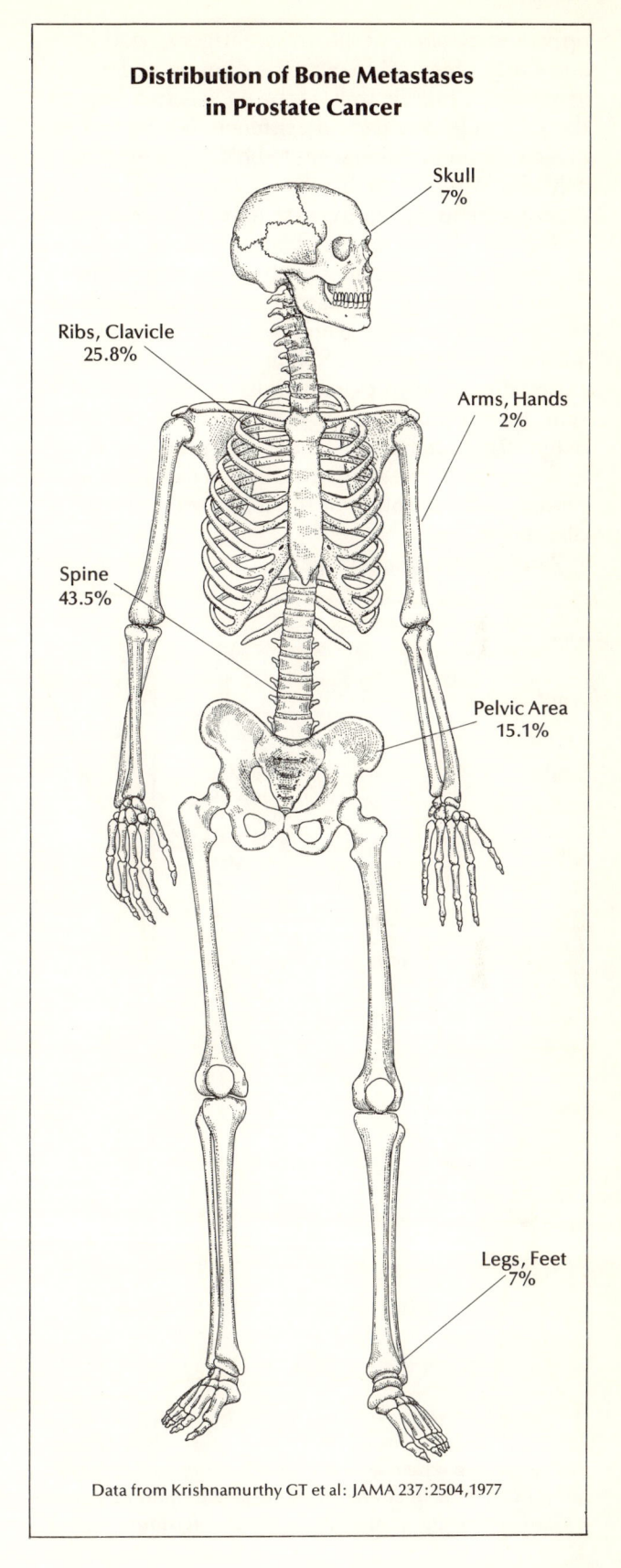

Distribution of Bone Metastases in Prostate Cancer

Skull 7%
Ribs, Clavicle 25.8%
Arms, Hands 2%
Spine 43.5%
Pelvic Area 15.1%
Legs, Feet 7%

Data from Krishnamurthy GT et al: JAMA 237:2504, 1977

opsy, and cytology of the urine. Surgery, irradiation, and drugs often fail to cure the disease, and if it has invaded the muscle wall, recurrence is frequent and the patient leads a painful existence. New drugs employed in combination seem to hold some promise.

Multiple myeloma has been recognized with increasing frequency in the past 30 years; in one review 80% of the patients were over 50 years of age. Men are more likely to be affected than women. This malignant proliferation of plasma cells in the marrow often presents as bone pain, pathologic fractures, or advanced osteoporosis. Solitary plasmacytomas occasionally occur in extramedullary sites such as the skin, the oropharynx, and near the spinal cord. The diagnosis is established by demonstrating an abnormal protein in the serum or urine in the presence of plasma cell infiltration of the marrow or of multiple plasmacytomas.

Anemia, thrombocytopenia, hypercalcemia, and infection occur as marrow is destroyed. The characteristic accumulation of large amounts of abnormal immunoglobulin proteins can damage the kidneys (myeloma kidney) and is accompanied by a decrease in the quantity of normal immunoglobulins, which adds to the propensity for infection. There is also interference with coagulation. The excess of proteins may bring on blood hyperviscosity, followed by obliteration of small vessels in the eye and central nervous system. This is a medical emergency that can be treated immediately with plasmapheresis. Spinal cord and nerve root compression must be detected early by radiographic means and treated quickly by irradiation. In recent years, palliation with antineoplastic drugs has extended survival for up to four years or so of useful and pain-free life in many patients. Those who respond to the drug mephalan have a median survival of 40 months, whereas those who do not respond usually succumb to the disease much sooner.

Although the press has given the public the impression that leukemia is a childhood disease, in reality it is another cancer primarily of older patients. Mortality rates for groups over the age of 45 have always been higher than for those under 15. The childhood form is acute lymphocytic leukemia, and its incidence peaks at age five. Chronic and acute myelogenous leukemia show an increase with age, but by far the predominant form in older adults is chronic lymphocytic leukemia, and men have a much higher death rate than women.

Patients with chronic leukemia may have no symptoms and are often discovered through a high white blood count on a routine physical examination or when blood is drawn at a "health fair" or similar event. In chronic myelogenous leukemia the spleen is usually considerably enlarged and serves as a reservoir for the entrapment and replication of leukemic cells. Characteristically, the patient develops a very large spleen, and the first symptom may be a feeling of weight in the left side of the abdomen. Usually the patient is not anemic or thrombocytopenic. This form of the disease may be controlled with such drugs as busulfan, hydroxyurea, or dibromomannitol, but these apparently do not significantly delay the transformation of chronic into acute leukemia, in which the blast crisis is frequently the terminal event.

Chronic lymphocytic leukemia has a long and usually benign asymptomatic progression. It is characterized by an accumulation of long-lived immuno-

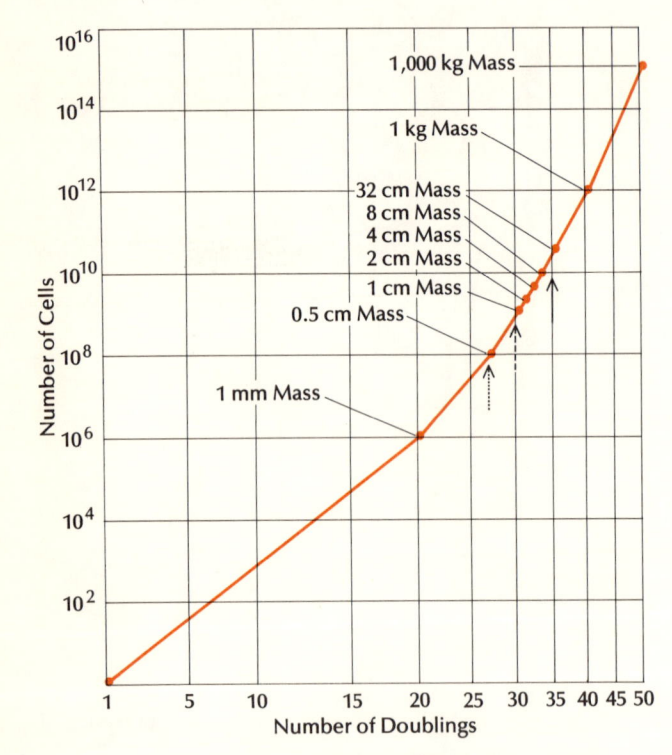

↑ Tumor First Visualized on X-Ray (27 doublings)
↑ Tumor First Palpable (30 doublings)
↑ Tumor 1 Foot in Diameter (35 doublings)

As theoretical data from studies by Silver et al and Collins et al show, the number of neoplastic cells is extremely high by the time a lesion is detectable by either x-ray or palpation. This of course explains why it remains so difficult to detect cancer in its earliest, curable stages.

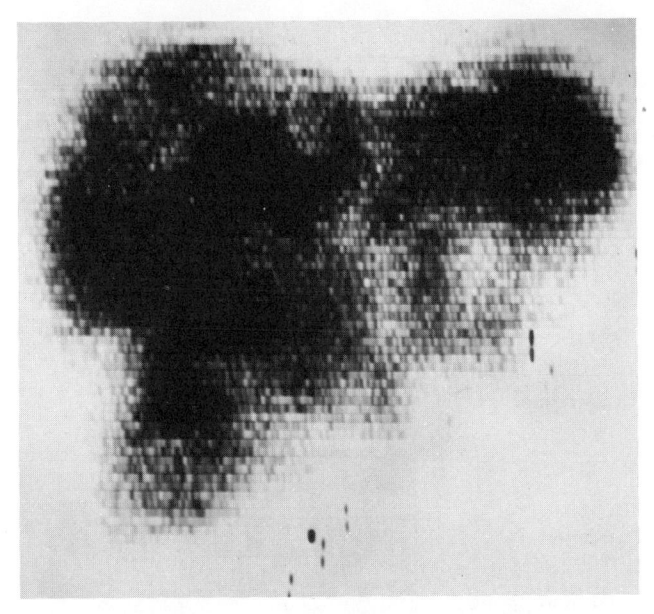

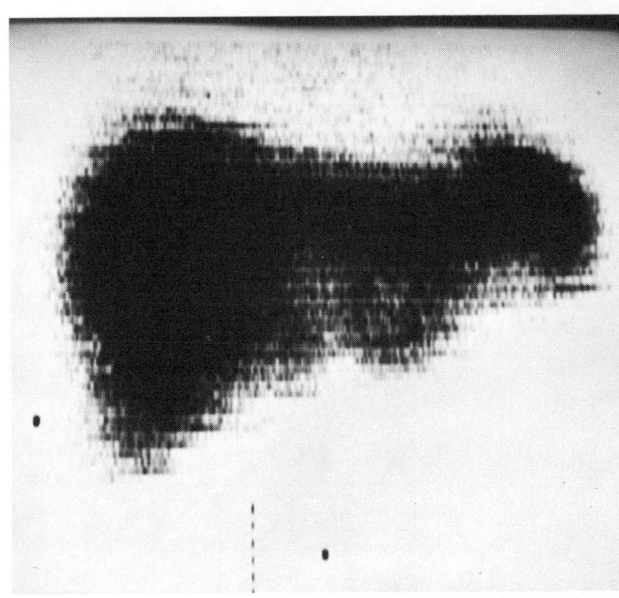

Liver scan at left above was made in male with metastatic melanoma; after five weeks of multidrug therapy (right) enlargement regressed, defects in tracer uptake disappeared. Below left: leg sarcoma metastases all but obliterated lungs in female; after six months of combined drugs, lungs appeared almost free of tumor (right).

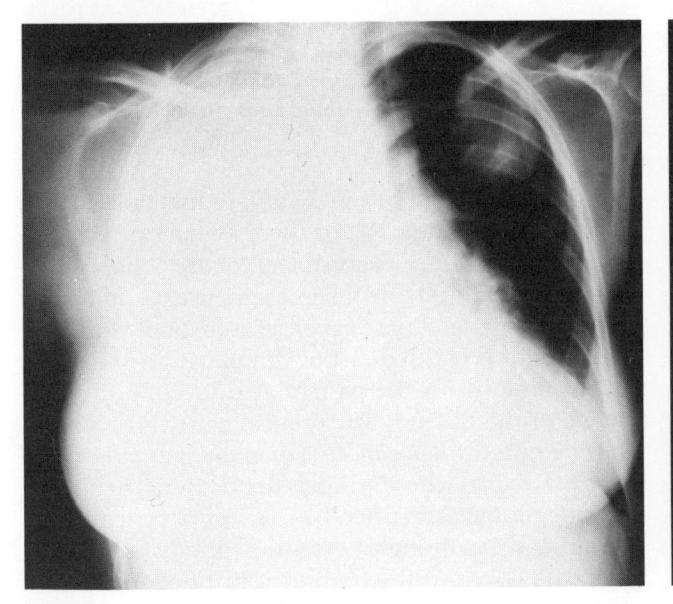

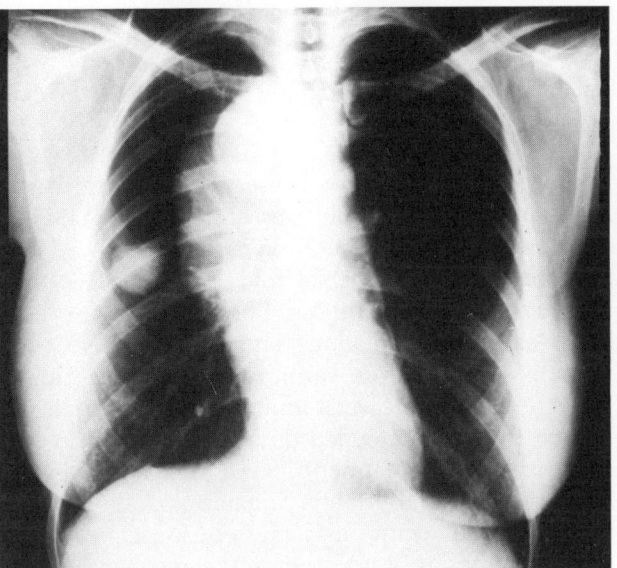

logically incompetent small lymphocytes in the peripheral blood, marrow, and lymph nodes. Some compromise of marrow function occurs, and generalized peripheral and central adenopathy and enlarged spleen are seen. Antiviral and other immune defenses become impaired, and production of an abnormal immunoglobulin sometimes results in an autoimmune hemolytic anemia and occasionally thrombocytopenia. Because the disease remains asymptomatic for so long, aggressive general therapy is avoided, since it can further impair the immune response. Localized adenopathy can be treated with an alkylating agent. Generalized nodal enlargement and the splenomegaly normally respond to localized irradiation. Corticosteroids are indicated for the acquired hemolytic and thrombocytopenic manifestations. However, there is no proof that therapy alters survival time. After some years patients tend to succumb to an infection.

Skin carcinoma, again affecting more men than

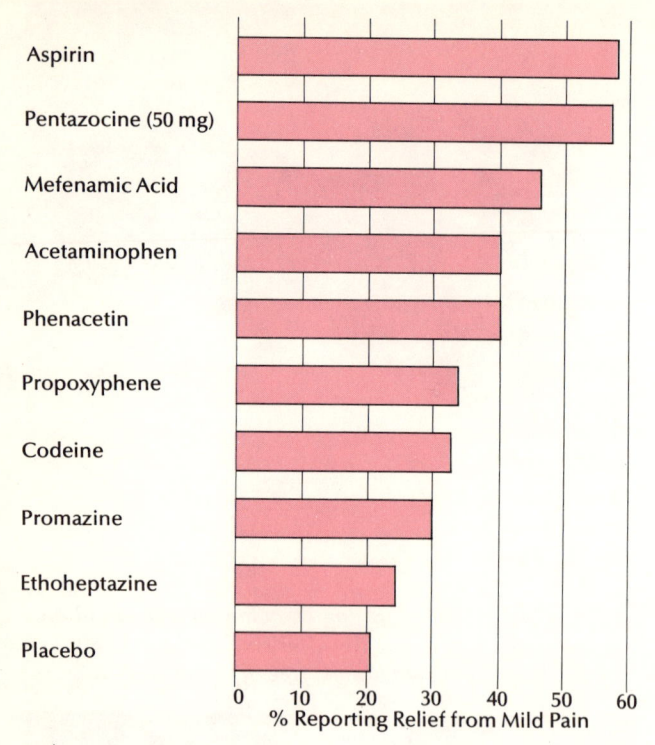

% Reporting Relief from Mild Pain	
Aspirin	~58
Pentazocine (50 mg)	~57
Mefenamic Acid	~47
Acetaminophen	~40
Phenacetin	~40
Propoxyphene	~34
Codeine	~32
Promazine	~30
Ethoheptazine	~24
Placebo	~21

% Reporting Relief from Severe Pain	
Pentazocine (100 mg)	~56
Levorphanol	~48
Meperidine	~47
Aspirin	~45
Morphine	~40
Anileridine	~37
Methadone	~36
Codeine	~32
Hydromorphone	~20
Placebo	~20

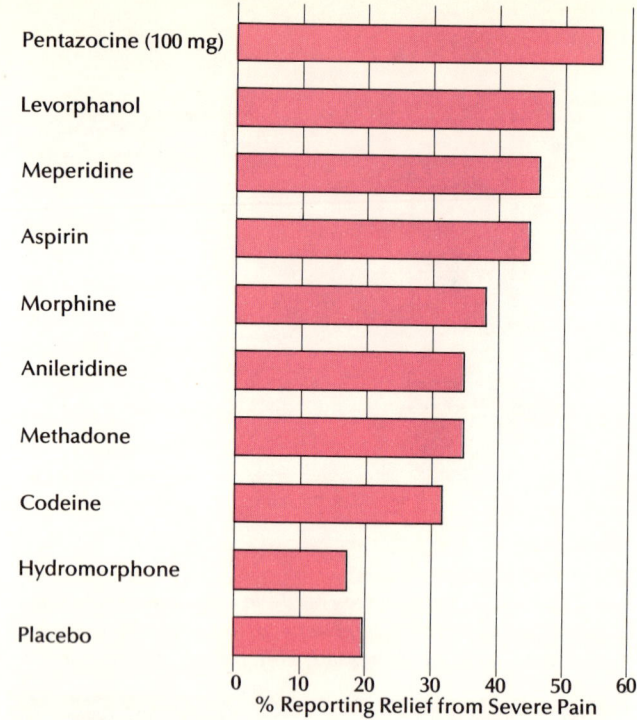

Pain relief experienced by two groups of patients after one dose of each of the analgesics cited above was evaluated by Moertel et al at the Mayo Clinic. Percentage benefiting from placebo is about same in each group.

women, is predominantly a disease of older persons. Exposure to the ultraviolet rays of the sun over many years causes tumors in such exposed areas as the face and scalp, the nasal labial fold, the bridge of the nose, and the inner canthus. These tumors are often best treated by irradiation. The elderly patient can tolerate as well as the younger the necessary high doses of radiation to such limited areas. Attempts to reduce the recommended dosages will result in recurrence, and retreatment increases the probability of morbidity and mortality. Squamous carcinoma of the scalp, if it recurs, may often be associated with cervical metastases, and the presence of these neck neoplasms reduces the cure rate fivefold.

Turning now to general considerations of treatment in older patients, I should like to emphasize again that the guiding principles are basically the same as those applicable in younger patients. Despite advanced years, the geriatric patient should be offered the opportunity for cure or relief of a potentially fatal disease. Chronologic age should never be the sole criterion on which a decision is made as to the ability of the patient to withstand a major operative procedure or a strenuous course of radiation or drug therapy. Also, one should not adopt the view that treatment will be too painful to inflict on the old patient, even though he or she may have a relatively short time to enjoy its possible ultimate benefits. Nor should the attitude be taken that the expenditure of time, money, and medical effort is just not worth it if the patient is old. No cost or complication of therapy is as ominous for the patient as extension or recurrence of the disease. Today most patients of all ages can be cured *when cancer is diagnosed at a localized stage.* Patients whose cancers are detected at a more advanced stage can often be relieved of pain and suffering and can enjoy an extension of satisfactory life. In other words, if the therapy is justified in terms of the possibility of cure or better survival of the patient, it speaks for itself and should be employed regardless of the patient's age.

Today new therapies and the combined modality approach make possible more aggressive treatment than was true five or 10 years ago. The surgeon, the new specialist in medical oncology, and the radiation therapist can work together to combine primary and adjuvant therapies. As a result, cure can be sought in many types of cancers formerly held to be incurable.

For example, it is not the breast cancer per se that kills the patient but its dissemination to the lungs, liver, brain, bones, etc. We now make the assumption that even after radical surgery there may be microscopic foci of the disease elsewhere, and so prophylactic drug therapy seems a reasonable approach. Similarly, carcinoma of the stomach or bowel will often extend into the nodes or throughout the entire organ wall, and patients will have a high recurrence rate even after "curative" surgery. Current multiple trials with adjuvant therapy employing drugs and combinations of drugs only recently available may prove to be successful in the old as well as the young.

While we can seek cures in a great many more patients today than in the past, the fact remains that only about one third of cancer patients are cured (in terms of a given disease-free survival time) and two thirds are not. This is not so much a failure of therapy as of detection of cancer when it is in a stage amenable to local therapy with surgery or irradiation. For the two thirds of patients we do not cure, we must keep in mind the natural history of cancer in its progression from local site to multiple distant sites. Treatment for pain and discomfort should also follow this progression. It should concentrate initially on the local lesions that cause pain and progress to control of the regional pain and then the rare generalized pain. Pain from localized disease may be amenable to palliative surgery, or to regional nerve block, or neurosurgical interruption of its sensory supply, or to irradiation. Pain from bone lesions is usually best treated by irradiation. Multiple lesions causing discomfort, pressure symptoms, or organ derangement may be treated by palliative chemotherapy, and most patients with advanced cancer should at least be considered for this modality.

Drugs are the most obvious form of pain control. In a study at the Mayo Clinic (see graphs, page 116), patients were divided into those with mild and those with severe pain, and 20% in both groups responded to placebo. Aspirin produced the best overall response. Some patients did not respond to any drug while some responded to many. It may be that the attitude of the physician in giving the drug is more important than which drug is given. He can provide better relief of pain when he keeps in mind that there is not only physical pain but the fear of pain and painful anxieties, all of which need relief. It also helps the patient if the physician tries to alleviate as best he can the anxiety of the patient's family.

Finally the point is reached when many cancer patients must face death. Half of our patients today die in the impersonal, mechanical atmosphere of the hospital, attached to monitoring, respiratory, feeding, and other devices, whereas 50 years ago they died at home, surrounded by family instead of physicians, nurses, and laboratory technicians. I think we have an obligation to our patients, when they are about to depart, to let them go in peace, "with dignity," as the current phrase has it, preferably at home.

To do this is often difficult for the physician, who may not be able to acknowledge the imminence of death. For many young physicians who have not been exposed to the natural history of cancer while in medical school, anxieties that they share with the laity about the "dread" disease have not been replaced by professional attitudes, and studies have shown that physicians as a group have a higher than average fear of death. Nearly everyone has a special fear of cancer (which prevents patients from coming to a doctor with a cough or lump), and the disease still carries a heavy stigma that heart disease, for example, does not. Yet the latter is far more common.

It should be kept in mind that the average period of survival in an untreated patient with breast cancer or lymphoma, for example, greatly exceeds that of patients with bleeding varices, stroke, or even myocardial infarction. It is necessary to remember that pain is seldom a major symptom of cancer and that increased comfort and worthwhile survival are easier to achieve for most patients with advanced cancer than for those with many nonmalignant diseases, whether the patients are young or old.

15

The Prostate in the Elderly Male

ALESSANDRO BASSO
Johns Hopkins University

Benign prostatic hypertrophy and adenocarcinoma of the prostate are among the most common urologic problems of the aging male. They are the common cause of prostatism, the clinical syndrome that is associated with abnormalities causing bladder outlet obstruction.

At times, prostatism can be insidious, with symptoms so minor that the patient does not seek medical attention. It is not uncommon during a workup for anemia or anorexia to find an elevated blood urea or creatinine that signals the presence of a urinary tract problem. Such a patient often has a chronically distended bladder and bilateral hydronephrosis detected during radiologic investigation of the urinary tract ("silent prostatism").

More often, however, the symptoms are overt, with decreased force of the urinary stream, hesitancy, frequency, nocturia, urgency, urge incontinence, and, at times, hematuria. Usually progressive, these symptoms may culminate in acute urinary retention. Sometimes this painful and frightening condition is precipitated by drugs that increase the bladder neck tone (such as a decongestant for the common cold), or ones that decrease the detrusor tone (such as anticholinergic drugs and certain tranquilizers).

Because the patient has a persistent residual urine after voiding, he is subject to urinary tract infections that at times may be associated with bacteremia and septic shock, in most instances due to gram-negative organisms.

Prostatic enlargement is not the only cause of these symptoms in the elderly male. Urethral strictures can be responsible for a similar clinical picture. However, in this situation, the symptoms frequently start after an episode of gonococcal urethritis or a traumatic lesion of the urethra.

Another condition that can be found in the uncircumcised older man is chronic balanitis, which may lead to distal urethral stenosis and cause severe urinary difficulties.

Prostatitis may produce symptoms of prostatism and be confused with a pathologic obstruction of the bladder outlet. The presence of an insignificant postvoid residual associated with infected urine and prostatic secretions will help in making the differential diagnosis. This is a condition occurring more often than not earlier in life, a point that should also be taken into consideration. Certainly infection can aggravate symptoms of prostatism even when obstruction is present.

Whatever the cause of bladder-outlet obstruction, the consequences can be severe not only for the bladder but also for the upper urinary tract and the kidneys. Once hydronephrosis occurs, it may be followed by renal insufficiency, with potentially fatal consequences.

The bladder wall becomes trabeculated, with formations of cellules and diverticula. Diverticula are noteworthy because they can serve as reservoirs of pathogenic organisms; they can also be a site of transitional cell tumors. Usually, these have a poor prognosis because of the absence of a muscular wall to serve as an effective barrier against the invasion of surrounding tissues (Kelalis and McLean).

Benign Prostatic Hypertrophy

One important contribution the family physician can make to lessen the anxieties of the patient with prostatic obstruction is to explain what the prostate is and what it does. Many patients believe the gland is essential to potency and that symptoms connected with it herald the end of sexual function. They are often surprised to learn that the prostate can be operated upon without necessarily endangering sexual function.

Patients will understand better the indications and type of surgery if they are told that the prostate surrounds the urethra and that the benign prostatic hypertrophy is an overgrowth of the inner part of the prostate (periurethral glands), which stretches the unaffected outer part, or the prostate proper.

Symptoms are not necessarily related to the size of the prostate. A median bar or a hypertrophic medial lobe can at times produce a more severe obstruction than can large hypertrophic lateral lobes.

The classic symptoms of prostatism almost invariably accompany hypertrophy. Upon rectal examination, the prostate feels uniformly enlarged, smooth, and elastic. One should keep in mind, however, that if either a median bar or a hypertrophic medial lobe is present, the prostate may appear to be of normal size.

The *etiology* of benign prostatic hypertrophy is only partially understood, although it is known that prostatic growth is influenced by hormones of the hypophysis, testes, and adrenals. Correlation between testes and prostate has always been suspected. In fact, in the nineteenth century castration was performed, with some frequency, in order to control prostate enlargement. This operation has been abandoned, at least for benign prostatic hypertrophy, but the reports have stimulated a long series of studies to elucidate the hormonal control of prostatic growth.

Attempts have also been made to control this growth by hormonal manipulation. Recently interest has been focused on antiandrogens. These are substances capable of competing with dehydrotestosterone in the nucleus of prostatic cells, blocking the DNA synthesis.

Scott and Wade at the Johns Hopkins Hospital have reported favorable results in treating benign prostatic hypertrophy with the antiandrogen cyproterone acetate. It is of interest, however, that although this compound has a very definite effect in curbing the growth of prostatic acini, it does not affect the fibromuscular stroma of the prostate. For

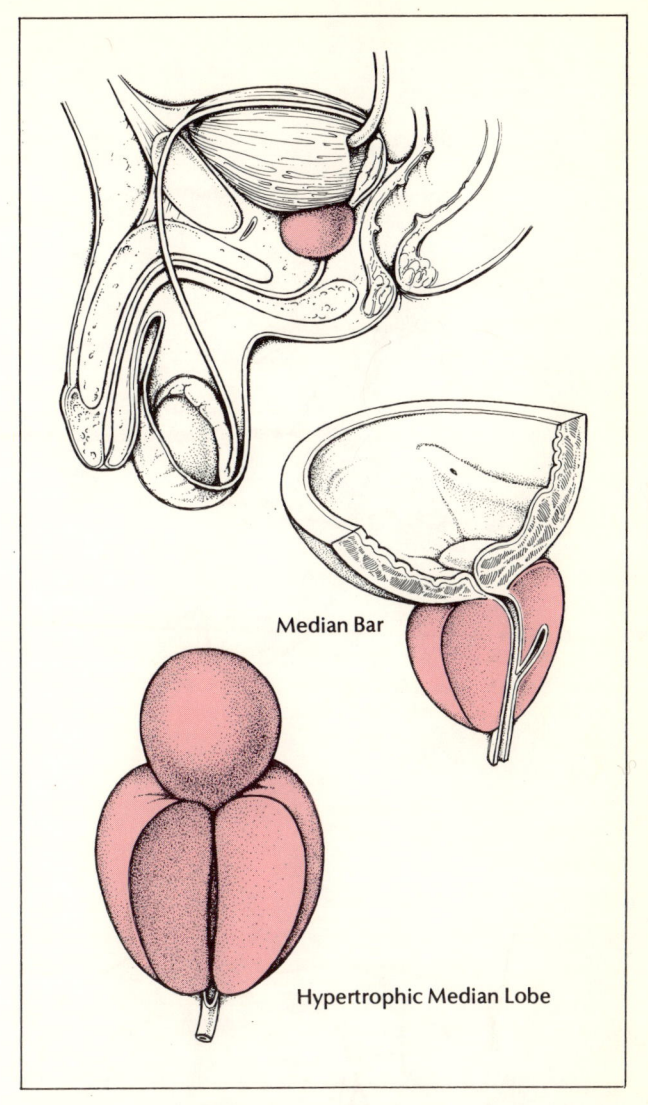

If either a median bar or a hypertrophic median lobe is responsible for the symptoms of prostatism, the gland may appear to be of normal size and contour (drawing at top) when examined rectally.

this reason its effect on prostatic hypertrophy is only partial.

Although advances in medical treatment of benign prostatic hypertrophy seem to be promising, they have not yet reached the point of real practical value. The treatment of choice is surgical, the so-called prostatectomy. The patient should be advised that this term is really a misnomer. In fact, what is excised is the periurethral adenoma, not the entire prostate. Since the prostate proper remains, and since this is where cancer originates, "prostatectomized" patients, as well as men who have not had

CHAPTER 15: BASSO

TRANSURETHRAL RESECTION (TURP)

SUPRAPUBIC

RETROPUBIC

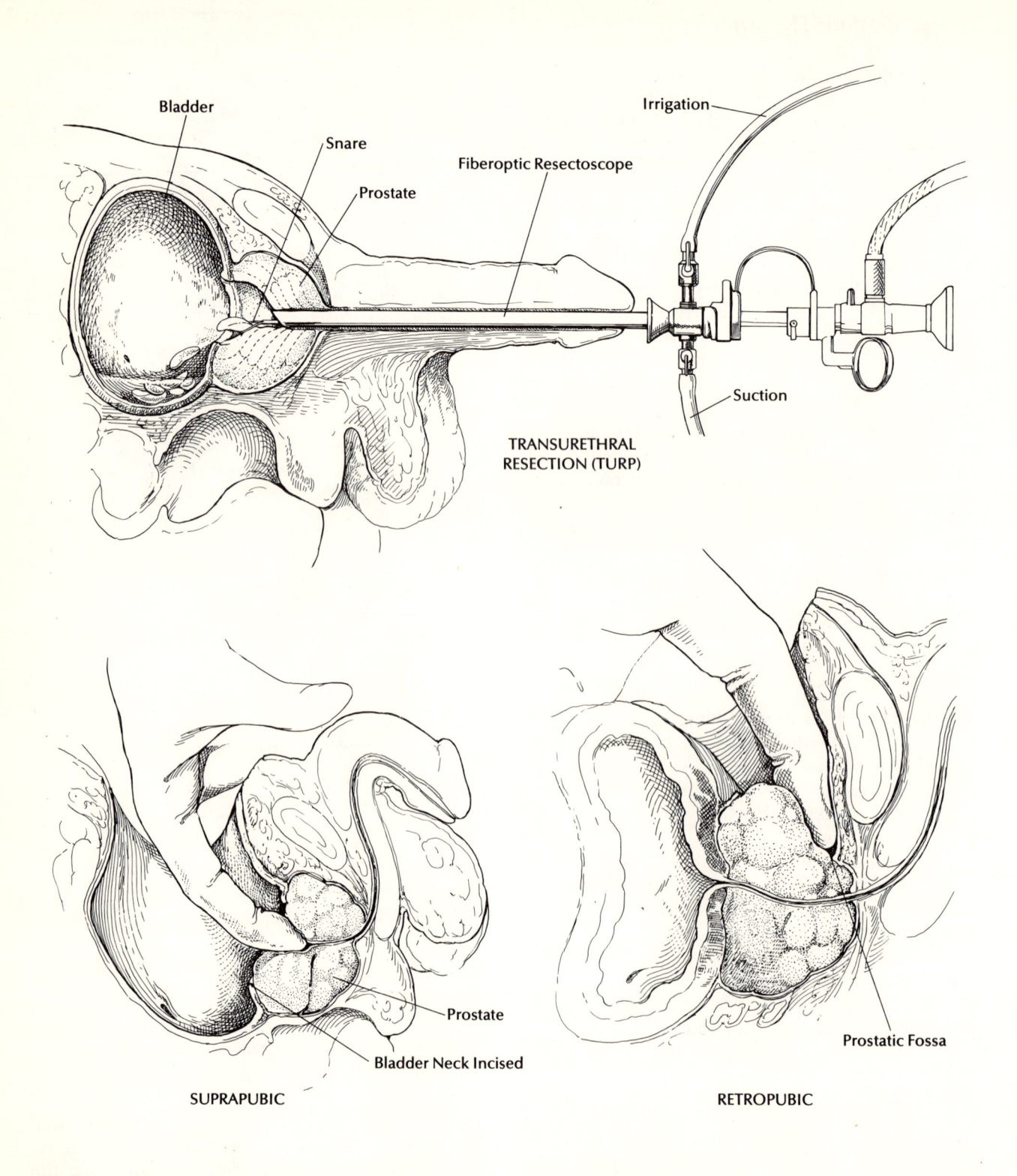

Illustrated above are some of the currently used approaches to resection of the prostate. The perineal approach to resection, not shown above, is used much less frequently than the TURP, suprapubic, and retropubic; although it may be anatomically more reasonable, it frequently causes impotence.

prostatic surgery, need to be periodically checked for malignant prostatic tumors. In fact, perhaps the most valuable role that can be played by this chapter is placing emphasis on the value of routine urologic monitoring of the geriatric patient. At least an annual checkup, which should include a rectal examination and a complete urinalysis, is recommended. If the patient has symptoms of prostatism, measurement of postvoid residual urine and determination of serum creatinine are indicated.

The measurement of postvoid residual is generally done by the urologist. It can give important information in deciding whether surgery is indicated in benign conditions. Generally, a residual of less than 50 ml in a patient with moderate symptoms of prostatism is acceptable.

Catheterization is also important in uncovering urethral strictures. When a large residual is suspected to result from long-standing obstruction, which is not infrequently associated with uremia, the procedure is best done in a hospital setting so that the patient can be monitored carefully. There is a danger that postobstructive diuresis sufficient to cause severe water and electrolyte imbalance may occur.

When frequency, nocturia, urgency, and urge incontinence are present, the possibility of an uninhibited neurogenic bladder – which is not infrequently encountered in patients with cerebrovascular insufficiency – should be considered. This evaluation is done by the specialist and is based upon the findings of a cystometrogram, plus the effects of administering such anticholinergic drugs as propantheline bromide (Pro-Banthine) and oxybutynin chloride (Ditropan). These drugs ensure relief from frequency and urge incontinence in unobstructed patients with neurogenic bladder who otherwise might be obliged to have an indwelling catheter.

When surgical treatment is indicated, it is important for the physician to explain to the patient that the procedures most often used to excise prostatic adenoma (transurethral resection and supra- or retro-pubic "prostatectomy") do not disturb innervation of the erectile system, and only rarely result in impotence (about 5% after TURP, according to Finkle and Prian). Indeed in many patients, postoperative impotence is psychogenic, particularly in the case of the older man who is convinced that the need for this operation confirms his senescence. One easily understands how important counseling may be in such situations (see Chapter 16, "Sex Counseling," by Glover). In contrast, however, perineal enucleation of prostatic adenoma frequently causes impotence. This is the main reason for its decreased popularity, in spite of the fact that this operation is more anatomical and less traumatic than other modalities of "open" prostatectomy.

Physicians should keep in mind that transurethral resection of the prostate (TURP), and suprapubic and retropubic prostatectomy will produce some degree of incompetence of the bladder neck with consequent retrograde ejaculation. While this will not interfere with erection and ejaculatory sensation, it will produce sterility.

The surgical procedure used most frequently is the TURP. If the prostatic enlargement is massive or if vesical lesions such as calculi or diverticula are present, the preference is for open procedures.

The current mortality rate for these procedures is less than 1% (Grayhack and Sadlowsky), even though many patients are poor risks because of their age and cardiopulmonary status.

The limitations on the use of TURP are associated primarily with the size and the configuration of the hypertrophic tissue. There is no general agreement on the prostatic size that is "ideal" for a TURP: the training and the skill of the urologist are important factors in this decision. Obviously, the configuration of the gland is important and also the presence or absence of urethral strictures, or, as already mentioned, of vesical lesions.

In general, it is important to limit the resection time to 60 or 90 minutes at the most. If the resection is any longer, chances of complications, such as hemodilution from absorption of irrigating fluid or late strictures, are much higher.

The resection should be complete in order to prevent bleeding, postoperative infection, and delayed healing of the prostatic fossa. Tunnel resection, sometimes used in high-risk patients with large prostates, is to be avoided whenever possible.

Whatever the procedure used, spinal anesthesia is preferred by many urologists not only for the lowered risk in patients with various forms of pulmonary insufficiency but also because the immediate postoperative course is much more comfortable, with fewer bladder spasms and less pain. Furthermore, with a TURP this type of anesthesia is a must because it will allow the patient to report abdominal pain should the bladder be perforated (an event that occurs in less than 1% of cases).

Generally, recovery is much quicker after TURP, as opposed to an open procedure. This is due mainly to the fact that an external incision is not necessary. After a TURP, the patient retains an indwelling cath-

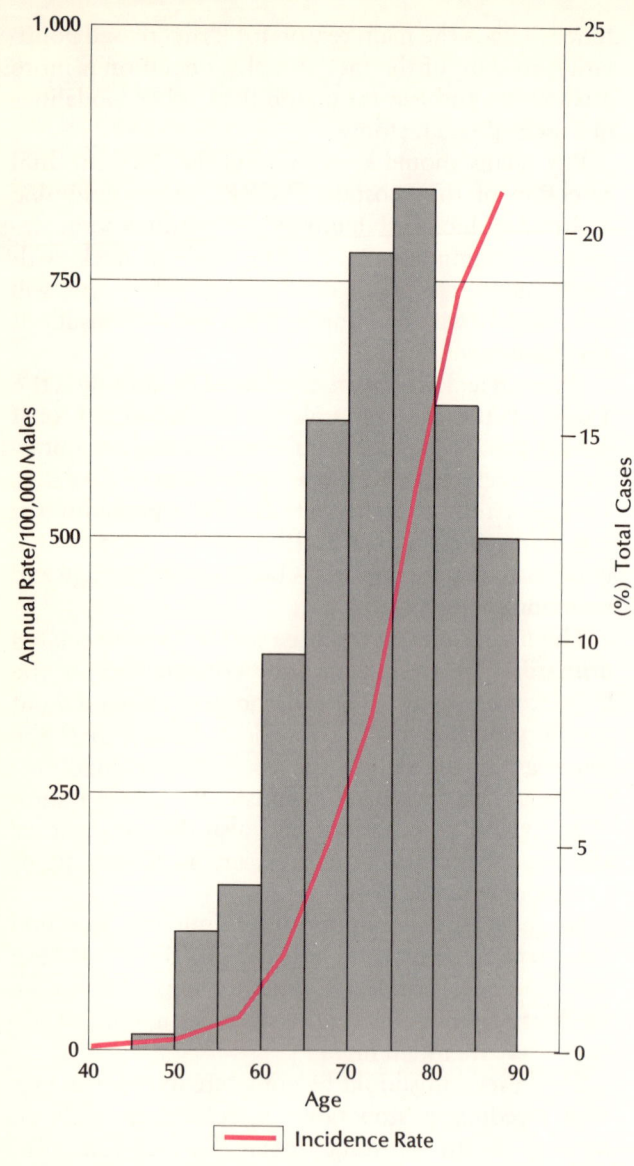

Adenocarcinoma of the prostate is especially prevalent in older men, with sharp acceleration in incidence after age 60. This carcinoma is the third leading cause of cancer deaths in men (data from Silverberg).

eter for about three days. By then gross hematuria has usually cleared, and the patient is able to urinate on his own. He will be ready for discharge a few days later.

After the catheter is removed, it is not infrequent for some degree of urgency and urgency incontinence to be present. This is transitory and the patient should be so informed. The incidence of *true incontinence* after surgery for benign prostatic hypertrophy is low (0.5% or less, according to Bergman et al, Millin et al, O'Connor et al, etc.).

When impotence occurs despite psychologic preparation, continued explanation and sexual counseling, and if the possibility of an organic cause exists, a prosthesis may be recommended for the patient who is well motivated to use it.

At the present time there are two types of prosthesis most commonly used. A pliable silicone rod that is inserted into each corpus cavernosum in order to create a permanent erection (Small-Carrion prosthesis) is one type. The other is a hydraulic device: when erection is desired, the patient manipulates a subcutaneous pump, and fluid is released into the two-cylindrical prosthesis inside the corpora cavernosa producing an erection; the content of the prosthesis is drained by activating another pump, thus ending the erection (Scott-Bradley-Timm prosthesis).

The Nonsurgical Patient

Thus far we have considered the patient who is willing to undergo surgery and whose lesion is operable. What about the patient who does not accept a surgical procedure or whose disease is inoperable? An indwelling catheter can afford him relief from obstruction, but there are risks of urinary tract infections, calculus formation, and recurrent encrustation of catheters, with subsequent obstruction.

One should keep in mind that this patient eventually will develop bacteriuria. Also, attempts to sterilize the urine or to prevent infections with suppressive drugs are futile and sometimes dangerous, because colonies of highly resistant bacteria will develop and will make the control of sepsis, if it occurs, much more difficult. Only symptomatic infections will need treatment with appropriate medications.

This type of patient will do better if care is taken to use catheters made of inert material, such as silicone. Most important of all, a closed system with good flow should be provided together with meticulous meatal care, good lubrication, and removal of encrustations.

The size of the catheter is also important. Generally a No. 16 or 18 French will suffice. A larger catheter may allow better flow, but because of the tight fit against the urethral wall, it will prevent drainage of urethral secretions, increasing the risk of acute infection and bacteremia.

Patients with indwelling catheters need specialized care, and one should not forget that the mortality from gram-negative septicemia is far higher than the mortality from surgery. Thus the decision to employ the catheter should be taken after careful and exhaustive clinical evaluation, and never solely for the convenience of the personnel who must care for the patient.

Adenocarcinoma of the Prostate

This carcinoma is the third leading cause of cancer deaths in men, according to Silverberg. While the incidence of benign prostatic hypertrophy rises after age 50, prostatic carcinoma is more common in the seventh decade of life and later. Geriatric patients may have both diseases at the same time.

As noted earlier, the prostate in benign hypertrophy feels uniformly enlarged, smooth, and elastic at rectal examination. By contrast, a circumscribed or diffuse induration is generally characteristic of carcinoma. Naturally, the clinical suspicion of cancer must be confirmed by biopsy. This is most commonly done by means of special needles introduced into the suspected area transperineally or transrectally; less frequently, an open biopsy by a perineal route may be necessary.

Since prostatic carcinoma usually originates from the prostate proper or the periphery of the gland, the symptoms of prostatism occur only when the tumor is far advanced locally. The early-stage carcinomas, which are amenable to successful long-term therapy, are generally detected in the asymptomatic patient during a routine physical examination.

How should the prostatic carcinoma be treated? This is a very difficult question to answer, as witness the disparity of opinions that are expressed in the urologic literature.

Without any question, carcinoma of the prostate is a serious disease and should not be considered lightly. Treatment depends mostly on the stage of the lesion and on the age of the patient. Tumors have little invasive potential in patients in their late seventies or eighties.

The staging system most commonly used at the present time was introduced by Whitmore in 1956. It is based on digital examination of the prostate and on the presence or absence of metastasis that can be

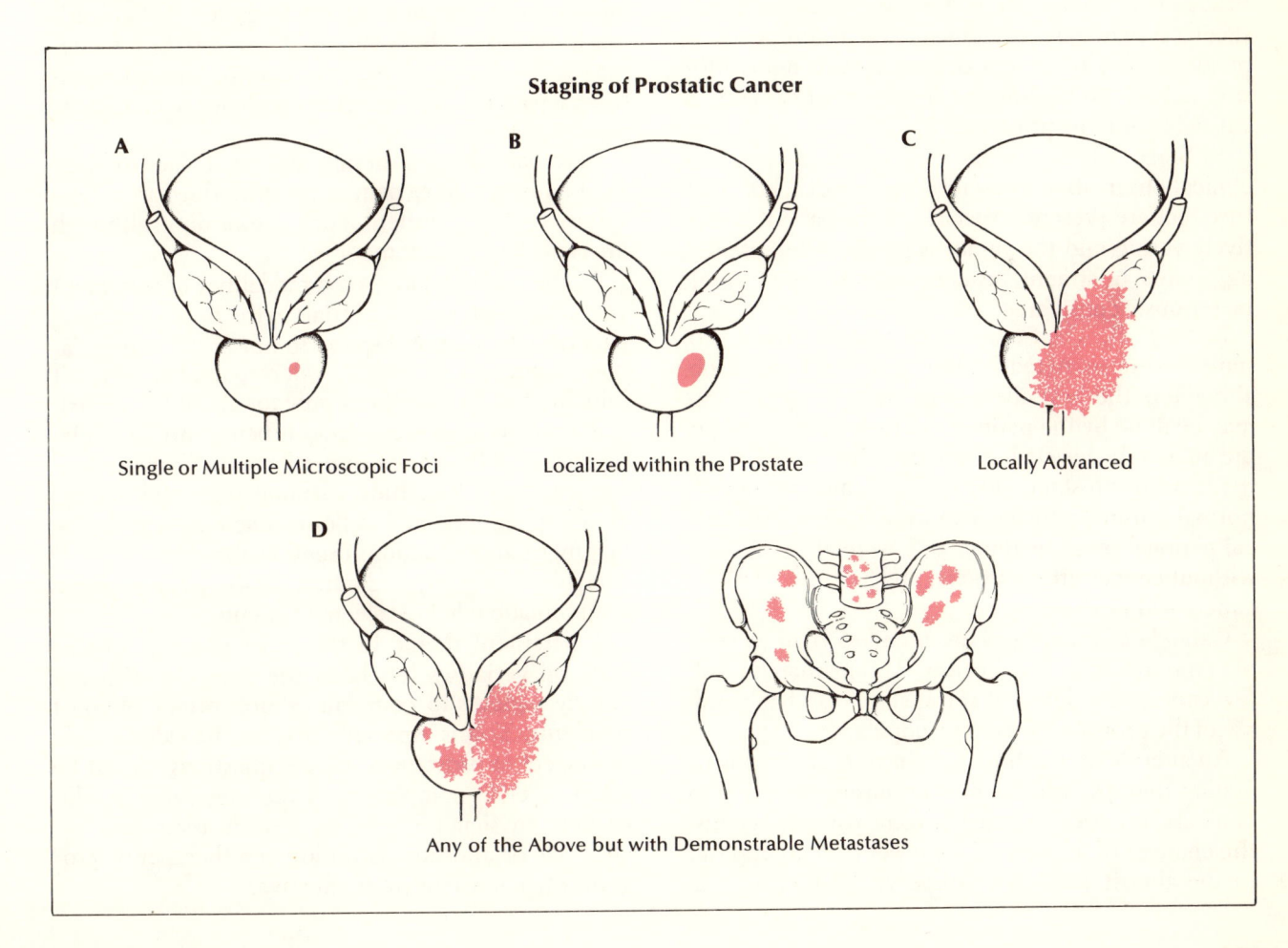

Staging of Prostatic Cancer

A — Single or Multiple Microscopic Foci

B — Localized within the Prostate

C — Locally Advanced

D — Any of the Above but with Demonstrable Metastases

demonstrated clinically by radiography, serum acid phosphatases, bone scan, etc.

Stage A represents the clinically unsuspected cancer identified during microscopic examination of prostatic tissue removed to relieve obstruction. In Stage B the cancer appears localized within the prostate; in the more advanced Stage C, the tumor extends beyond the prostatic capsule, but as in Stages A and B, there is no clinical evidence of metastasis.

The hallmark of Stage D is demonstrable metastasis. The prostate, although in many instances diffusely stony hard, irregular and nodular, could have any of the above noted characteristics at a rectal examination.

It should be kept in mind that this classification is purely clinical, and does not take into account the presence or absence of node metastasis, which can be accurately evaluated only by pelvic node dissection. The surgical staging does not necessarily correspond to the clinical one. Between 8% and 45% of Stage B tumors (Nicholson et al; Wilson et al) and 50% to 75% of Stage C tumors (McLaughlin et al; Bruce et al) have node metastasis. Thus a different staging system may be adopted in the future, because prognosis and treatment of tumors with node diffusion is likely to be different from that of cancers localized within the prostate.

In Stage A tumors when only one focus is noted, clinical observation alone is recommended; but if diffuse foci are present, especially if the patient is relatively young and the tumor is poorly differentiated, aggressive treatment, usually radiotherapy, should be seriously considered.

In Stage B, when only a well circumscribed prostatic nodule is noted, radical prostatectomy probably offers the best chances of cure; this procedure may be done by the perineal route or with a retropubic approach. Jewett has reported that out of 86 patients with prostatic nodules and microscopically normal seminal vesicles who were treated with radical perineal prostatectomy, 33% were alive and well without cancer after 15 years, and 43% died without cancer within 15 years.

Candidates for surgery are men less than 70 years old who are otherwise healthy. Unfortunately, only few cancers are detected at this stage – probably only 5% of the prostatic carcinoma population.

An alternative treatment in Stage B patients is radiation therapy, which offers promising results (Ray et al) and is better accepted by some patients because the chances of impotence are fewer (30% as opposed to the almost 100% after surgery). Neither does irradiation cause incontinence, which is present in about 5% of the patients treated surgically. Radiation therapy may also be administered by interstitial implantation of ^{125}I (Hilaus, Whitmore, Grabstald, and Batata).

When the cancer is locally advanced (Stage C), radiation therapy is generally recommended. At this stage, also, results are encouraging (Ray et al).

Finally, in Stage D, when metastases are present, hormonal manipulation (estrogens and castration) appears to be indicated. The prognosis for these patients is not good, since only a small percentage, according to Nesbit and Baum, will survive five years from the time of diagnosis. However, a distinct group of these patients may enjoy a perfectly normal life and many will experience relief from symptoms.

As a rule, only patients with symptomatic metastasis should be treated, because it has been demonstrated that the effects of hormonal therapy are not permanent, and the physician treating an asymptomatic patient with hormonal manipulation may have nothing to offer at a later stage, when symptoms appear. Also, it should not be forgotten that according to results of the Veterans Administration Cooperative Urological Research Group, the estrogen-treated patients have a higher incidence of cardiovascular problems.

External radiation therapy also has a place in Stage D, mainly to relieve pain in circumscribed areas. Response to this treatment is often rewarding, although life expectancy is not modified.

At the present time, new modalities of treatment are being used in clinical trials in the hope of helping patients who do not respond to hormonal manipulation (about 70% of patients will respond to treatment initially, but 80% of them only for about two years). The evaluation of these drugs is being carried out by the National Prostatic Cancer Project. From preliminary results of this study, estramustine sulphate, cyclophosphamide, and 5-flourouracil appear to be helpful in such situations (Scott et al).

Hypophysectomy and adrenalectomy can produce symptomatic relief in selected patients.

A persistent theme in the other chapters of this book on geriatrics has been the reticence of many elderly patients to complain about serious physical problems. This is especially true for the elderly male in respect to prostatism. Direct questions should be asked to elicit complaints. A routine review by the primary physician may either provide assurance that all is well or indicate institution of a therapeutic program when it will be most effective.

16

Sex Counseling

BENJAMIN H. GLOVER
University of Wisconsin

That sexual desire and expression are normal in the elderly is commonly appreciated by physicians today. But, unfortunately, this appreciation is not necessarily translated into clinical practice. When an elderly patient presents with a problem that may be wholly or partially one of sexual expression, the opportunity for helpful discussion and counseling is too often missed. The patient's denials (of either sexual difficulties or interest) are let stand, or there is a referral which, in effect, surrenders the long-term rapport most favorable to patient-physician communication.

Why does this happen? Perhaps a discussion with the patient on the subject of sex is imagined to be mutually uncomfortable, not worth the time in a busy office practice, or something that simply is not done with patients older than the physician or of a different sex. Perhaps the physician realizes that, beyond general knowledge, he or she has little specific information concerning what is appropriate sexual activity for the elderly. Or perhaps the physician is unfamiliar or uneasy with the approaches to eliciting information and/or to providing counseling in the primary care setting.

It may be that on both sides of the consulting room desk are nonperformance fears: the patient's problems may arise out of fear of the embarrassment attendant upon disclosure of failure of sexual performance; the physician fears inability to perform as counselor on sexual matters. I am convinced there is much the primary physician can do that is helpful in giving the elderly patient an appropriate perspective on her or his sexuality. As a matter of fact, most elderly patients do not have such deep-seated sexual problems that referral to a specialist is necessary. Nor does the primary physician need an extensive background in sex counseling or therapeutic techniques. What is essential is the application to sexual problems of approaches characteristic of good family practice in general: promoting discussion, listening in a sympathetic, nonjudgmental way, and offering compassionate advice.

Physicians themselves possess the best practical approaches to breaking through blocks or "hang-ups" in dealing with sensitive subjects. I know of no better way than through exchange of views and information between the physician and the person or persons involved. In what follows, I would like to encourage an atmosphere of casual, practical exchange about sex-related problems as the physician may find them in 1) the elderly male, 2) the elderly female, 3) the elderly couple, and 4) the elderly patient with coronary or other disease.

The Elderly Male

Let's consider the case of an elderly patient who presents no specific symptoms but complains generally about occasional headache, backache, and skin changes that he fears may be cancer. He mentions his prostate and some vague abdominal pains. The physical examination reveals nothing unusual. The physician prescribes a lotion and tells the man to come back in six months.

But the man is back in two weeks, with the same

CHAPTER 16: GLOVER

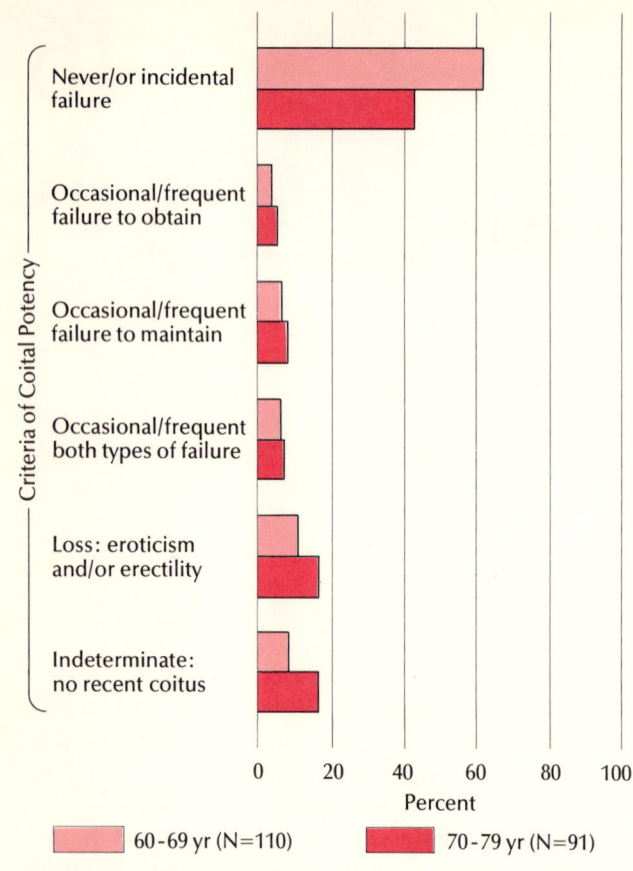

Graph of data from Martin, collected during interviews of men participating in Baltimore Longitudinal Study, shows that in seventh decade more than 60%, in eighth decade more than 40%, report retaining coital potency.

vague complaints. His visits become more frequent. The physician begins to see him as a lonely old man who is, or is becoming, hypochondriacal. For the man's apparently intensifying depression, and partly to give him "something," the physician prescribes a mild tranquilizer and dismisses him. Sensing rejection, the elderly man is not likely to come back. He probably will seek out another physician who, he hopes, will know what to do.

If he is lucky, he may find a physician willing to initiate a discussion of sexual problems. This physician may recognize that within the rambling, nonspecific complaints are clues: reiterated questions about the prostate (in the absence of discernible disease, which must be systematically sought) and complaints of vague abdominal pain are often attempts to draw attention to that region of the body.

The examination now turns to sexual function, approached in a relaxed way to encourage responsiveness. The physician puts down his pen, leans back, and says, "You know, you've never told me about your sexual function, Mr. Smith. [He does not use "granddad" or any title that may be regarded as patronizing or impersonal.] Are you having any trouble at all?" The patient, typically, denies, but the denial is telling: "I don't do that any more." The physician is not deterred by the patient's fear of being found abnormal in wanting sexual activity "at his age." He must steer the conversation back to sexuality and pose such specific questions as: "Are you having your usual amount of sexual activity? Are you getting good, solid erections, or do you find at times you have only partial erections, or sometimes you just don't succeed at all with your partner?"

He also inquires about morning erections, wet dreams, and frequency of masturbation. If present, wet dreams and morning erection indicate capacity for full potency. These physical signs can be used to reassure a patient who believes himself impotent that he is, in fact, capable of functioning with a partner. Masturbation shows that the patient can at least satisfy himself. This may be all he really wants. And the physician's observation that he can function may be enough to encourage him to venture into the social atmosphere of sexual experience. But to minimize the risk of further frustration, the patient may need to be released from the destructive attitude that good sex equals nothing less than a solid erection and vigorous orgasm every time.

I have found that many elderly patients, despite first denials, do want to talk about their sexual problems. *They welcome discussion.* Taking the sexual history may be in itself therapeutic. The physician has a good chance to perform a most important service: to reassure the patient that occasional failure to achieve erection is not a sign of impotence and that sex is more than achieving orgasm. I find I am telling such patients what they know intuitively but want affirmed: as people age, the intimacy of the sex act – the sharing, closeness, and caressing – have a meaning and pleasure that may be exquisitely real whereas achievement of orgasm is largely symbolic. With age, caressing and touching become far more satisfying as reassurances of sensory adequacy, because the sense of touch (especially in the fingertips and other highly sensitive areas) is attenuated. For this reason, oral as well as manual stimulation is of profound gratification to the elderly. Similarly, perfumes as well as pheromones tend to enhance sexual excitation via the olfactory pathways. Just lying in another person's arms may bring greater satisfaction in old age than in

SEX COUNSELING

youth. The elderly patient may be highly receptive to these observations as affirmations of his normality. Only a small number of males lose all interest in sex and the ability to function as they age.

History-taking may reveal the origin of psychogenic impotence. It may arise from any event or sequence that virtually suspends sexual activity. For example, a man who has experienced the slow death of his wife from cancer and has had no sexual activity during her illness may be offered affection, including sexual relationship, by a neighbor. Because of his memories and guilt, he is unable to function. The encounter, instead of helping to relieve the widower's depression, intensifies it. The fear of being unable to perform becomes a self-fulfilling prophecy.

The physician in our hypothetical case, while acting to open up discussion, has *not* taken certain actions. He did not refer the patient immediately to a urologist; the physical examination did not justify that. Indeed, had an unjustified referral been made, negative findings by both primary physician and specialist probably would add to the patient's despair. Interestingly enough, patients often are cheered when told that a physical cause has been found for their impotence and that they are being referred to be helped. If it is benign prostatic hypertrophy, a transurethral resection, which rarely impairs potency, is performed, and physicians must make sure that this is understood. If it is a problem requiring relearning of sexual behavior, the patient can be told that relearning is possible at any age and that the therapy may be effective within a matter of weeks.

Nor did the physician prescribe psychotropic drugs as a means of ushering the patient out of the office. For the otherwise healthy patient with sexual depression, there is nothing helpful in such tranquilizer prescriptions; they reduce sexual drive and raise the chance of further nonperformance. Moreover, when a patient is suspected of having sexual depression, an assessment must include a thorough drug history, in-

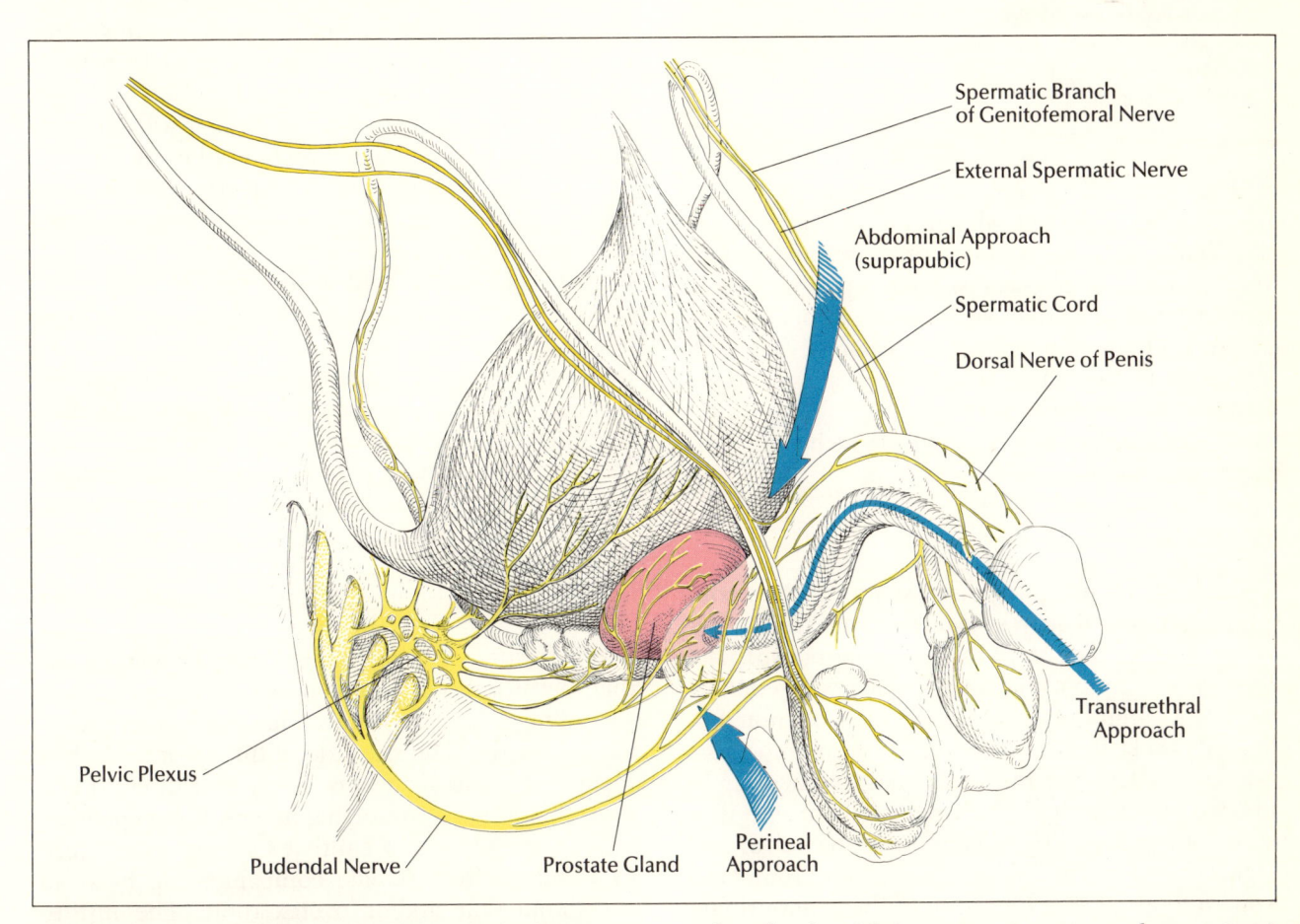

As drawing shows, surgery for benign prostatic hypertrophy by the transurethral route avoids local nerve fibers and is thus less likely to impair potency than perineal or abdominal approaches.

> **Frequent and Common Causes of Sexual Dysfunction in Males**
>
> Trying too hard
> Drugs
> Diabetes, adrenal tumors, hypothyroidism, Friedreich's disease, etc.
> Arteriosclerosis – severe
> Neurologic disease – multiple sclerosis, muscular dystrophy, stroke, brain injury
> Psychologic or psychiatric disorders – depression, manic states, anorexia nervosa, anxiety, phobias, conflicts, serious psychotic states, performance fears
> Hematologic anemias, fatigue states, physical exhaustion, cardiorespiratory embarrassment
> Toxins
> Injuries and painful states – amputations and deformities, colostomy, enterostomy, blindness, deafness, intersex states, dyspareunia and vaginismus, spinal cord injuries (though reflex and psychologic erections and/or ejaculation and potency are possible in many cases)
> Infections, febrile reactions
> Operations – prostatectomy (perineal and less often transurethral resection or suprapubic)
> Obesity, bulimia

cluding intake of alcohol, a sexual depressant. Not infrequently, a patient who has drifted into hypochondriasis may list a dozen or more medications from a variety of physicians. Such a personal pharmacopoeia may include an astounding mix of tranquilizers, tonics, stimulants, antihistamines, etc., all adding up to a crushing attack on potency. The patient may not realize that in resorting to drug stimulation to enliven a dull retirement life he has generated sexual dullness.

The Elderly Female

Much of the foregoing discussion of factors contributing to sexual depression in the male also applies to the female. The steps in evaluating nonspecific, depressive symptoms having possible sexual etiology include a careful physical examination. As noted by Dr. Glowacki in his discussion of postmenopausal women (see Chapter 13), sexual performance can be affected by such physical changes as increased dryness, thinning, and bleeding of or in the vulvar and vaginal mucosa. Painful intercourse may prompt the woman to avoid sex. Infections of the genitourinary tract also may initiate the woman's sexual withdrawal. The patient probably will be relieved to hear that these conditions are eminently treatable by topical creams, ointments, lubricants, and other measures.

The physician can use the occasion of a vaginal examination to develop a sexual history, again in a sympathetic, nonjudgmental, and specific manner. An elderly woman often is embarrassed about the strength of her sex drive vis-a-vis men of her generation; she also may be embarrassed by wrinkling and loss of breast contour; a male's nonperformance may be interpreted as her failure. For these and other reasons, masturbation is common among elderly women. About one woman in four over age 70 masturbates, and it may be the only outlet for the woman who has no male partner. Nevertheless, women tend to be more inhibited than men in accepting masturbation or even in discussing it. One gambit to open discussion is to note that a great many people masturbate, and some find it better than seeking out a partner. From her experience, does she think this is true? If the physician can persuade her to discuss her problem, the opportunity may occur for advice on how to use a vibrator and other means of enhancing masturbatory satisfaction. This may be all the patient wants and needs. I have found this to be a healthier and less dangerous method of dealing with depression and hypochondriasis than prescribing drugs.

For many elderly women, the recognition that they may have to be the one to invite or initiate a sexual encounter is very difficult. Sexual manners of a bygone era may be hard to dislodge. As with men, not only is there fear of nonperformance but grief and loneliness may have so altered sexual response that individuals feel themselves to be impotent. Women should be encouraged to talk about the fact that they have lost husbands, that their male friends have died, that lack of heterosexual opportunities has driven them into hypochondriasis, depression, homosexual relationships, or that they try to attract younger males.

If such "confessions" are forthcoming, the patient should be told that she need feel no guilt about efforts to survive emotionally. It may be pointed out that, because women outlive men by eight years on the average, they may indeed have to be more sexually aggressive. The sex ratio of three women to two men in the late sixties gives way to a three to one ratio at later ages. In nursing homes, the preponderance of women is so great that some men are forced to withdraw from female companionship to avoid overstimulation and/or overexertion. The institutional response often is to attempt to control the women with tranquilizers.

The elderly woman may benefit from being told that males of her age require patience in achieving erection and ejaculation. If the male appears to have difficulty, she can help in such ways as stuffing the flaccid penis into the vagina, by stimulating and massaging, and by giving verbal encouragement. She should be told that, as men age, they enjoy the texture of fabric and skin, the odors of perfume, and conversation about old times – all of which can be employed to enhance the enjoyment of sex. She may be counseled, along with the male, that there is nothing wrong with exploring different sexual positions, so that excitement and comfort are attained. Nor is there anything perverse about a sexual encounter that gives one partner an orgasm while the other enjoys the intimacy without orgasm. The woman should be told that failure of a partner to have orgasm is no basis for a feeling of guilt or inadequacy on her part.

The Elderly Couple

Couples who have grown old together often adapt their sexual activity naturally, changing their earlier athleticism to something less strenuous but appropriately satisfying.

However, some couples find sex alienating or impossible because of chronic conflicts, communication difficulties, and different appetites. The extended refractory period of the male in achieving erection may lead to nonperformance fear and limitations on coitus, to the wife's distress. (By calling attention to the disorder and telling him to see the doctor, she may exacerbate it.) Similarly, the elderly woman with increased vulvar irritability may find the penis abrasive and resist her husband's advances. Dyspareunia and vaginismus can result. The failure of sexual activity may produce conflicts and withdrawals in what had been a warm relationship.

Many failures in sexual activity may have nonsexual origins – in guilt about the way children turned out, or in fault-finding about missed business or social opportunities. Failure of the couple to maintain communication and enjoyment of each other often is manifested in sexual avoidance. The physician is told that because the partner is uninterested in sex, the patient is planning an extramarital affair. The patient is seeking the physician's approval. Care should be taken to make no overt judgment of the patient's plans; the professional concern is not the sanction of a style of living but the maintenance of the patient's stability. The time may be ripe for bringing the partners together to communicate.

Once the door is opened, the elderly are grateful to have a discussion over why their rapport is dying. If communication can be restored, the couple often finds renewed enjoyment in sexual activity. The prognosis depends on a couple's style in meeting the stresses of life, and this is often well estimated by the physician who has attended them over the years.

Drugs Often Used by Elderly That Tend To Suppress Libido

Antispasmodics-Anticholinergics
- Diphenhydramine
- Propantheline bromide
- Atropine
- Trihexyphenidyl

Sedatives
- Barbiturates
- Antasthmatics
- Alcohol
- Flurazepam

Narcotics
- Codeine
- Meperidine
- Oxycodone
- Heroin

Antihypertensives
- Chlorothiazide
- Guanethidine
- Hydralazine
- Rauwolfia alkaloids
- Pargyline
- Methyldopa

Antianxiety Agents (in large doses causing CNS depression)
- Meprobamate
- Diazepam
- Chlordiazepoxide
- Oxazepam
- Clorazepate dipotassium

Antidepressants
- Tricyclics
- Monoamine oxidase inhibitors (MAOI)

Stimulants
- Epinephrine
- Amphetamines
- Caffeine (small amounts)
- Anorexic agents
- Methylphenidate
- Ephedrine

Tranquilizers
- Phenothiazines
- Thioxanthenes
- Butyrophenones
- Dihydroindolones
- Haloperidol

Evaluating Sexual Problems in the Elderly

```
Patient Complaints
─────────────────
"Nerves"
Fatigue, lassitude, general weakness
Indigestion
Nonspecific abdominal pains
Urinary tract complaints with findings
Backaches and headaches
Loss of interest in anything
Weight and appetite loss
Irascibility, querulousness
Excessive sleep in daytime
Loss of sexual interest, function, or contact
            │
            ▼
  Drug History and Dosages
            │
            ▼
 Physical Exam Including Genital Exam
       │             │
       ▼             ▼
Obtain sex history    If physical and
and ascertain pres-   genital exam suggest,
ent sex practices     refer to specialist
       │                    │
       ▼                    ▼
Relationship to:       Urologist
Complaints             Gynecologist
Consultations          Psychiatrist
Social limitations     Proctologist
Religious and          Cardiologist
other constraints      Internist
       │                    │
       ▼                    │
Office counseling or referral to specialist
```

The same familiarity may put the physician in the best position to provide information and advice as well as to discern functional behavioral disorders in one or both partners. These may well be treatable through modalities available to the primary physician (see Chapter 4, "Functional Psychiatric Disorders," by Joffe).

Patients with Physical Disability

Patients with chronic illness may forego the pleasure of sex unnecessarily because they have never been informed that sexuality can be expressed safely within limits. For example, patients with cardiac disabilities may stop sexual activity for fear of dying or having precordial pain during intercourse.

The fact is that the sex act is not extremely stressful to the body. Documented instances of death during intercourse are rare. The average energetic sex act is estimated to require only 150 calories. The heart rate is much higher during treadmill testing of cardiac patients, and the death rate in these circumstances is only 1 per 10,000 tests. The average pulse rate in intercourse is about 117, with a high of 144, a low of 90, and a very rapid return to preactivity levels. (Masters and Johnson have reported a high of 180 and a low of 110.) The heart may beat faster, longer, during a brisk walk or an angry discussion.

Unfortunately, cardiac patients may get little of this information and little or no advice on resuming intercourse. The general rule is resumption three months after myocardial infarction. The level of sexual activity is restored to precoronary status in one third of patients following this rule, while two thirds sustain some permanently reduced level. Patients can be told that energy demands can be reduced by lying on the side or by having the partner on top and doing the oscillations. Coronary and angina patients, if they feel the slightest strain, can rest a while and resume. Nitroglycerin to prevent angina may be taken before intercourse. Even Grade IV and some Grade III coronary patients, who should avoid exercise sufficient for orgasm, can enjoy sexual activity in modified form: the closeness, warmth, and other sensory experience that augments intimacy. (Advice to have sex in this form also may be appropriate to patients impotent because of neural pathology in diabetes, spinal cord trauma, or other disease.)

In general, patients may assume invalidly that they must restrict sexual expression because of the common infirmities of old age. It may be quite helpful for the physician to make a point of telling the elderly patient that a particular condition need not eliminate or reduce sexual activity. Arthritis and osteoporosis, for example, unless unusually crippling, present no sexual problems. In such instances, or in cases of partial paralysis, satisfaction may be achieved through oral or anal stimulation. Many elderly patients do not readily accept this, of course, but I have often seen this attitude change.

Adaptations of conventional sexual stimulation may be advised on a temporary as well as a permanent basis. The patient with a recent hernia repair may have to refrain temporarily from coitus because of discomfort. The patient should be reassured that the discomfort will disappear, and that other forms of sexuality can be enjoyed until healing is complete. For patients with fractures, the physician can recommend positioning and other aids to sexual function.

Accommodations in chemotherapy also may be necessary. I have pointed out the enhancement if not production of sexual depression by tranquilizers and other psychotropic drugs. Many medications used to treat cardiovascular diseases, including hypertension, can have sexually depressing effects, too. The physician faces a conflict when a patient, burdened by fear of sexual nonperformance, requires such drugs. One must separate the pharmacologic from the emotional. Often, the dosage really is insufficient to inhibit sex (as witnessed by the patient's report of an occasional morning erection), and equally often, the dosage can be reduced or a substitute drug can be found that controls the disease without impairing sexual function.

Adaptations in chemotherapy may be based on timing of the dose. For example, tricyclic drugs are often prescribed to be taken in one dose at night; this timing may interfere with sexual expression and could be altered to an afternoon dose. Alternatively, the physician could advise the patient to have intercourse at a time when the drug's effect is weak, as in the first hour or so after ingestion of a psychotropic drug or after the fifth or sixth hour of a sedative.

The sexually depressing effects of drugs or diseases should be made clear so that patients do not confuse pharmacologically induced performance failures with true impotence.

Referrals

Patients should be referred when their impotence has been unresponsive to treatment, when they have severe dysfunctions (i.e., unusual dyspareunia and vaginismus), and when they demonstrate destructive tendencies or compulsions. Included in the last category is masturbation by insertion of pins, sticks, and other objects into the genitourinary tract. The obsessive group includes persons who feel they are destined by some deity to inseminate the world or to save it by attracting males. The persons whose chronic neurosis manifests itself in an uncontrollable need to masturbate constantly should be managed by a specialist. Patients with strong suicidal views – who indicate they have taken steps to end a life that seems to hold nothing for them but more loneliness and failure – should not only be referred but taken to the consultant at once for therapy and protection. Some child molesters (nonviolent) are often very inadequate people who have serious communication problems with their own age group. The destructive molesters are a far more serious group, usually psychiatrically very ill. Both groups usually require long and difficult individual and family therapy.

Referrals may be made to known and qualified marital or sex counselors as well as to appropriate medical specialists – urologists, psychiatrists, gynecologists, etc. Unfortunately, financial considerations may deter an elderly person from seeing a specialist or attending sex clinics for counseling, training in sensate focus, relaxation exercises, and so on.

When symptoms of sexual depression reveal an extended history of untreated venereal disease or other genitourinary tract infection, the patient should be referred to a specialist immediately. In eliciting this history, the physician should try to minimize any guilt the patient might feel by noting that anyone can acquire an infection of the genital tract (and avoid the term "venereal disease"). Ordinarily, the primary physician can deal with genital, including prostatic, infections. In the case of sexually related symptoms of chronic prostatitis, a referral of the patient for urologic evaluation connected with possible intrusive procedures should be made with precautions. Whether the patient asks or not, he should be told explicitly that a procedure does not produce untoward sexual effects; otherwise, the patient may make the assumption – silently – and become impotent. Likewise, the woman referred for genitourinary surgery should be told, if the facts justify it, that there probably will be no untoward sexual effects.

When it is a younger male physician treating an elderly woman with a genitourinary problem, it is all the more important for a truly nonjudgmental attitude to be conveyed. The necessary search for a venereal contact is a matter of delicacy, of course, in patients of both sexes. My approach is to say, "You

Q&A* for Physicians on Sex in the Aging
(More than one answer may be correct)

1. The most vulnerable male sexual function with increasing age is:
   a. homosexuality
   b. ejaculation
   c. erection
   d. refractory period
   e. tactile sensation

2. Improving the institutional setting to maintain sexual experience for the aged includes:
   a. ensuring privacy
   b. providing double beds
   c. encouraging social permissiveness
   d. retraining for an understanding staff
   e. all of the above
   f. none of the above

3. Control of female sexual behavior in the institutionalized aged exists largely because:
   a. of strong childhood and adolescent taboos
   b. of fear of social ostracism from peers
   c. lesbianism is illegal
   d. masturbation does not occur in this age group
   e. none of the above
   f. of staff functioning as wardens

4. Regular sexual activity for the aged can:
   a. maintain sex hormone levels
   b. extend sexual functions throughout life
   c. satisfy only if with a consenting partner
   d. delay social and personal deterioration
   e. be salutary in those with moderate cardiopulmonary diseases
   f. require less work than climbing a long flight of stairs

5. Impotence in the aged:
   a. may be related to the incest taboo of the young
   b. is commonly associated with performance fear in the female
   c. is normal for males over 62 years
   d. is to be expected in postmenopausal women
   e. need not be a consequence of prostatectomy
   f. occurs in two thirds of males following cardiac disease
   g. can be restored by injections of testosterone
   h. all of the above

6. Practicing physicians working with the aged:
   a. need only facts to treat sexual disorders
   b. must be able to elicit fears of patients
   c. have found group discussions effective in exploring sexual problems
   d. often need to reeducate staff as well as patients in institutional settings concerning sexuality
   e. should not stress orgasm as a goal in enrichment of life

7. *Match*

a. single-again performance-guilt sexual dysfunction	1. use-or-lose rule
b. expectation-demand block	2. death-in-the-saddle
c. coronary death with illicit sex	3. widower's syndrome
d. continued sex activity for life	4. malcommunication
e. greatest cause of sexual incapacity	5. "performance" inadequacy

*For answers, see opposite page

---

have an infection that we must take care of, for your sake and the other person's. If it is likely to spread, we have to find that individual. We won't use your name, of course." It is important to avoid reactions of scorn or hostility that will deter patient compliance with medications and follow-up. To encourage cooperation, the physician should be calm and casual, emphasizing health needs of the patient and staying away from religious and social judgments.

Whether for medical or other reasons, the manner of making a referral is crucial. The patient must recognize that he or she is not being fobbed off. The best maneuver is for the physician to contact the specialist by telephone in the patient's presence and set the tone for an appointment at a time agreeable to patient and specialist. Simply handing the patient the name of a specialist may be useless; patients often do not follow through and may never return to the primary physician.

It should be kept in mind that some older persons have been socially withdrawn much of their lives and do not wish to improve their sexual adaptations. They are difficult to work with because they deny that anything needs to be done. Such individuals, nonetheless, may be willing to see a specialist at their physician's urging. If they follow through to an appointment, there may be a chance of benefit.

Physicians can do much to promote the idea that

sexual relations among the elderly are natural and to be encouraged. They can be of profound help in maintaining mental, physical, and emotional well-being. However, the elderly have their own ways of making love; these may have nothing to do with the sexual prowess of youth but rather focus on intimacy and sharing of each other's body and mind.

Many sexual problems of the elderly are amenable to the interventions of the primary physician. Some elderly persons abstain from sex, lose potency unnecessarily, and show no untoward symptoms. Those whose well-being is damaged by sexual depression may ask for help in the language of hypochondriasis and nonspecific complaints. They should be recognized and assisted.

To do this, the physician has to overcome misconceptions about sex in old age. The view that sexual behavior inexorably vanishes with old age is not true. To the contrary, sexual behavior is a learned pattern; it can be badly learned and perpetuated; it can be thrown out of gear; it can be relearned and improved upon – at any time in life – if the individual is freed of taboo and misconception. The last place the patient should find disapproval or dismissal of his or her struggle against performance fears, myths of sexual termination, and social disparagement of sex in old age is in the office of the primary or family physician. Total functional loss is unnecessary at any age, in male or female.

Answers:

1 c, 2 e, 3 a, b, f, 4 a, b, d, e, f, 5 a, e, 6 b, c, d, e, 7 a-3, b-5, c-2, d-1, e-4

17

Skin Care and Problems

DEREK J. CRIPPS
University of Wisconsin

As with other organs, how the aging process affects the skin will ultimately depend on its inherited vulnerability to the stresses of the environment, one example of which is sunlight. Typically, the skin gradually becomes dry, yellow, and wrinkled in the old, with lentigines, seborrheic keratoses, and other unwelcome blemishes, while the hair becomes gray and often sparse. Yellowing and thickening are likely to be prominent on areas exposed to sunlight and are caused by the degeneration of elastic and collagen tissue in the dermis. Production of sebum and sweat is often reduced in the elderly, and the epidermis in particular is often thin and atrophic. While the pathophysiology of aging in the skin is poorly understood, generalized changes such as atherosclerosis of dermal arterioles may be one of the factors involved.

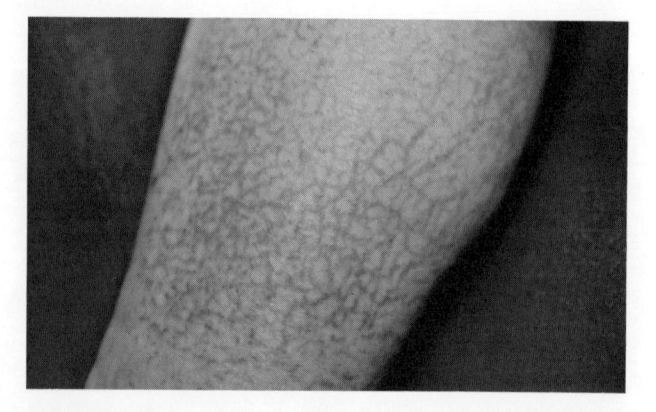

Severe xerosis (erythema craquele) of the lower leg shows typical reticulation and rhomboidal scaling.

Pruritus is one of the more common symptoms in the elderly, and although internal disorders may be responsible and will be discussed, pruritus is usually related to dryness. Desiccation of the stratum corneum, the outer keratin layer of the skin, occurs in conditions of lowered humidity, such as are produced by central heating, desert climates, or drying cold winds. Pruritus that occurs in the fall and winter is described by dermatologists as pruritus hiemalis. Pruritus usually appears on the limbs, particularly on the lower legs, and in severe xerosis a typical pattern of reticulated erythema and rhomboidal scaling has been aptly described as erythema craquele. Control of environment can be achieved not only by living in (or moving to) coastal regions where humidity is higher, but by making sure that the house or the place of work or leisure is adequately humidified with an attachment to the heating system or by using separate room humidifiers to modify the winter dryness of the ambient air.

Recognition of pruritus hiemalis can be made by direct observation or from a history that itching increases when the patient first gets into bed and that he is troubled by the presence of static electricity. While bathing of the skin will achieve hydration of the stratum corneum, shortly afterward the water evaporates and the result is that the skin is further dried. Patients should not be told to avoid bathing but rather to lubricate the skin immediately thereafter with an ointment such as Aquaphor (95% petrolatum), which traps the moisture. Creams, which can be defined as water with oil droplets, are not sufficient to relieve dryness unless the condition is very mild. Bathing in water that is too hot or using detergent soaps, bubble baths, or sodium bicarbonate will aggravate dryness. A common mistake in bed bathing of the elderly is the use of soapy water. If it is not adequately rinsed off, the soap that remains on the skin intensifies the dryness. Subsequent lubrication with an ointment is also indicated. Instead of using soapy water, mineral oils can be added to the bath water; these usually contain a surfactant that makes the oil miscible with water, and this may be sufficient for cleansing. (Example: Lubath, Alpha-Keri bath oil.) Cotton underwear, which should not be wrinkled, is useful to protect the skin from irritation by woolen garments or synthetic fabrics.

Sometimes an allergic contact dermatitis may result from wearing clothing that contains dyes such as paraphenylenediamine, or from the formalin in permanent press fabrics, rubber, the dichromates in leather, and metals such as nickel. Such contact dermatitis is more likely to be recognized by the physician and patient than an allergic reaction to topical medications, particularly if the latter are initially used to treat the dermatitis. Such offenders include the caines (i.e., benzocaine and cyclomethycaine [Surfacaine]), neomycin, preservatives in creams such as methyl and ethyl parabens or ethylenediamine. These causes of dermatitis are not limited to the elderly, nor are other exogenous causes such as scabies or lice, which may well occur in institutions or nursing homes.

Following is a summary of therapeutic suggestions in xerosis:

1. Soak with cool baths daily if the patient prefers.
2. Avoid detergent soaps, bubble baths, and sodium bicarbonate and use only mild superfatted soaps, such as Oilatum.
3. Trap skin moisture with Aquaphor after bathing. Once the dryness has been relieved, Eucerin, which is equal parts of Aquaphor and water, may be used.
4. Avoid moisturizing creams or lotions, which are too dry.
5. Relief of pruritus can often be achieved if ¼% menthol is added to Eucerin. If corticosteroids are used, 1% hydrocortisone is usually sufficient.
6. Wear smooth unwrinkled cotton next to skin.
7. Ensure that the atmosphere is adequately moist either by modifying the central heating system appropriately or by adding a bedroom and/or living room humidifier.
8. Avoid situations that contribute to poor sleep, since increased awareness of itching at night may not

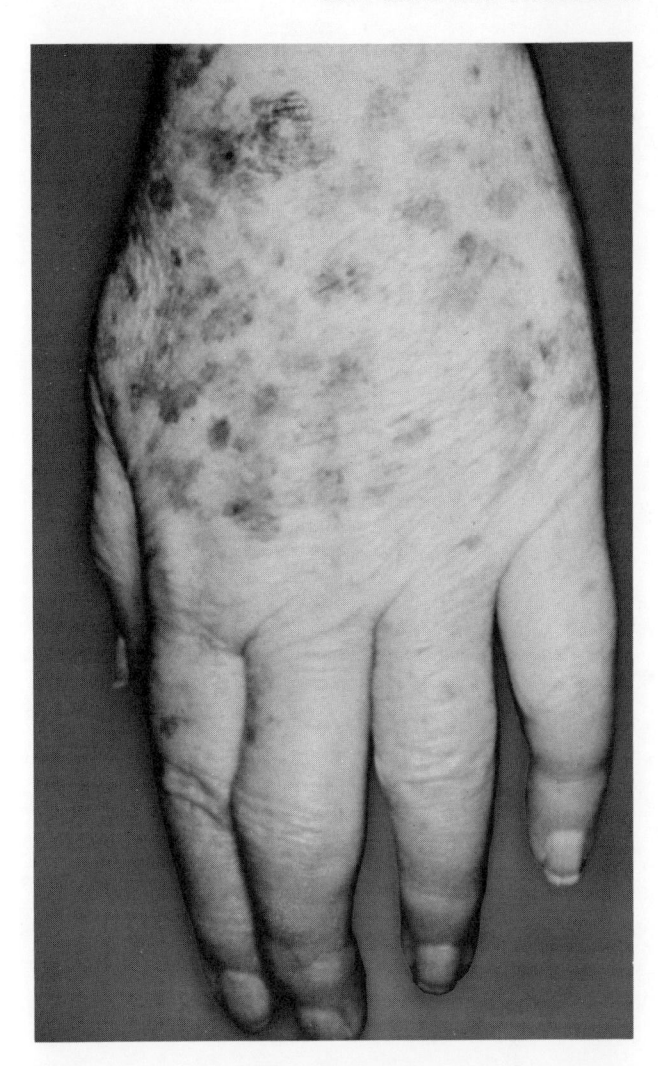

Senile lentigo and actinic keratosis occur most often on exposed areas, such as head, neck, and upper limbs. Sunscreens may prevent precancerous keratoses.

only result from the xerosis but be aggravated by insomnia. It is unnecessary here to specify the causes of poor sleep, but one may suggest to patients that they avoid excessive caffeine (coffee or cola products) after the midday meal.

Sometimes pruritus is the result of endogenous diseases. Among those so associated are diabetes, myxedema, and gout. A table summarizing signs and symptoms and the appropriate diagnostic studies appears on page 140.

Localized pruritus may also occur in persons under stress, such as worry over retirement. Common sites include perianal areas (where the problem may be worsened by poor hygiene), the back of the neck, ears, wrists, ankles, hands, and flexural areas such as the cubital and popliteal fossae. Excoriations and subsequent rubbing produce a dermatitis, which in itself causes itching. Topical fluorinated corticosteroids may be of help, but their long-term use may cause atrophy of the skin, and hydrocortisone cream is preferable.

Solar (Actinic) Degeneration

The degree and severity of the skin changes resulting from sunlight depend on the duration and intensity of exposure. The changes appear on areas such as the V of the neck, the extensor aspects of the arms, the dorsa of the hands and face, the back of neck, etc. Solar degeneration can be recognized by wrinkling, atrophy, hyper- and hypomelanotic macules, telangiectasia, yellowish plaques, and keratoses. Elastic degeneration on the back of the neck presents as a thick yellowish plaque with accentuated skin markings known as cutis rhomboidalis nuchae from their geometric shape. Changes are more likely to be seen in the rufous Celt and fair-haired, blue-eyed Scandinavian than in persons of Mediterranean background, and are least often seen in the black. Persons who are sensitive to sunlight and who sunburn easily should take particular care to protect their skin from sun by wearing a hat and suitable protective clothing. The most effective sunscreens are PABA (para-aminobenzoic acid) and alcohol emollients such as PreSun or Pabanol lotions, but these have a tendency to stain clothes somewhat. Less sun-sensitive patients may obtain adequate protection from creams containing PABA esters (Sea and Ski) or other creams that contain menthyl anthranilate and cinoxate (Maxafil), benzophenones (Uval), etc. Protection of the skin may prevent actinic keratoses, which are precancerous.

Rosacea and Seborrheic Dermatitis

Increased vascularity in the center of the face, most often seen in those who blush easily, may lead to rosacea, with a corresponding increase in soft tissue, sebaceous gland hypertrophy, increase in the size of the nose (rhinophyma), and secondary acne. Seborrheic dermatitis may occur alone but is more common when mild rosacea is present as when there is mild erythema with scaling on the bridge of the nose, eyebrows, eyelids, alar nasi, and behind the ears. Seborrheic dermatitis is aggravated by stress and is seen in some neurologic diseases.

The treatment of rosacea is removal of any substance that perpetuates the erythema, such as ingested alcohol or spices. In addition one should prescribe oral tetracycline (250 mg daily), abrasive soaps, and topical applications of 1% to 2% sulfur in 1% hydrocortisone cream to the areas of seborrheic dermatitis. (The sulfur may be prescribed as Fostril or Sulfacet.) Comedones or sebum that block the large sebaceous glands are mostly observed on the face and temples. RETIN-A Brand tretinoin gel is applied once daily until the comedones are removed and then twice weekly for maintenance, if required.

Some other skin lesions common in the elderly include *seborrheic keratoses,* on trunk and temples and between the breasts in women, which present as elevated, greasy-brown scaling papules. There is a hereditary predisposition to this problem. Treatment entails removal with a sharp curette (without local anesthetic if small), followed by application of a styptic such as Monsel solution. *Cherry angiomas,* small 1 mm to 4 mm raised vascular papules, require no treatment.

Skin tags are most frequently found on the sides of the neck, on the axilla and on the inner surface of the upper part of the thighs. The patient is often overweight and shows a hereditary predisposition to

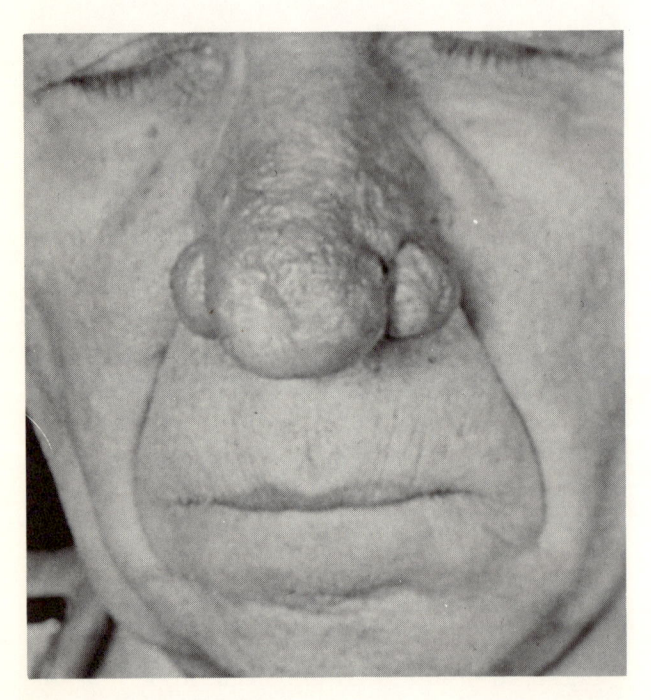

Rosacea and rhinophyma, with increase in soft tissue, sebaceous gland hypertrophy, and secondary acne may result from increased vascularity in center of face.

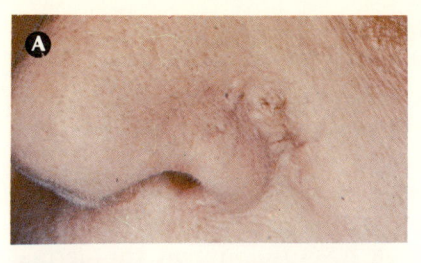

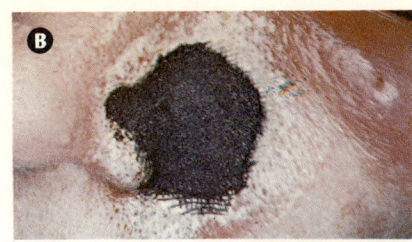

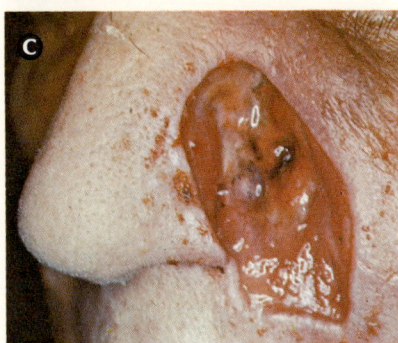

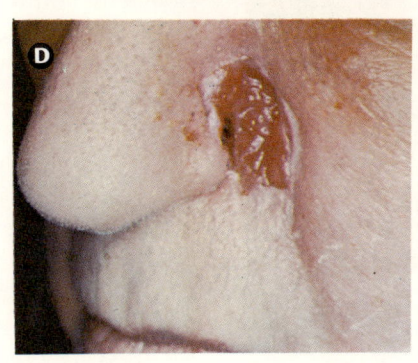

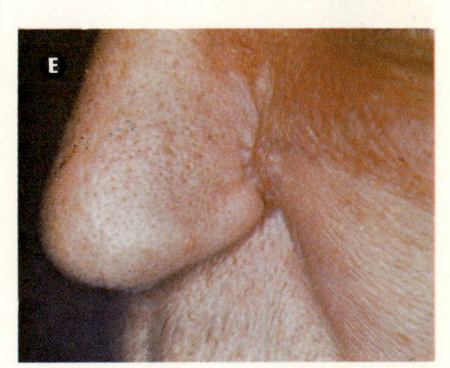

SKIN CARE AND PROBLEMS

Patient with basal cell carcinoma (A) is treated by Mohs' chemosurgery, dichloracetic acid and zinc chloride paste (B), and excision. Frozen sections are taken and studied until lesion is eradicated (C). Two weeks later (D) ulcer has diminished; two months later (E) site is healed.

form skin tags in pressure areas. These may be removed with small curved scissors, without local anesthetic, after which styptic may be applied.

Spider angiomas, central arterioles with projecting finger-like telangiectasia, are usually 2 mm to 3 mm in size and are most commonly seen in women and in patients with liver disease. Treatment consists of light electrodesiccation of the central arteriole.

Dermal *nevi* may be pigmented or flesh-colored and may have been present for many years. They generally do not require any treatment (unless cosmetic considerations make removal desirable).

Milia are small (2 mm) keratin-filled cysts; the face and eyelids are a common site. They also occur on

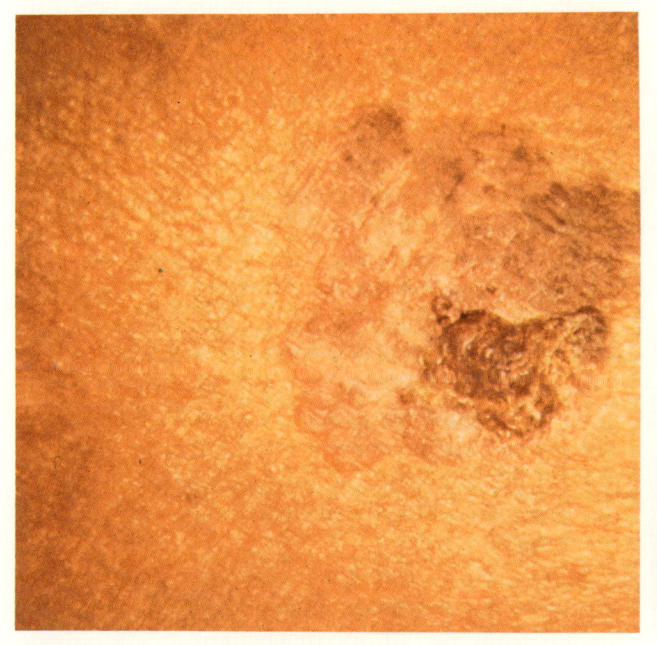

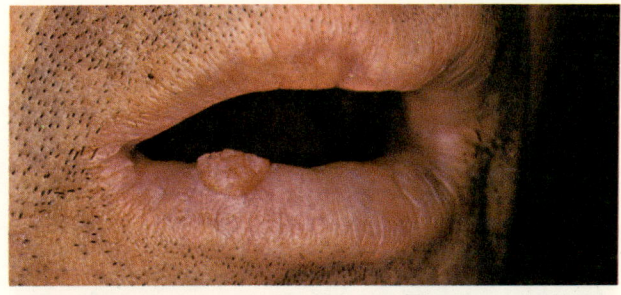

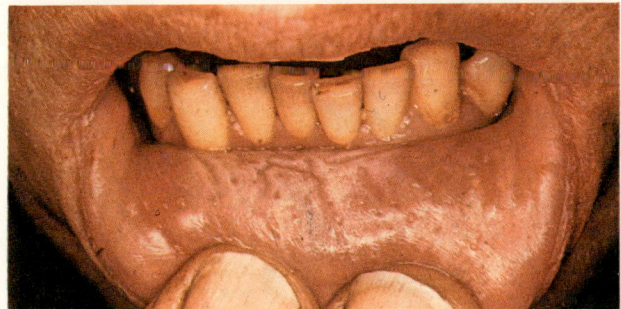

Bowen's disease (left), hard to distinguish from superficial basal cell epithelium, may be associated with visceral malignancy. Squamous cell carcinoma (top) may arise from leukoplakia (bottom) or actinic keratosis.

CHAPTER 17: CRIPPS

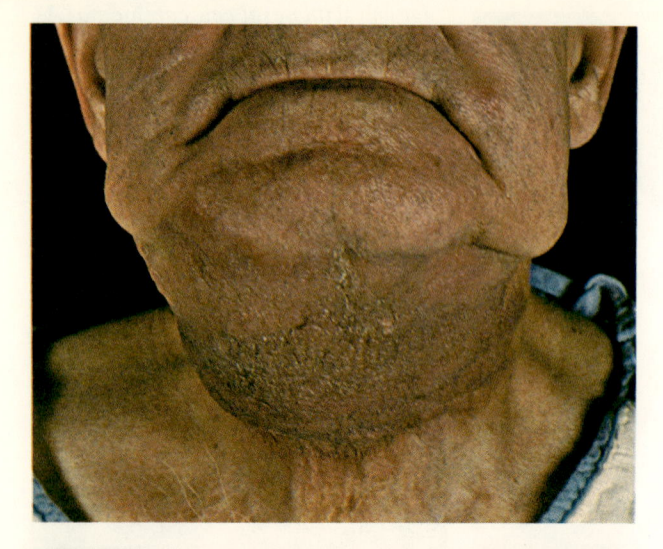

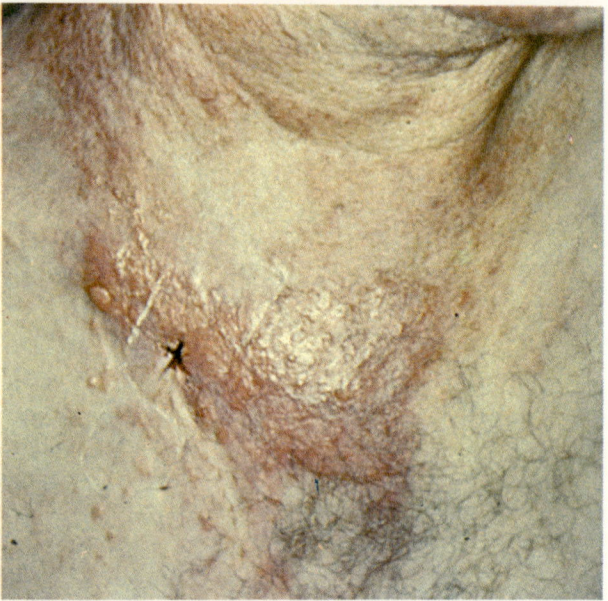

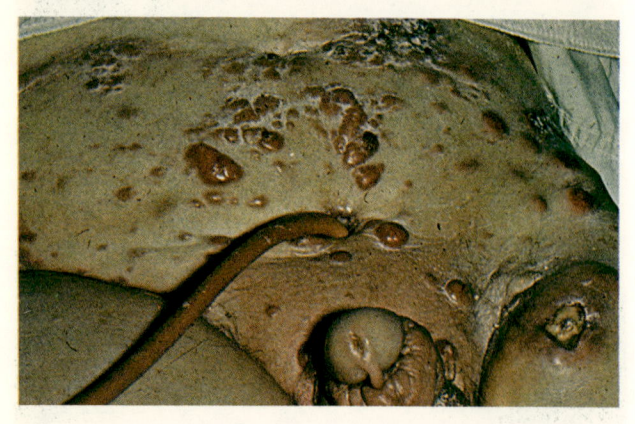

The cutaneous manifestations shown are, from top to bottom, related to metastases from primary malignancies of the stomach, a parotid gland, and the prostate.

the scrotum, where they may be mistaken for enlarged sebaceous glands. They can be removed by gently puncturing the part with a scalpel and expressing the contents by gentle pressure with a comedo extractor.

Senile purpura is most often observed on the arms and is associated with atrophic, lax skin. There is not sufficient connective tissue to support the dermal blood vessels, and no treatment is available.

Malignant Dermatoses

Let us begin our discussion of this group of lesions with *actinic keratoses,* which are sometimes called precancerous keratoses and occur most frequently on the exposed skin of face, neck, ears, and forearms. These are small, persistent, scaling keratoses on an erythematous base, and if left untreated, after many years often develop into squamous cell carcinomas. There are several choices of treatment, particularly if lesions are multiple. The first is to apply 5-fluorouracil in a 1% or 5% solution or a 5% cream (e.g., Efudex) twice daily for two to four weeks. The medication serves a diagnostic as well as therapeutic purpose, since the initial effect is to produce inflammation of the keratoses, which makes them easier to recognize. Single lesions are simply treated by electrodesiccation and curettage or by application of mono-, di- or trichloracetic acid.

Basal cell carcinomas are more likely to occur on the face and may present in several forms. The rodent ulcer, with rolled pearly border and central ulceration, is easily recognized, but thickened plaques such as the morphea-like basal cell or pigmented basal cells present more difficulty in diagnosis. Their presence is confirmed by biopsy. Superficial multicentric basal cell carcinomas may present as a scaling patch with an advancing, thin, raised glistening border, which may be mistaken for a patch of psoriasis or eczema. Treatment varies from ionizing radiation or simple excision and pathologic evaluation to curettage, electrodesiccation, and treatment of the base with dichloracetic acid (Sherwell's technique). The Mohs' chemosurgical technique, which is removal under microscopic control, is particularly useful for recurrent basal cells near vital areas (see photos at top of page 137).

Squamous cell carcinoma may arise from precancerous actinic keratoses, leukoplakia of the lower lip, or long-standing chronic ulcers. The treatments include ionizing radiation, excision with or without irradiation, Mohs' technique, or cryotherapy.

SKIN CARE AND PROBLEMS

Malignant melanoma in the elderly most commonly presents as a lentigo maligna (malignant freckle), which is a hyperpigmented macule on an exposed area that, often after a number of years, becomes darker and nodular as it increases in size. The treatment of choice is wide excision. Electrodesiccation and curettage or x-irradiation is usually not the treatment of choice.

Paget's disease of the nipple may be found in women who present with a unilateral dermatitis around the nipple that fails to respond to topical steroids. They should be carefully examined for induration or retraction of the nipple; the cause usually is an underlying duct adenocarcinoma, and the condition should be treated as breast cancer.

In *Bowen's disease*, a small, scaling, red, raised patch with an irregular surface and edge is present; it may be difficult to distinguish from a superficial basal cell epithelium. Excision is the preferable treatment, and it should be noted that the presence of a cutaneous Bowen's carcinoma may be associated with increased incidence of a visceral malignancy.

In addition to malignant dermatoses, several internal malignancies display cutaneous manifestations, some of which are general and nonspecific, while others are highly specific. Thus pruritus, particularly of the lower legs, is common (30%) with Hodgkin's disease and with lymphocytic lymphoma. Urticaria and bullous diseases (such as erythema multiforme, pemphigoid, and herpes zoster or shingles) should alert the physician to look for an associated cause. Finger clubbing (hypertrophic pulmonary osteoarthropathy) may suggest carcinoma of the bronchus or the pleura. Arsenical keratoses are not in themselves malignant, but inorganic arsenic that may have been ingested a number of years previously is carcinogenic.

The specific manifestations include *malignant acanthosis nigricans*. This light-brown discoloration, which feels like velvet on palpation, may be observed in the perineum, groin, and axilla. Not seen except in adults, this sign is invariably associated with internal malignancy, mainly of the gastrointestinal tract (95% stomach).

Dermatomyositis is a less universal sign of internal malignancy, which will, however, be found in 15% of dermatomyositis patients on an overall basis with the incidence rising to almost 50% after middle age (45 to 50 years). The condition is manifested by proximal muscle weakness and tenderness, and heliotrope color with edema of the upper eyelids. Pink patches with scaling over the knees, elbows, and dorsa of the

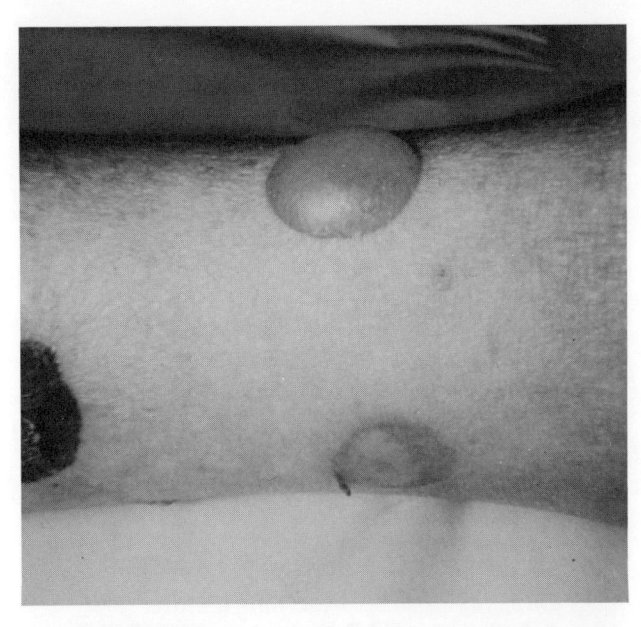

Pemphigoid, shown above in the lower leg, with possible subepidermal bullae, may be observed in the elderly. Another problem that requires aggressive treatment is venous stasis dermatitis and ulceration (below).

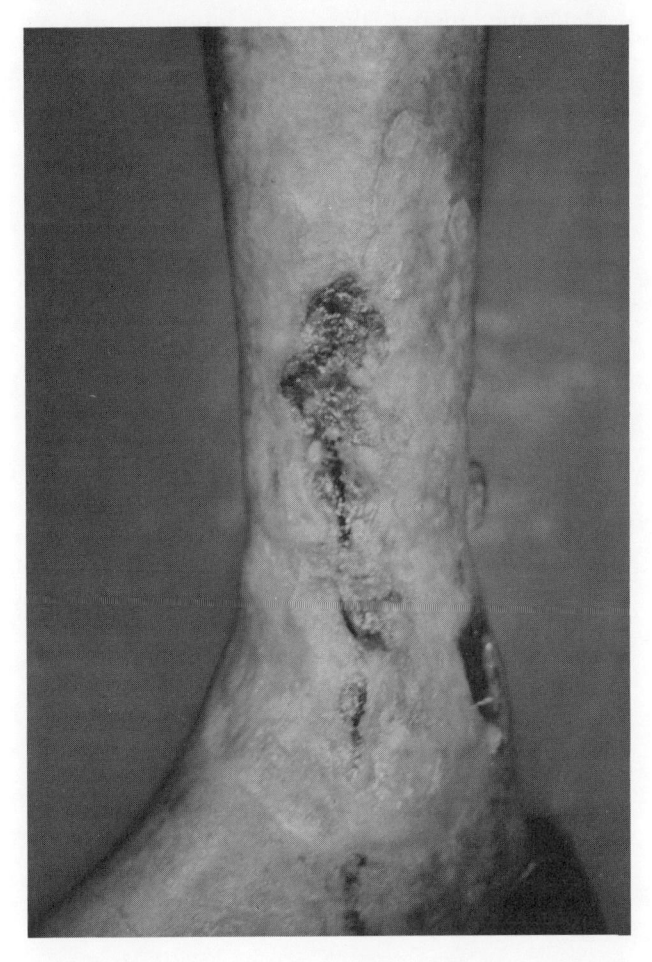

CHAPTER 17: CRIPPS

Pruritus Caused by Endogenous Disease

Primary Disease	Signs & Symptoms	Laboratory Tests
Diabetes	Weight loss, thirst	Urine, blood glucose
Myxedema	Sluggishness, coldness, deafness	Serum cholesterol, T_3, T_4
Gout	Arthritis, tophi	Serum uric acid
Liver disease	Jaundice, spider angiomas	Liver function
Blood diseases and reticulosis	Anemia, splenomegaly, lymphadenopathy	Blood count, marrow and tissue biopsies
Visceral malignancy	Appropriate localized signs, weight loss	Chest x-ray, barium meal, etc.

finger joints may also be presenting features.

Bowen's disease and Paget's disease of the nipple have already been described. Erythema gyratum repens (serpiginous scaling erythema) and carcinoid are rare.

Metastatic lesions to the skin are found, in order of frequency, in breast cancer (50% of women patients), stomach, uterus, lung, large intestine, kidneys, and prostate. Their presence should alert the physician to the most likely primary site.

Skin Ulcers

Ulcers, particularly of the lower legs, are quite common and represent not only a diagnostic but a therapeutic problem. The physician should be aware that ulcers may be not only of vascular origin, such as venous stasis, arterial insufficiency, and vasculitis, but may also have a hematologic basis, such as anemia or proteinemia. Other causes include collagen disease, fungal or bacterial infection, syphilis, tumors, metabolic disorders, pyoderma, gangrenosis, and drug toxicity – such as bromides and iodides.

The treatment will depend on the cause, but for the purpose of this chapter the discussion will be limited to venous stasis and decubitus ulcers.

If the dermatitis is acute and eczematous, a secondary irritation or allergic sensitivity to topical medications such as neomycin should be considered, and the offending substance eliminated. Simple compresses moistened with Burow's solution 1:20 or 1:40 (aluminum acetate) or saline 0.5%, and applied for 30 to 60 minutes three to four times daily, are initially helpful to soothe the dermatitis and cleanse the ulcer. Hydrocortisone cream 1% can be used to relieve the dermatitis, but it is essential to reduce edema by elevating the leg or by wrapping it with Ace bandages or by having the patient wear suitable supportive stockings. If an ulcer has developed, debridement with compresses and topical antiseptics, such as povidone-iodine (Betadine) and 1% gentian violet, can be employed. When the ulcer is clean, it is covered with the same antiseptics and absorbable gelatin powder (Gelfoam) or fine mesh gauze. The leg, including the ulcer, is then covered with Unna's boot (zinc gelatin) from the foot to below the knee. It is preferable to change the boot at 24 hours initially because of the exudate and then gradually increase the intervals between changes so that they go up from 48 hours to seven to 14 days. The purpose of the boot is not only to reduce and control the edema but to protect the ulcer. There are many other successful methods, such as applying gold leaf directly to the ulcer, but this material is difficult to handle, and the treatment is not an easy one to utilize.

Pressure sores are frequently seen in bedridden, debilitated patients in the older age groups, particularly if they have neurologic problems. The skin of such patients must be watched constantly for erythema and the patient turned every two hours while awake. Sheepskin, foam rubber pads, air mattresses, and even warmed water beds can be used in more severe problems. Use of a Stryker frame makes it much easier to turn the patient. Wrinkled and damp sheets are a common cause of irritation. Once the decubitus ulcer has developed, there is no single panacea, and the physician should use whatever program he considers most helpful. However, the ulcer should be kept clean with a suitable antiseptic, as described above. Exposing it to a heat lamp for 15 minutes every three to four hours at a distance of 12 to 15 inches helps to promote healing.

18

Visual Loss in the Elderly

ABRAHAM L. KORNZWEIG
Jewish Home and Hospital for Aged, New York City

Whether the changes that occur in the eyes with advancing age should be considered "normal" senescence or pathology is an open question, but at least two positive statements can be made: First, some decrease in visual acuity can be expected in almost every aged individual. Second, a surprisingly high percentage retain good to adequate vision to age 90 and even beyond. There are also a number of general medical diseases common among the elderly that have harmful effects on vision. Thus any discussion of vision problems in the geriatric age group must be concerned with both the problems arising in the eye and those associated with systemic disorders. As in other chapters in this book, emphasis will be on the role of the family or primary physician in the (ophthalmologic) management of the elderly patient.

"Don't wait to be told." Perhaps that should be the physician's first principle in the ophthalmologic context. Fear of blindness is widespread among the elderly, as is the belief that failing sight is a natural and inescapable concomitant of growing old. Together these cultural factors cause many to remain silent about changes in sight. Withdrawal from favorite activities, depression and other personality changes, even accidents and trauma may be the end result of such silence. For these reasons it is important that the family physician incorporate a regular, albeit rapid, visual evaluation into the routine physical exam even in the absence of a specific vision complaint by the patient. In order not to alarm the patient, the physician should explain that performing an eye examination is part of good preventive care at any age and does not imply that something is wrong. This may well elicit a response by the patient and open the way to a dialogue in which the patient can be given not only reassurance but specific information as to the various approaches through which visual disability can be helped and eyesight preserved.

That the vast majority of the elderly continue to have useful vision throughout life is not just pep talk. About 20 years ago my associates and I made a survey of visual acuity among more than 1,000 elderly institutionalized patients (they ranged in age from the 60s through the 90s, with the largest number in the group from 70 through 79). About 85% of the entire group were found to have visual acuity entirely adequate for their needs. Specifically, more than 70% were characterized as having "good to useful" vision (15/15 to 15/40), another 15% had "fair to adequate" vision (15/50 to 15/70), and only 15% were considered to have "poor" (15/100 or less) or "very poor" (15/200 or less) vision. Very few (about 1%) had no light perception, and very seldom did vision loss serve to immobilize the individual. When we broke the data down according to whether subjects were under or over age 80, close to 80% of those over 80 were found to have fair vision or better (see graph on page 142). Expectedly, the percentage in the "good" category declined with each decade of age.

As is implied above, although visual acuity diminishes with age, the sight elderly people retain is al-

CHAPTER 18: KORNZWEIG

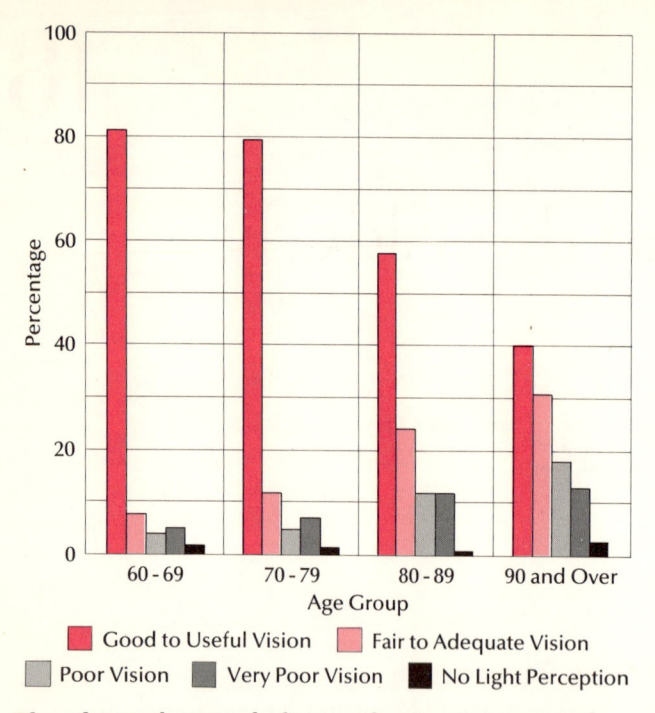

Though visual acuity declines with aging, it remains adequate or better in most cases. Graph is based on author's study of 1,000 residents of a home for aged. More than 900 of the subjects were between 70 and 89 years old.

most always adequate for the more limited range of activity that characterizes their time of life. The primary physician may feel confident that the assurance his elderly patients seek is not that their vision will be as good as it was in youth but that they will continue to be able to take care of themselves and do the things they want to do, such as keep house, pursue a hobby, drive a car, or go about some business in which sharpness of vision is not essential. The primary physician is in a much better position, thanks to knowledge of the patient and his or her personal environment, to give such assurance than most specialists, although referrals are sometimes indicated.

It is for this reason that I strongly recommend that the eyes be tested at least annually in the course of the regular physical checkup. In the standard vision test, using Snellen's eye charts, each eye should be tested separately, and if the patient wears glasses, with the glasses on, since it is important to ascertain whether any impairment is correctable optometrically. If a new or different Rx appears desirable, referral should of course be made, since few generalists are trained in refraction. A bedside eye test chart can also be obtained that can be carried in a physician's bag or pocket. In addition, a few other tests will screen the geriatric patient for a wide range of primary and secondary ocular problems. For example:

• A check of the pupillary reflexes for direct and indirect reactions to light will show whether the pupil reacts to direct but not to indirect light, or vice versa, implying some interruption in the reflex system. Further investigation to determine whether the break is of neurologic, ocular, vascular, or other origin is then indicated.

• A confrontation test, with the patient looking straight ahead as the physician moves his fingers in from the side, is a simple means of ascertaining whether the patient has lost peripheral vision in one or both eyes. The possibility of hemianopsia is supported if, on questioning, the patient tells of being unsteady on his feet or of frequently bumping into people, and is further strengthened by an eyes-closed equilibrium or finger-to-nose test. With such indications referral to a neurologist is called for.

• A check of the eyes for uniform movement in all directions is another means of checking neurologic as well as muscular adequacy.

• A check for intraocular pressure should be done, preferably using a Schiotz tonometer. The technique involved is detailed later in the discussion of glaucoma and can easily be learned in one or two sessions with an ophthalmologist. If no tonometer is available, an approximate estimate can be made by ballottement, using the index finger of each hand on the upper lid of the patient, as he looks down. The fingers are pressed down alternately against the eyeball and an evaluation of the resistance is made. It can be compared to that in the physician's own eye, if his is normal. This method is valuable especially if one eye is congested and feels more rigid than the other. Acute congestive glaucoma, an eye emergency, may be present. If it is, treatment can be started immediately by the primary physician – 2% pilocarpine drops every 15 minutes or half hour for several doses (as discussed in more detail later) – before the patient is seen by the ophthalmologist.

• Dilatation of the pupils and ophthalmoscopic examination of the fundus may provide evidence of renal disease, hypertensive or diabetic retinopathy, macular degeneration, and, occasionally, tumors. This test should be done whenever possible, using a 10% solution of phenylephrine hydrochloride, or cyclopentolate hydrochloride ophthalmic solution 1%.

Only a few minutes are required to carry out these tests, but if they are consistently performed, the primary physician may feel confident that many problems will be caught early enough to provide help for the elderly patient and preserve useful vision. I will discuss some of the specific problems in more detail later on, but one more maneuver is worth mentioning at this point: if there is reason to suspect the presence of an aneurysm in the cerebral vessels, it is worthwhile to listen for a bruit with the bell stethoscope placed right up against the closed eye. Advance warning of an impending stroke may occasionally be obtained in this way.

Clearly, any ophthalmologic studies have to be fitted into the context of the patient's general medical history. One component is the patient's medication history and current drug profile, since a substantial number of drugs may have untoward effects on the eyes. For example, compounds containing atropine and atropine-like substances dilate the pupils and may raise intraocular pressure and as such are an obvious hazard to patients with glaucoma. Examples of such drugs are phenylbutazone (used in arthritis), which contains homatropine, and trihexyphenidyl (used in Parkinson's disease), which contains an atropine-like substance. Corticosteroids used in arthritis for prolonged periods may produce posterior subcapsular cataracts. In older patients, the problem for the primary physician often requires making a trade-off, weighing the therapeutic needs relevant to systemic disease against the risks to the patient's ocular function.

Let us turn now to a) some of the threats to vision that arise within and around the eye, including methods of treatment; b) a brief discussion of the role played by eye signs and symptoms in the diagnosis of systemic disease; and c) what can be done for the patient whose vision cannot be improved or retained.

Problems Arising in the Eye

Cataract: With age, the lens fibers lose their transparency and become yellowish and cloudy, and vision gradually worsens. It has been said that anyone who lives long enough will show evidence of cataract formation. In the study of 1,000 institutionalized persons cited earlier, more than 60% had some evidence of cataract.

Little can be done to prevent cataract formation, but surgical removal of the lens can now be carried out successfully in 95% to 98% of cases and there need be no hesitation in recommending it even to the very old. Surgical techniques have been greatly improved recently. Fine silk, chromic catgut, and nylon sutures are used to close the incision, allowing the wound to heal firmly with less postoperative bleeding into the anterior chamber. Local anesthesia is usually sufficient, though general anesthesia may be indicated if the patient is unduly apprehensive. Ambulation is usually possible on the first or second postoperative day, minimizing pulmonary and vascular complications.

Only in rare instances should surgery be withheld because of age or collateral disease. Several studies have shown that aged persons withstand cataract surgery well and have a good expectation of recovering functional vision. As a rule, if the patient is ambulatory, is well oriented, needs surgery, and desires it, it should be done. Those who fear the operation can be assured that the hazards are very few and the percentage of good results very high with modern methods of treatment. Nor is there any reason to wait as was once customary until the cataractous lens is "ripe" or "mature." Today's improved methods permit cataract removal as soon as the patient is handicapped in his or her ability to read, write, sew, and so forth. If a patient has senile macular degeneration, the operation for cataract removal may have to be deferred until such time as the patient is more severely handicapped and loses his peripheral as well as his central vision. In rare instances, a very elderly patient will develop postoperative confusion or even psychosis. Where there is any suspicion of emotional imbalance that might become worse after surgery, a preoperative psychiatric consultation is advisable.

A relatively recent technique that may be particularly valuable in the geriatric individual is the intraocular lens implant. The hyaline capsule of the lens is cut open, the cataractous lens extracted, a plastic replacement lens inserted, and the flaps of the capsule closed over it. Or the capsule may be removed and the insert held in place with tiny projecting feet or sutured to the iris or the sclera. Problems with the implant do arise, however, from difficulties of keeping it in place, secondary infection, clouding of the cornea, secondary glaucoma, and sometimes immunologic rejection. Because of these there is a complication rate of about 15% to 25%, in some series, which is unacceptable in younger patients but not necessarily so in individuals with a shorter life expectancy. One may risk these for the advantage of attaining the nearly natural restoration of sight the implant can afford. Minimal, if any, correction by glasses is needed after a successful implant. If complications do occur, the implant can be removed and the patient is usually no worse off than if she or he had had the conventional lens extraction first.

CHAPTER 18: KORNZWEIG

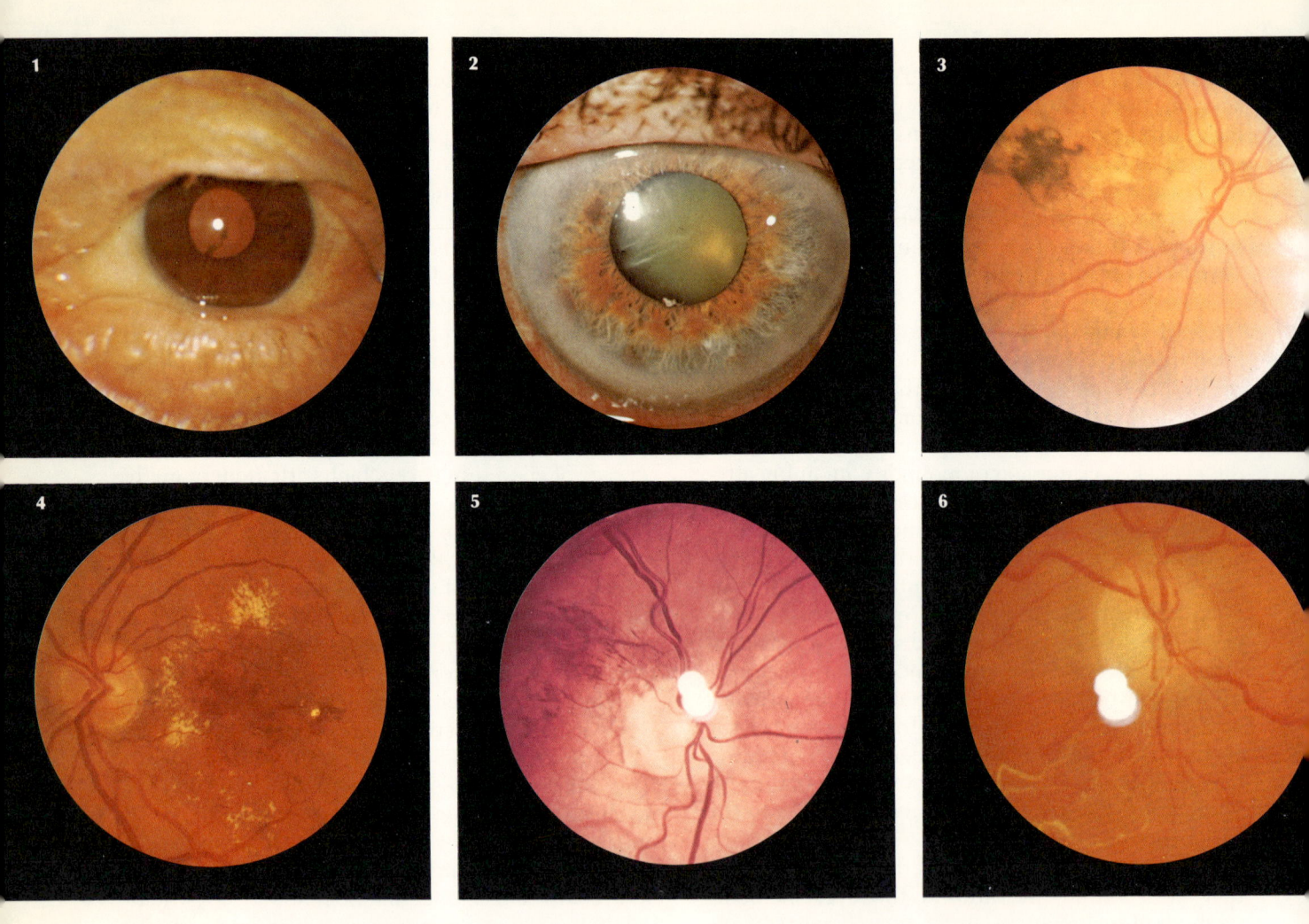

Eye pathology in the aged includes: 1) early cataract in pupillary area, which resembes a spoke; 2) cataract formation in pupillary area, with conjunctival congestion; 3) pigmentary changes in macular region, an early sign of degeneration; 4) diabetic retinopathy, with numerous exudates and hemorrhages in and around macula (pinpoint hemorrhages are capillary aneurysms); 5) sector hemorrhage in retina from occlusion of central retinal vein branch; 6) hypertensive and arteriosclerotic retinal arterioles (white lines are occluded vessels).

More experience can be expected to solve some of the remaining problems with the implant and make its use more widespread. Perhaps 1% of the half-million cataract operations performed annually in the U.S. are now being done by this method. It takes longer – an hour or thereabouts as compared with 15 or 20 minutes for the conventional techniques – and of course requires special training.

Macular degeneration: About 30% of the elderly sustain a gradual loss of central vision from this cause while retaining peripheral vision. Such persons can be confidently assured that they will not go blind. While their ability to read, to write, and to watch television or a movie may be severely impaired, they will continue to see well enough to take care of themselves and to move around.

Of the many systemic diseases affecting the macula, most are well known – hypertension, diabetes, nephritis, central nervous system disorders, and vascular thrombosis. Of these, the most important is diabetic retinopathy. Patients who have had diabetes for more than 10 years begin to develop hemorrhages and exudates in the retina that can affect vision and in extreme cases cause blindness. Amebic dysentery and histoplasmosis also damage the macula, as may lifelong exposure to such bright lights as the welder's arc. Alcoholism, especially when combined with smoking, affects central vision indirectly as a result of malnutrition and vitamin B complex deficiencies. The maculo-papillary bundle of nerve fibers is mainly involved and central vision is impaired and eventually lost. In the absence of specific causes, the etiology of macular degeneration is little understood, although some investigators postulate a hereditary predisposition. Familial clustering has been noted. Considerable research on this disease is now in progress.

Treatment is far from satisfactory. Vigorous treatment of such underlying causes as diabetes or hypertension occasionally yields some improvement of central vision or, at least, retardation of the degenerative process. For most patients, low-vision aids are the best that can be offered, and these will be described later in the chapter.

Glaucoma: The abnormal increase in intraocular pressure is usually caused by some obstruction to the outflow of the aqueous humor. The outflow is in the angle of the anterior chamber, through the trabeculae and into Schlemm's canal, from which the aqueous goes into the scleral veins and back to the general circulation. The chief problem remains detection before the increased pressure, which is transmitted to all areas of the eyeball including the optic nerve and retinal vessels, leads to such irreversible changes as optic atrophy and loss of visual field and vision. The incidence of the disease rises from age 40 to about 65, after which it tends to level off; prevalence in the age group over 65 is from 5% to 10%, depending on the population studied.

While the person with acute congestive glaucoma seeks help immediately, the person with wide-angle glaucoma is usually asymptomatic, and vision loss may occur insidiously before trouble is perceived. This is why it is so important for primary physicians to check the intraocular pressure periodically. This is best done with a Schiotz tonometer. The procedure is briefly as follows: With the patient reclining, a drop of local anesthetic is instilled in each eye; the patient's hand opposite to the eye being tested is elevated and the patient told to fix his gaze on it. The physician separates the eyelids so the cornea is exposed (without pressing on the eyeball) and the plunger of the tonometer is put directly on the cornea, in as perpendicular a position as possible. The position of the indicator arm on the millimeter scale is noted, and then converted to millimeters of mercury.

The average normal intraocular pressure is 18 mm Hg, with variation between 13 and 20 mm Hg considered normal. Pressure between 21 and 25 mm Hg is considered suspicious, or early glaucoma. Any pressure above 25 mm Hg is definitely abnormal, and indicates true glaucoma.

However, as in all human indices, the variations can be quite large. Patients with normal pressure, but with evidence of cupping or pallor of the optic disc and some defect in the visual field could have the rare low tension glaucoma. On the other hand, a patient with higher pressure, even as high as 30 mm Hg, but with no evidence of cupping of the optic disc and no field defect, may very well be an ocular hypertensive, and have suspected glaucoma. Such patients have to be observed several times before a correct diagnosis can be made.

Another test used by ophthalmologists to help in the diagnosis of glaucoma is to measure the rate of outflow of the aqueous from the anterior chamber of the eye. This test, called tonography, is similar to tonometry; but it differs in that the instrument is left on the cornea for four minutes and the change in pressure is recorded on an electric galvanometer. This can be converted to a coefficient of outflow (C). The average C varies from 0.20 cu ml of aqueous to 0.35 cu ml per minute. Any value of $\dot{C}$ below 0.17 cu ml per minute is an indication of increased resistance to outflow. A C value of 0.1 or 0.05 is a definite added indication of glaucoma.

Also, the appearance of the optic discs should be noted; increased cupping of the disc or temporal pallor are important signs. In addition, visual fields have to be taken, for signs of enlargement of the blind spot or paracentral scotomata.

The choice of clinical strategy has been aided considerably by the classification of glaucoma into wide- or narrow-angle types. The determination is made by gonioscopy, in which a special prism contact lens is placed on the anesthetized eye and the angle of the anterior chamber examined with a binocular microscope under direct illumination. Most chronic, asymptomatic cases are of the wide-angle type. Current practice is to avoid surgery in these patients as long as possible but to place them on treatment with drugs that diminish the formation of aqueous humor and improve aqueous outflow. The carbonic anhydrase inhibitors (e.g., acetazolamide) are valuable for short-term use, though patients should be watched for possible side effects. These drugs should not be employed in those with marked renal or hepatic dysfunction. Another useful group of drugs are the long-acting miotics. These are the anticholinesterases such as ecothiopate iodide, a drop of which, in a concentration as low as 0.06%, will contract the pupil for 12 to 18 hours and prevent loss of visual field.

Helpful for the busy or forgetful patient who re-

CHAPTER 18: KORNZWEIG

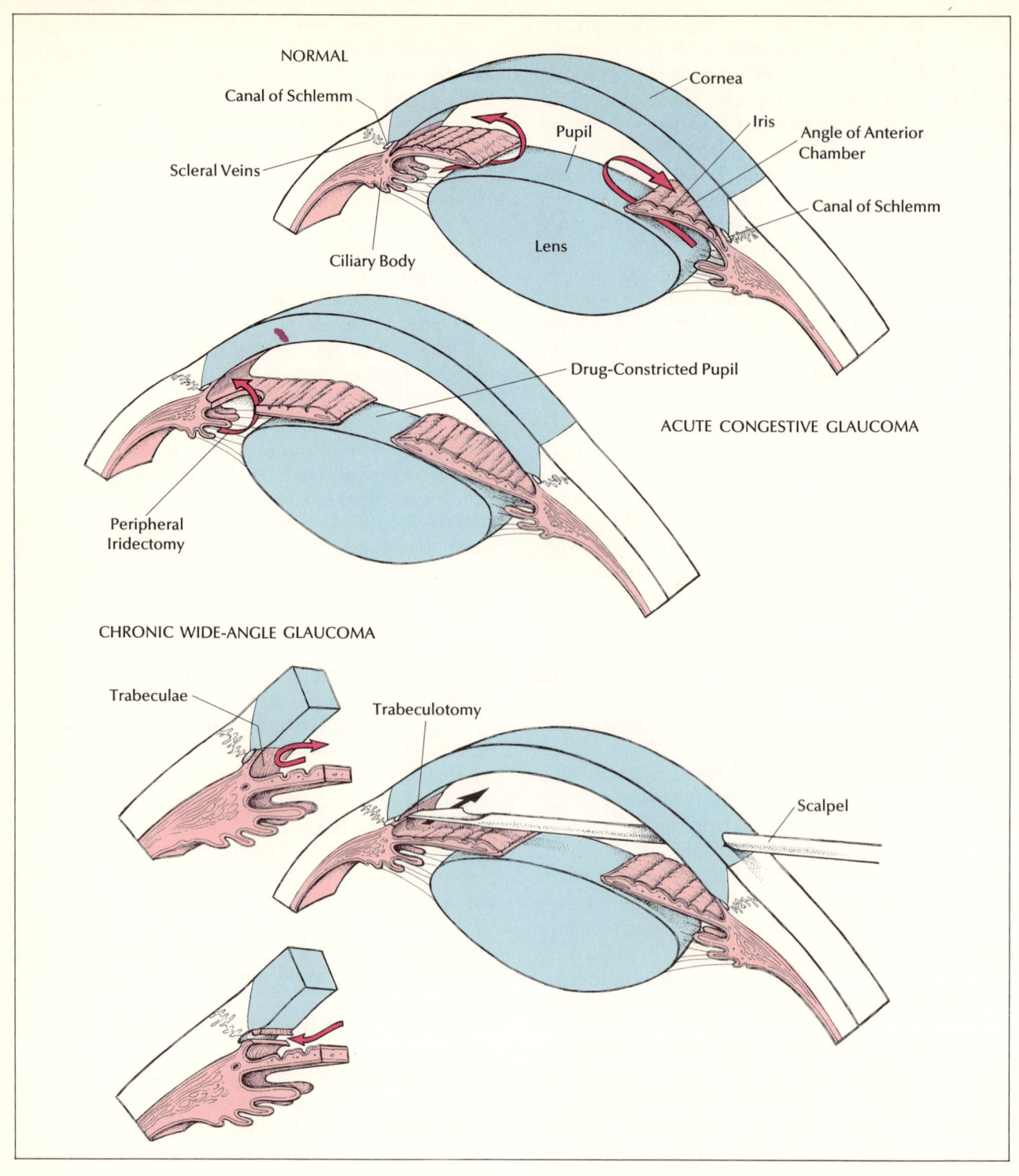

In normal eye, as shown at top, aqueous produced by ciliary body flows through canal of Schlemm to return to general circulation. In acute congestive glaucoma, angle of anterior chamber is too narrow or blocked and aqueous cannot enter canal. Treatment (center) includes use of miotics to constrict the pupil and widen the angle and peripheral iridectomy to provide a supplementary channel. In chronic wide-angle glaucoma (bottom), the problem is that the aqueous cannot penetrate the trabeculae to enter the canal. When drug treatment is no longer effective, trabeculotomy may be performed to improve the aqueous outflow by enlarging the canal.

quires prolonged treatment is the new "ocusert" method of administering medication such as 1%, 2%, or 4% pilocarpine hydrochloride. Rather than instill drops every three or four hours, the patient places a medicated polymer membrane into the conjunctival sac. The medication is released osmotically for a week, after which the membrane must be replaced. At present the cost is a drawback: about $30 a month, or five or six times what eyedrops cost.

Narrow-angle, or acute congestive, glaucoma typically presents as an emergency (as noted earlier). Formerly, when therapy for reducing pressure was not effective within 24 hours, surgery was considered obligatory to save eyesight. The emphasis today is on lowering intraocular pressure by administering carbonic anhydrase inhibitors (orally or intravenously), often in combination with agents that raise the blood's osmotic tension and draw fluid from the eye (examples are urea or mannitol intravenously or glycerin in orange-flavored water by mouth). Local miotic drops, such as pilocarpine hydrochloride (2%) every half hour and eserine salicylate (0.5%) every hour for six hours, also help improve aqueous drainage. These measures generally make it possible to avoid operating until high intraocular pressure and marked vascular congestion have been mitigated.

The preferred operation today for chronic wide-angle glaucoma is trabeculotomy, also called goniotomy, in which an opening is made into the trabeculae of the anterior chamber to enlarge the normal outflow channel. The result is more physiologic and also less arduous for the patient than the older trephine technique (in which a hole was made in the eye from the outside and covered with a flap of conjunctiva). If trabeculotomy is not effective or judged by the ophthalmic surgeon to be inadequate, a more extensive procedure is considered – a trabeculectomy, in which a portion of the trabecula is removed completely.

The importance of early detection of glaucoma cannot be overemphasized, especially in persons with a family history of the disease and in diabetics.

Diabetic retinopathy: Because improved management has prolonged the lives of diabetic patients, the incidence of diabetic retinopathy has gone up to the extent that it is now responsible for about half the blindness encountered among the aged. Whether it can be prevented is uncertain, but good medical care of diabetes is an obvious need, together with drug and dietary treatment of associated hypertension and atherosclerosis. The best hope of therapeutic success lies in early diagnosis and photocoagulation of retinal bleeding points. Photocoagulation can be effective in the early stages, but results are equivocal later. Photocoagulation appears to stabilize vision for longer periods than other procedures do. A relatively new procedure – vitrectomy – has been successful in a number of cases in which the eye was filled with blood and vision was lost completely. In this procedure, the vitreous gel is replaced with a clear saline solution.

Vascular disorders: Occlusion of the retinal circulation is another possible complication of diabetes, hypertension, renal disease, and atherosclerosis. On examination of the retina, arterial occlusion is manifested as stenosis of the retinal arteries and local edema or, when the central retinal artery is involved, a cherry-red spot in the macula. Venous occlusion is marked by large retinal hemorrhages in a single area if a branch is involved, or by hemorrhages over the entire retina if the central vein is affected. Macular lesions are identified by edema, pigmentary disturbances, or hemorrhages.

Small or minute emboli from atheromatous plaques in the aorta or internal carotid arteries may cause transient ischemic attacks in the retina or the brain. These are called small strokes if the cerebrum is involved, amaurosis fugax if the retina is affected. One should, in this case, suspect narrowing of the internal carotid artery. Such a vascular narrowing could be further verified by ophthalmodynamometry, which measures the diastolic pressure in the ophthalmic artery, in order to detect a difference in the two eyes. The ophthalmodynamometer is applied directly to the temporal sclera of the eye, while the observer watches the retinal circulation through the dilated pupil. As soon as arterial pulsation is noted, the instrument is removed and the diastolic pressure is read on the plunger. A repeatable difference between the two eyes of more than 15 mm Hg indicates a significant difference in blood flow in the arteries. This in turn could be followed up by angiography of the internal carotids and possible surgical removal of the atheromatous plaque in the affected artery.

Arterial occlusion is an ocular emergency and requires immediate measures to dilate the retinal vessels and restore circulation before six hours have passed, especially if it is the central artery or branch supplying the macula that is blocked. An eye deprived of its blood supply for more than six hours will lose its sight completely and permanently, even if circulation is reestablished later. The retina does not survive prolonged ischemia. Treatment is with amyl

CHAPTER 18: KORNZWEIG

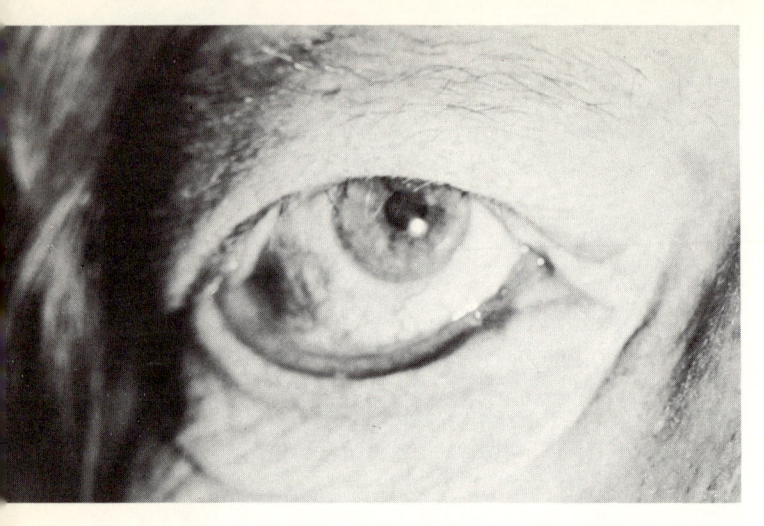

In senile ectropion of the lower lid, exposed conjunctiva is at risk of infection, which can usually be minimized by topical medication or other palliative measures.

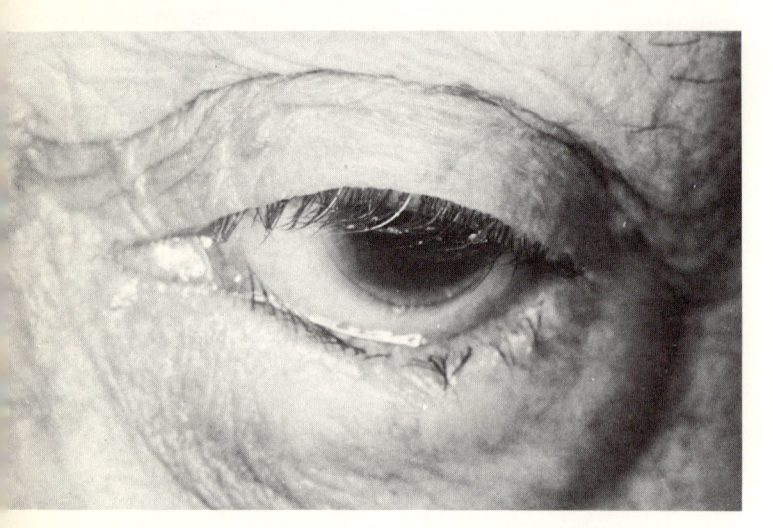

In entropion, eyelashes rub against cornea and conjunctiva, causing irritation. Lashes may be taped out of the way or epilation performed to remove an ingrowing lash.

nitrate inhalation, retrobulbar injection of acetylcholine, and intravenous papaverine hydrochloride. Another simple emergency treatment that can be given by the physician is rebreathing into a paper bag. This increases the CO_2 content of the inspired air and may help to dilate the retinal arterioles sufficiently to permit the embolus to travel further up the arterial tree away from the macular area. It may also relieve an arteriolar spasm.

In venous occlusion, the main symptom is visual loss, but the prognosis is less grim. Anticoagulants have been effective when occlusion is confined to branches of the retinal vein but rarely when the central vein is completely blocked. Therapy should begin upon diagnosis and continue for at least several months.

One of the newer methods for study of the retinal circulation and the macula is called fluorescein angiography. A solution of a sterile, neutral dye, 5% or 10% fluorescein, is injected into the median cubital vein at the elbow. The patient has been positioned in front of a camera equipped with special filters to enhance the observation as the dye reaches the retinal circulation in about eight seconds. The pupil of the affected eye has been widely dilated. As soon as the dye is seen by the observer, photographs are taken in rapid succession at 0.8 second for one or one and a half minutes and then at longer intervals of two, five, 10, or 15 minutes, if necessary. In this way the dye can be seen entering the arteries, proceeding to the capillary bed and leaving the retina through the retinal veins. Much has been learned about the retinal circulation by this method.

It has helped in the treatment of some cases of macular disease, diabetic retinopathy, venous occlusion, and in differential diagnosis. If the fluorescein dye is seen to leak from the vessels into surrounding tissue, the area is treated by a laser beam and the leaking vessel is sealed off. This is of special importance in patients with macular edema resulting from such a leak. The edema is absorbed and vision improved. It is also being used in cases of diabetic retinopathy, where such leaks and small hemorrhages are common.

The side effects of this diagnostic procedure are minimal, less than 0.5%, consisting chiefly of nausea and occasional hives. An allergic background would be a contraindication.

Problems Around the Eyes

Let me turn now to a group of conditions that, in the main, can and should be handled by the family physician. This is not only less costly but of course is more convenient and comfortable for the elderly patient and his family.

Senile ectropion and entropion: As the elastic and fibrous tissues of the eyelids atrophy and sag with aging, eversion of the lids often occurs; ectropion of the lower lid exposes the conjunctiva to chronic infection. Although surgery is the definitive approach, palliation often suffices in many patients. The family physician should try to train the patient to dry the tears with an up-and-inward motion of a cloth (or tissue), rather than the down-and-outward instinctive habit of mopping the eyes. Topical astringents and antibiotics also may be helpful, such as zinc sulphate solution 0.25% or sodium sulphacetamide solution 10% or 30%, depending on the infection's severity.

Senile entropion may lead the patient to complain that he feels a foreign body in the eye; this is because the lashes rub against the cornea. Adhesive strips attached to the outer corner of the lid and anchored on the cheek may be used to prevent this irritation. If a foreign body is indeed present, it may be removed by everting the lid to brush or irrigate it away. If an eyelash is growing the wrong way, epilation can be performed in the office. Referral is indicated if a foreign body is deeply embedded in the cornea.

Conjunctivitis: This common geriatric problem is readily apparent; the conjunctiva and eyelid margins are usually congested and inflamed, and one can see secretions in the conjunctival sac and crusts on the eyelids. Before initiating treatment the physician should use a sterile applicator to obtain culture material from the conjunctiva and lid margins. Colonies (most often of staphylococci) will usually grow out within 24 hours. Drops of sodium sulfacetamide solution (strength and frequency varying with severity of the infection) and bathing with a weak boric acid solution will alleviate the condition until antibiotic sensitivity results permit switching to more specific treatment.

Dry eyes: Also a common geriatric problem, xerophthalmia, or keratoconjunctivitis sicca, is difficult to diagnose by inspection. The patient complains of a burning or sandy feeling in the eyes. An objective test calls for inserting a strip of litmus paper between the lids at the outer canthus and having the patient keep the eyes closed for five minutes. Normally tears will moisten the paper for a distance of at least 10 mm; if less than 5 mm becomes wet, the test is positive. Treatment consists of providing artificial tears: having the patient or family member instill two or three drops of 0.5% solution of methylcellulose into the conjunctival sac of each eye three or four times a day.

Herpes simplex of the eye: Generally the infection involves one eye, which is painful and partly congested but without purulent secretion. Tearing is common. The patient feels as though a foreign body were in the eye. Flashlight examination may show a grayish area on the cornea, but the best way to demonstrate the lesion in the early stages is to touch the conjunctiva with the tip of a fluorescein-stained sterile paper slip and then irrigate the tissue with sterile solution. Affected epithelium will retain the stain, outlining the dendritic corneal ulcer. The condition responds quickly to drops of 0.1% idoxuridine solution, instilled into the conjunctival sac hourly for a few days. The drug is available as an ointment for overnight use. Corticosteroid ophthalmic preparations are contraindicated in herpes simplex; indeed, their use in this condition may aggravate it.

The Eye as Systemic Window

The retinal vascular conditions discussed earlier as ocular problems may also of course give clues to trouble elsewhere. We all know that the cardiovascular patient's increased risk of thrombotic and embolic disease may be manifested in the retinal circulation, and that occlusive cerebrovascular disease may become evident through transient blurring of vision, diplopia, homonymous hemianopsia, and blindness. Peculiar changes in visual field – such as an altitudinal hemianopsia in which upper or lower fields are absent in one or both eyes – may reflect pressure on the optic nerve tract by calcified or sclerotic carotid arteries.

A few other examples may be cited to show how wide a range of bodily systems may be implicated in eye disorders. A slight retinal hemorrhage accompanied by moderate albuminuria should lead to a consideration of nephritic disease. Ocular muscle paralyses may require comprehensive medical and neurologic investigation, since possible causes include diabetes mellitus, brain tumor, myasthenia gravis, cerebrovascular accident, and trauma. Unilateral proptosis suggests an orbital growth or invasive meningioma; bilateral or unilateral proptosis, thyroid disease. An increased sedimentation rate in an elderly person with unexplained vision loss may be the clue to acute phase temporal arteritis.

In sum, the family physician investigating vision problems may encounter neurologic, metabolic, oncologic, renal, cardiovascular, and other etiologies – all the more reason for emphasizing that visual complaints in the elderly should not be taken lightly even when the patient tends to accept his ocular disability.

But there are times when limited vision is beyond help by medical or surgical means. The task, then, of the family physician is to help the patient do the best he can within his or her own environment. He may need little more than instruction in dark adaptation (learn to wait a few moments after passing from a light into a dark setting, as when entering a movie house) or he may need low-vision aids. Basically, low-vision aids are magnifiers of various types. Some attach to spectacles for close-up activities such as reading and playing cards. Telescopic aids help in watching television or even in driving a car. Some are hand-held, some supported on a tabletop or other fixture for reading or dialing the telephone, and many are wired for illumination. Large-print newspapers and books are of course well known.

Closed-circuit television has been used institutionally for persons who wish to study. Reading matter is placed before a television camera and magnified up to 10 times on a screen the patient observes. The cost per circuit may be $1,000 or more.

Catalogues of low-vision aids are available from chapters of The Lighthouse (N.Y. Association for the Blind) or from low-vision clinics of hospitals and eye institutes. A list of such clinics is available from the National Society for the Prevention of Blindness, 79 Madison Avenue, New York, N.Y. 10016.

At the Jewish Home and Hospital for Aged in New York City, we established a low-vision clinic after realizing that many of our elderly residents needed more than the services the regular eye clinic could provide. Some residents, especially the most aged, tended to conserve their eyesight, fearing that it might otherwise be exhausted and they would become blind. They needed to be persuaded that this is not the case and that they should try the low-vision aids. Patients with multiple handicaps and depression were the least responsive. But those with an eagerness to read or to participate in social activities often learned to adapt quite well. Constant encouragement was necessary. Patients had to be reminded of the need for good illumination and for holding reading material at the right focal point.

What were our results? In a little over a year, we treated 83 patients aged 71 to 101; their visual acuity ranged from 20/100 in the better eye (51 patients, most of whom had macular degeneration) to the bare ability to perceive hand movements or light (two patients). In 62 of the 83 patients, some improvement in ability to do desired activities was recorded. In 46 of the 62 the improvement stemmed from a change in reading glasses to incorporate a magnifying element. A +6 diopter addition provides an enlargement of 1.5%, a +10 addition, 2.5%.

Help also can be offered to geriatric patients who are blind or virtually blind, so they can help themselves in their own homes and in institutions. At the Jewish Home, we are training volunteer aides to teach blind patients to clothe and feed themselves. The aides are shown how to teach a blind person a variety of self-help methods, such as hanging clothes systematically in a closet in order to know where the brown suit or the black dress is. Family members can also be given such instruction.

Often, a small improvement in a patient's vision yields a major change in outlook on life, mobility, and self-esteem. It is hard for a person with good vision to realize how much it means to be able, once again, to read a letter or to sign one's own name in the right place. There is no better argument for the timely intervention of a physician than the achievement of such meaningful improvements.

19

Otolaryngologic Problems

ROBERT J. RUBEN
Albert Einstein College of Medicine

Of the nation's 22 million elderly persons, about one in four has a significant hearing problem, according to the U.S. National Health Survey. As one might expect, well over half the elderly with hearing problems are 75 years or older. An undetermined number of the elderly have other problems that affect their ability in speech as well as in hearing.

In perhaps no other area of geriatrics can more good be done for more patients – in terms of maintaining or improving quality of life – than by attention to communicative disorders. This chapter focuses on diagnosis and treatment of hearing disorders, allied problems, and head and neck tumors – all of which may or do interfere with communication.

The family physician should be generally familiar with what the specialist can do in diagnosis and treatment. None of this special knowledge will be brought into service for many patients unless the primary care physician recognizes the need and, when appropriate, makes a referral. Such recognition must be early enough for the patient to obtain maximum benefits. Certainly, one cannot afford to indulge in thinking wishfully that the hearing loss will go away or that it is being exaggerated in the context of multiple geriatric burdens.

The danger is that a "trivial" complaint may go unrecognized even though it signals a serious underlying disease. For example, a man in his seventies who had been given throat lozenges, penicillin, decongestants, and other medications for persistent hoarseness was found in our clinic to have cancer of the larynx. In another case, an elderly woman came to us with a history of falls and fractures, with no hearing in one ear and a severe loss in the other. Ménière's syndrome of six years' duration was the diagnosis. Surgery was carried out to destroy the useless diseased ear and a hearing aid was fitted in the other. The woman now feels that life is worth living. She is no longer dizzy. She is able to converse with her friends and family.

By the time a geriatric patient presents with a speech or hearing loss, the situation is serious. The rule in these cases is a familiar one: the sooner treated, the better the prognosis. If the loss is moderate but progressive, the patient who comes to treatment early does better at handling further losses.

The diagnosis of a disorder affecting hearing or speech, or dizziness in the older patient, is often a complex affair. All the more reason why the family physician should maintain a low threshold of suspicion. What are grounds for referral? A patient who repeatedly falls should be asked if he or she experiences dizziness. If the answer is yes, an otologic and neurologic workup for central or peripheral vertigo is indicated.

In most cases, the patient will say he or she does not hear well, or that spouse, children, or friends are having trouble making themselves understood. Nonetheless, the patient shrugs this off, saying nothing is "really" wrong. Actually, the patient is likely to be in trouble.

Another manifestation of hearing disorder is withdrawal, often a subtle symptom but one to which the

151

CHAPTER 19: RUBEN

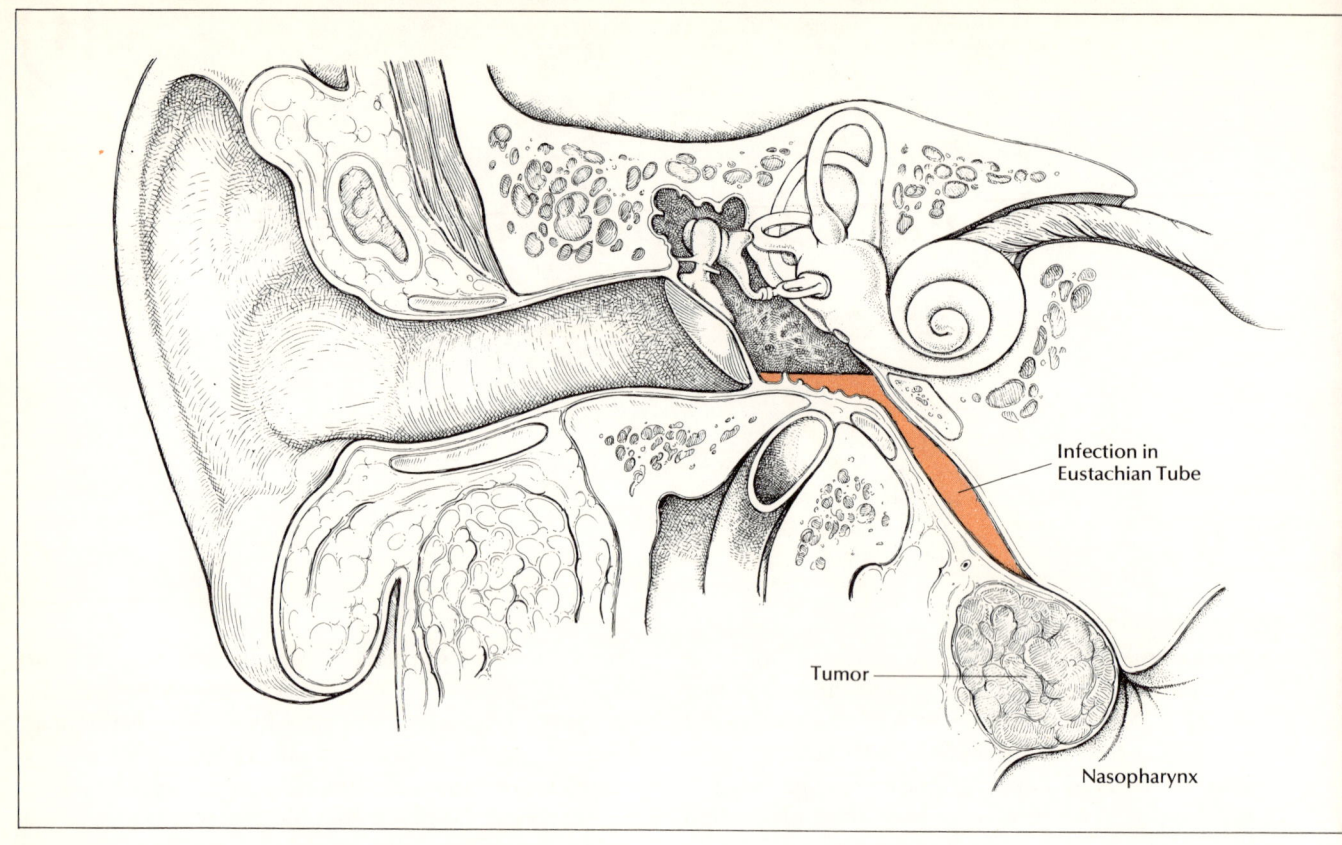

Possible involvement of the eustachian tube and nasopharynx is suggested when an ear infection with discharge develops suddenly in the elderly patient. Two of several possible etiologies are suggested in the drawings

family physician may be particularly sensitive. Of course, other factors often underlie withdrawal in elderly patients. However, the possibility that hearing loss is responsible for this (and other psychiatric manifestations) deserves prompt investigation.

As the illustration on page 154 shows, hearing acuity tends to decline with age. Generally, the lesion associated with this loss is degeneration of the inner ear in the area of the basal turn. This is reflected in high-tone losses, from 1,000 to 8,000 Hz. This decline, of course, is only one element in a spectrum of hearing problems, which I will now discuss in some detail.

Disorders of Hearing

In localizing auditory pathology, physical examination and audiometric testing are the diagnostic mainstays. The former will generally permit the physician to detect offending outer-ear factors. Audiometry can usually differentiate between middle-ear disease, most commonly manifested as a conductive hearing loss, and inner-ear problems that lead to neurosensory loss. Of course, neurosensory loss can, by definition, result from auditory nerve defects.

Outer ear: Among the most easily treatable causes of hearing loss is cerumen that occludes the external auditory canal. Generally the result is only a modest hearing loss. But if there already is other conductive hearing loss or neurosensory loss, the combined impediment may stifle communication.

Removal of cerumen usually is handled in the primary physician's office, by irrigation or by delicate removal with a wax curette. Irrigation should never be tried if a hole in the tympanic membrane is suspected, from, for example, evidence of mastoid operation or a history of otorrhea.

A relatively rare disease that can be devastating is malignant external otitis. Most external otitis, characterized by edema and discharge from the auditory canal, can be handled easily with debridement and such topical medications as cortisone drops containing antibiotics or a hydroscopic agent (Burow's solution). However, in diabetic patients, otitis externa

above: at left, a nasopharyngeal tumor blocks the pharyngeal ostium of the tube; at right, chronic infection of the paranasal sinuses provides a reservoir of organisms that travel to the pharynx by the pathways indicated.

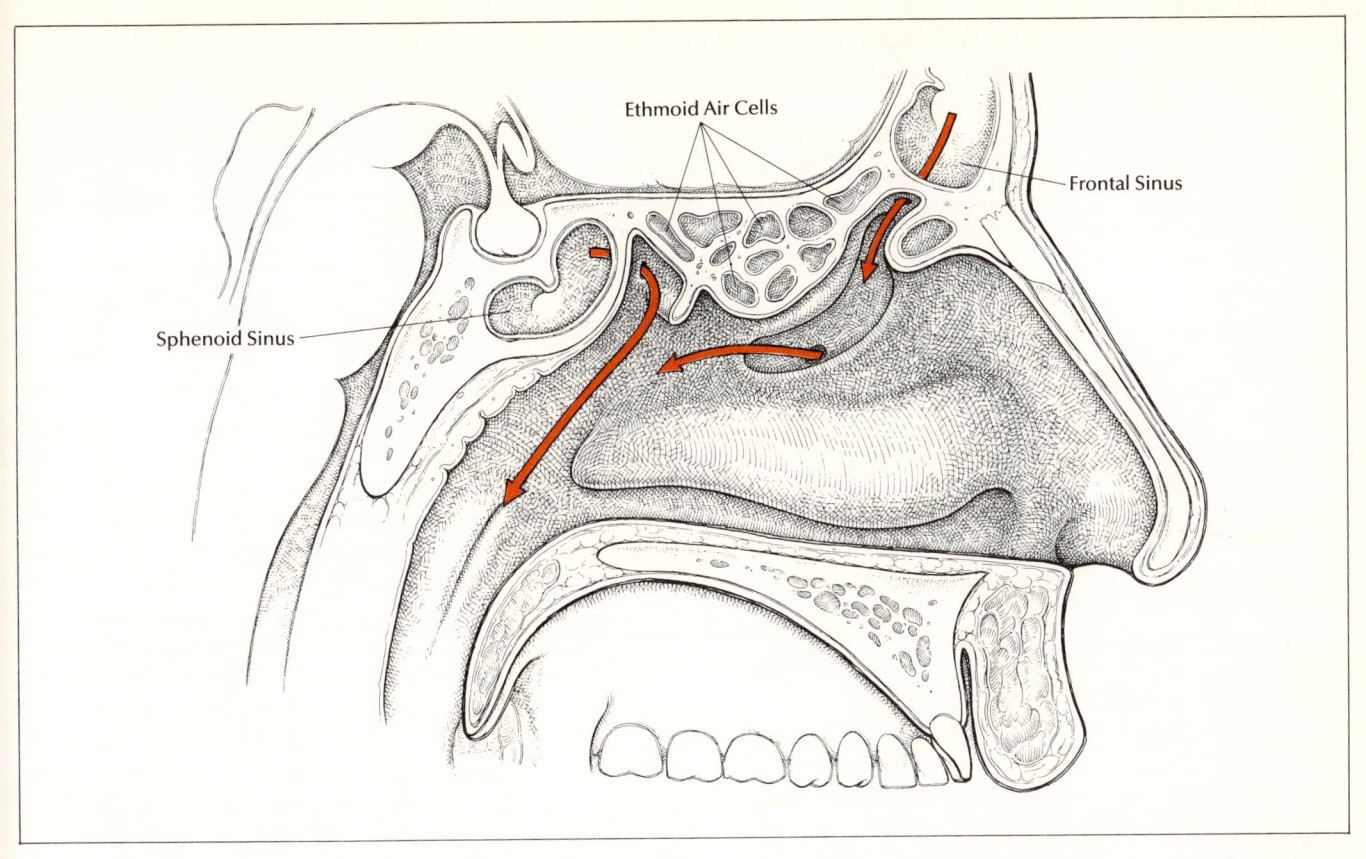

tends to become a runaway disease that can cause osteomyelitis of the base of the skull; hence the possibility is one to be kept in mind with such patients.

Middle ear: A fairly frequent cause of geriatric hearing loss is scarring of the tympanic membrane and/or the ossicular chain. This scarring may come about from the acquired condition known as tympanosclerosis. In tympanosclerosis, there is calcification of the tympanic membrane and a binding down, or scarring, that stiffens the drumhead.

Otosclerosis, a genetic disease transmitted as an autosomal dominant, is more prominent in the female than in the male. It causes fixation of the ossicular chain, especially the stapes, and affects the bony capsule of the inner ear. It may be a cause of neurosensory as well as conductive hearing loss. Paget's disease, a pleomorphic disease of bone that may become manifest in the ear, can also produce both kinds of hearing loss. In evaluating a patient with acquired hearing loss, Paget's disease should be ruled out radiographically and by laboratory test for increased alkaline phosphatase values.

The treatment of conductive hearing loss depends on whether or not a discharge is present. If there is no discharge, the treatment may be through surgery, which can be successful in the elderly. If there is drainage, the ear must first be treated either medically or surgically so that the drainage stops. The use of a hearing aid, especially in patients who are surgical risks, can be of great benefit. A hearing aid is not always accepted by patients, however, and may be inadvisable if the tympanic membrane is perforated and the middle ear is prone to infection.

If the middle-ear hearing loss is secondary to infection, combined surgical and medical management may be necessary. Infection in this area is a well-known threat, not only to hearing but also to the facial nerve, the sense of balance, and even to life itself. Infection may be associated with a cholesteatoma, which can erode the auditory ossicles and extend into the mastoid air cells. If the cholesteatoma is small and the patient is cooperative in that good follow-up can be achieved, surgery may be avoided. However, if involvement of vital inner-ear structures or the meninges is suspected, hospitalization for surgery is strongly recommended.

The sudden development of an ear infection with discharge should alert the physician to possible involvement of the eustachian tube and nasopharynx. There are several etiologies that should be considered: 1) nasopharyngeal tumors that block the tube's orifice; 2) chronic infection of the paranasal sinuses, with or without an allergic factor, which may be indicated by polyps; 3) a neurogenic problem, such as paralysis of the palate associated with physiologic dysfunction of the eustachian tube; 4) chronic middle-ear infection; and 5) tumors of the external or middle ear.

Inner ear: The cells of the inner ear undergo their last mitosis about the second month of fetal life and are never replenished. With the attrition that occurs during a lifetime, the ability to hear is compromised. There is less amplitude and more distortion in perceived sound. Congenital syphilis, leukemia, and macroglobulinemia may produce similar effects, as may central nervous system disease, especially of the brainstem. Late-onset genetic degeneration of the inner ear, for which there is no treatment, is seen.

An acquired cause of hearing loss – producing cochlear damage – is ototoxic medication. A brief list of some ototoxic drugs is given in a table on page 155. While I have not provided dosages for these drugs — some of them are quite controversial – most of this information is available in the *Physicians' Desk Reference*. Particular caution is indicated for all of these agents, especially for the aminoglycoside antibiotics, if there is any history or evidence of renal disease. The physician seeing a new patient with a hearing loss should take pains to elicit a drug history. Rheumatoid arthritis patients who are using perhaps as much as 1.5 to 2 gm of aspirin daily may experience neurosensory hearing loss, which is often reversible when another anti-inflammatory agent is substituted. It is wise to monitor audiometrically all patients on heavy aspirin regimens.

Unfortunately, except for aspirin, removal of the drug or other offending factor rarely reverses neurosensory loss. Nicotinic acid, other vasodilators, antidiuretics, and other medical treatments appear to have no more than a placebo effect. Consequently, patients with neurosensory loss should be considered for rehabilitation (with hearing aids and/or aural habilitation) after a complete medical workup. This should cover testing of middle and inner ear, eighth nerve, and CNS function.

Sound trauma is an environmental factor with neurosensory consequences. Superimposed on the inner ear's degeneration with age, sound trauma can have severe impact on the patient's communicative ability. Hearing loss possibly due to sound trauma should be documented thoroughly, since the patient may have a right to compensation from a current or past employer. One example may be cited: a retired

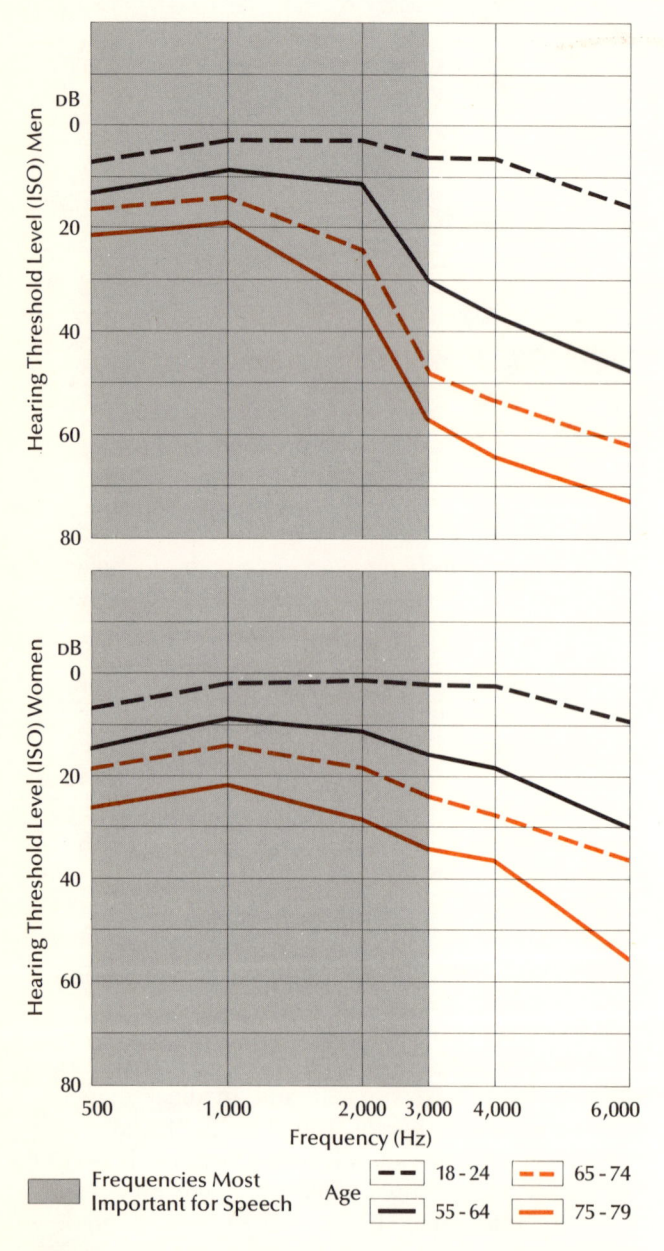

Graphs showing decline in hearing acuity with age are based on National Health Survey data. Values plotted are medians of composite audiograms for the better ear in men and women surveyed in 1960-62.

police officer who had worked as a pistol-range instructor for the police force was found at retirement to have a hearing loss much greater than expected for his age. With this fact documented, he was able to gain compensation for the disability. Occupations associated with sound trauma involve exposure to explosions, guns, and jackhammers in mills, foundries, mines, and factories.

No discussion of the inner ear can omit the problems of the *vestibular system,* although hearing loss may not be directly at issue. Patients who report unsteadiness or dizziness may have central or peripheral vertigo. Peripheral vertigo, the patient's sensation that the environment or the body is revolving, may be a sign of disease of the inner ear or eighth nerve. Central vertigo (vague unsteadiness for a moment or two) can be related to the eighth nerve or the brainstem. The differential diagnosis is by neurologic, audiometric, and vestibular examination. In routine testing, an atypical nystagmographic response (a fast component either to the right or vertically, rather than to the left or horizontally) strongly implies CNS disease. Such a response is among the earliest signs of aneurysm, arteriosclerotic occlusion of arteries, and other CNS vascular disease.

Eighth-nerve involvement: Suspicion should be aroused if patients complain of mild dizziness, which usually is not true vertigo, and inordinate difficulty in discriminating speech. The vestibular response on the affected side is diminished or absent. Special audiometric tests will pinpoint the location of the lesion, often an acoustic neuroma or other tumor. A radiograph (e.g., a CAT scan when available) of the internal auditory meatus is also an important part of the workup.

Whether or not the tumor should be removed is a decision involving the otologic and neurologic surgeon. The larger tumors must be removed because of an actual or imminent increase in intracranial pressure. The smaller tumors may carry little morbidity or mortality risk in the elderly patient.

Other diseases that may present with an eighth-nerve type of hearing loss are the demyelinating diseases such as multiple sclerosis (rare, of course, in the elderly). Assessments can be obtained at medical centers that have strong departments of otolaryngology and of hearing and speech disorders.

Tinnitus: A vexing disorder, tinnitus may be due to inner-ear or CNS causes. Unfortunately, in most cases a specific cause cannot be traced, and, similarly, specific therapy cannot be offered. However,

---

Commonly Prescribed Medications of Potential Ototoxicity

Aminoglycoside Antibiotics	Diuretics
Streptomycin	Ethacrynic Acid
Dihydrostreptomycin	Furosemide
Viomycin	**Antiprotozoal Agents**
Vancomycin	Quinine
Gentamicin	Salicylates
Capreomycin	
Tobramycin	
Neomycin	

Note:
Ototoxicity, in many instances, is dosage-related; for specific information, consult *Physicians' Desk Reference.* All these drugs, but especially the aminoglycoside antibiotics, should be used with particular caution when there is any history or evidence of renal disease.

---

there are several rare but important lesions that should be sought out. Patients should be screened by stethoscope to determine if there is an objective basis, such as an arteriovenous fistula. This life-threatening condition is amenable to surgical correction. Glomus tumors, or paragangliomas of the middle ear, can be surgically extirpated. Many times they present as a pulsating tinnitus in the heart's rhythm rather than as hearing loss.

Hearing Aids

Hearing aids are not always successful. In many inner-ear cases, not only is volume "turned down" or acuity lost but sounds may be significantly distorted. A slight gain in loudness may be intolerably exaggerated or, because of cochlear destruction, words become confused. Patients for whom English is not a native language have their problem compounded because it becomes more difficult than before to discriminate English words.

For patients who cannot accept a hearing aid, it may be in order to recommend training in lip reading (if vision is adequate) or in decoding the distorted signals. European countries, especially the Scandinavian, have centers for extensive habilitation of the elderly, but, unfortuntely, the United States lags in the provision of such habilitative services, though there have been excellent demonstration projects. Many hearing aids are sold today with little or no profession-

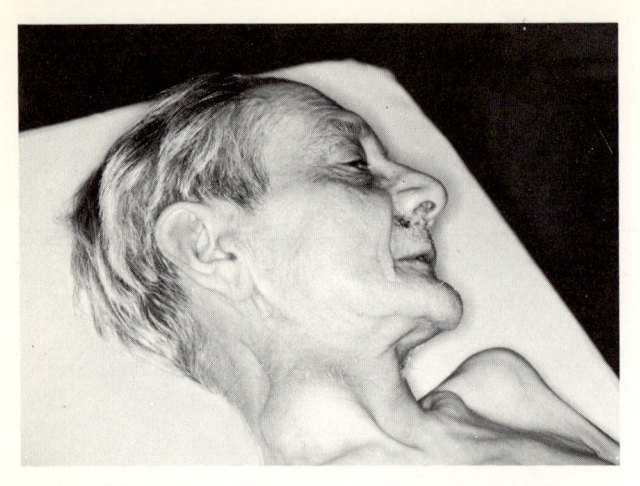

In this elderly patient the mass seen in the neck is a metastasis from a primary carcinoma of the pyriform sinus. A basal cell carcinoma can also be seen as a darkened area below the nostril. Head and neck tumors are much more frequent in the elderly than in younger groups.

al otologic or audiologic evaluation of their usefulness to the patient. In one study, patients' needs were correctly defined at a university hearing testing center before they were sent to hearing aid dealers; some of the dealers urged patients to buy quite unsuitable aids. However, the Federal Trade Commission recently decided that, effective in mid-August 1977, hearing aids may be sold only to persons who have had a medical evaluation, unless they waive examination.

The usefulness of an aid depends, in large part, on the patient's acceptance of it. The workup of a patient who may be a candidate for a hearing aid should include the following: The patient's hearing is tested, a complete otologic examination is performed, and tests are done to rule out significant and life-threatening diseases. At this point, a hearing aid evaluation is scheduled. Several aids are tested on the patient in a sound-treated chamber. The patient is then referred to a dealer for *rental* of the aid found to meet his or her needs. This trial is important because the aid is effective only to the extent that the patient finds it useful and comfortable in the home, workplace, and social environment. Patients require training in the proper use of an aid, including interpretation of its signals, and in supplementary use of visual cues.

Wholesale prescription of aids to nursing home populations has produced scandals in some state and local Medicaid programs. If the patient can communicate, the proper approach begins with routine testing. The patient who is aphasic or has other severe CNS disease is probably not a candidate for a hearing aid.

Head and Neck Tumors

The frequency of head and neck tumors is greater in the elderly population than in younger groups. This is so much the case that a physician should not assume that, in an elderly patient, a mass in the paranasal sinus is a polyp rather than a cancer. Signs and symptoms must be taken seriously, and suspicious cases should be referred as soon as possible to an otorhinolaryngologist.

The more common and significant presenting symptoms are proptosis (indicating tumor of the ethmoids, frontal sinus, maxillary sinus, or orbit); bleeding from the nose (carcinoma of the nose and/or paranasal sinuses); an ill-fitting denture that once fit properly (tumor of the antrum, palate, mandible, or floor of the mouth); an ulcer within the mouth; any slight change of voice or hoarseness (tumor of the larynx); and dysphagia (tumor of the larynx and upper esophagus). A paralyzed vocal cord should prompt a thorough investigation, including chest films, to make sure that the laryngeal nerves are not involved. Any neck swellings may indicate primary tumors of the neck, nasopharynx, and thyroid as well as metastases to the neck. Facial swelling may indicate parotid tumors.

The earlier detected, the earlier these tumors can be treated and the better the outlook. The physician and patient should not be deterred from the effort of a thorough workup in the erroneous belief that nothing can be done. Actually, experience with treatment of head and neck tumors in the elderly has been encouraging, provided the tumors are diagnosed early. The complexity of staging may be exemplified by carcinoma of the larynx. Tumors can be classified as supraglottic, glottic, and subglottic. Depending on origin, each carries a different prognosis and course of therapy. Referral to a specialist with experience related to the larynx and its tumor biology is indicated, for both workup and intervention.

Treatment of these tumors consists mainly of irradiation and surgery. Recently, the five-year survival rates (especially of patients with late-stage tumors) have been greatly improved by combined therapy. In addition, there have been significant technical innovations in resection and immediate reconstruction of head and neck areas. Large tumors of the pharynx and larynx and of the paranasal sinuses are now extirpated successfully, with reconstruction following so rapidly that the patient can often leave the hospital well launched on his rehabilitation program. Even the most extensive surgery of the head and neck region is well tolerated by the elderly in general.

A significant technique for certain small carcinomas is partial laryngectomy, which preserves the larynx as a speaking organ. However, if the larynx must be removed entirely, many patients regain vocal communication by esophageal speech and/or electromechanical devices.

The Anxious Patient

The approach to the anxious patient with a hearing disorder varies, of course, with the personality and the details of the illness. Basically, our clinic says to the patient: "We can do something to help you. While you may think your 'glass' is half empty, it is also half full and there is a lot you can do despite an impairment. But you have to try to help yourself as we try to help you."

Working with an elderly person who has a hearing impairment requires patience. Instructions and advice have to be repeated. The patient has to be asked if he or she really understood what was said. In areas of the country with polyglot populations, the physician may need some language skills for patients whose native tongue is not English. My essential point is that the patient must be approached on his or her terms.

The patient must be kept informed about what will happen in testing. I tell him or her that tests are being done to make sure nothing really serious is wrong. I explain what the tests are, that they won't hurt, and that the patient may have to return to the hospital once or twice for them. On a subsequent visit, the patient will learn the results of radiologic, audiologic, and clinical laboratory tests. I tell him or her: "We have found you don't have a tumor, or leukemia, or thyroid disease. You do have an inner-ear problem. This happens to many, many people, but you don't need an operation, and there are other ways of helping you." When patients hear that, they generally relax.

In explaining our procedure for trying a hearing aid, I will point out that we do not know for sure that an aid will work. I describe the testing and mention that the patient will be directed to a place to rent an aid to see how he or she likes it. "You're going to have to be the doctor yourself, to know whether it is really helpful," I will say. Some patients return and say they would prefer an operation. If the loss is neurosensory, I will tell them an operation is not possible. If otosclerosis is involved, I will explain that an operation has pros and cons, just as the hearing aid does. I will emphasize the values of a hearing aid. This is especially important in the older patient who is not a candidate for operation because of physical condition. The benefit of a hearing aid over an operation, because of the operative complications of dizziness that may lead to falling, must be brought out.

Candor combined with sympathy and patience is the best approach to patients with hearing and other communicative disorders. Considering the negative connotations that many sectors of our society attach to growing older, a patient may see himself or herself as making a devastating admission when exposing a hearing or speech problem.

To be old and to have a hearing problem is to be subject to a double discrimination. I would like to think that things are changing. But I wonder. Despite years of complaint, the federal tax laws continue to discriminate against the person with hearing loss. A blind person receives an extra tax exemption but one who is deaf does not. Deafness is a silent lesion – pun thoroughly intended. The deaf cannot communicate well with friends, relatives, and business associates; they need help in using their intellectual and social potential. While I am not confident that this message will leave a mark on the tax structure, I do believe that cooperation of family physicians and otolaryngologists can and will continue to help improve the quality of life for the elderly.

Surgical Management of the Elderly

PHILIP FERRIS
Franklin Square Hospital

The essence of effective surgery for the geriatric patient in the operating suite may be summarized briefly as "Do as little as necessary to solve the patient's problem." The preoperative and postoperative role of the surgeon is not so readily stated. In weighing the risks and benefits of surgery, one must bring into play knowledge, sensitivity, and judgment attuned to old age. A referring physician with deep understanding of the patient and family is a godsend to the concerned surgeon, especially when the patient is on a course that will require more and more cooperation between hospital and office.

Whether it is best to leave well enough alone, manage medically, or attempt surgery is a far more complex decision in the elderly than in other patients. Collateral problems – mental, physical, and social – may be more important than the primary disease process in their effects on the indications, timing, and extent of surgery. Among the factors to be weighed are 1) life expectancy vs the natural course of the disease; 2) comfort vs complications; 3) motivation vs chronic morbidity; and 4) risk of nonoperative management vs hazards of surgical failure.

An example of how the first pairing may produce a balance against surgery is the case of a 70-year-old patient with significant heart or lung disease who develops a thyroid nodule. Since the heart or lung disease carries a life expectancy of two or three years and the nodule, even if carcinomatous, may take up to 10 or 15 years to pose a serious threat, it makes sense to leave the nodule alone. The quality of the patient's remaining life would not be improved by incurring the pain and risks of operation. On the other hand, in a patient with angina so crippling that life is intolerable, coronary bypass surgery should be considered provided no other major disease is present – even though the operative risk is higher than in the first hypothetical case. The quality of life makes the risk worth taking.

In weighing comfort against complications, the risk to be judged is that complications in the elderly tend to escalate quickly to life-threatening proportions. The patient who develops a stress ulcer and bleeds following herniorrhaphy may require a second operation; the lengthened hospitalization increases the risk of thrombophlebitis, pulmonary embolism, and pneumonia. Several complications may be tolerated by younger patients but not by the elderly, who often lack physical reserves. Therefore, every effort must be made to avoid the first complication.

"Will to live," or "motivation," can play such an important part in controlling postoperative complications that its absence must be reckoned with preoperatively. The properly motivated patient will try to keep the chest clear, to ambulate, and in general to follow his doctor's orders. The patient who strongly associates illness with impending death may be an unreliable candidate for surgery unless his negative attitude can be decisively changed.

In assessing the advantages of medical vs surgical management, the referring physician as well as the surgeon should be acquainted with the behavior of disease processes in the elderly. Efforts should be made to ascertain age-specific morbidity and mortality rates by type of procedure; often the surgeon can provide such information. Carcinoma of the breast, for example, becomes nonaggressive in old age, and this is generally the case with other tumors, though malignant melanoma may be a controversial exception. The arteriosclerotic process seems to burn itself out in old age. For this reason the kinds of deterioration that may frustrate arterial bypass surgery in younger patients are unlikely in the elderly, and patency of grafts is maintained at a higher rate over the years. With abdominal aneurysms a similar situation pertains. Time from diagnosis to rupture in persons over 65 who refuse operation is almost twice that of persons under 65 (30 vs 18 months).

With respect to duodenal ulcer, the situation is a little different. In patients of all ages duodenal ulcer can usually be managed medically, but if a younger patient requires surgery it is generally on the basis of medical intractability, and the operation is performed on an elective basis. In contrast, the elderly patient who requires surgical intervention most often needs it because of bleeding (to a lesser degree, obstructive symptoms or perforation may be the indication). Accordingly, 85% to 90% of ulcer surgery in the elderly is performed on an emergency or urgent basis (see graph on page 162), whereas in younger groups this is the situation less than half the time.

In addition to the four factors cited above, the surgeon should assess the patient and family situation, keeping in mind that their receptivity to whatever measures – surgical or medical – are proposed is highly dependent on the surgeon's approach. Perhaps the single most important act of the surgeon outside the operating suite is to convince the candidate for surgery and the family that he or she will help them not only with the immediate surgical problem but in planning for aftercare as well, for example, in making plans to care for an infirm patient at home or by readmitting the patient, if necessary, or some other option. That understanding may be enough to enlist the family's acceptance of an active role. The change in family feelings spreads to the patient, and the tendency to hide symptoms and fears diminishes.

The value of candor and compassion was shown to me in the case of a patient who became despondent because of progressive bowel incontinence. Afraid to let his family know of the illness, this elderly man shuttled between a daughter in Florida and one in Baltimore whenever he sensed they were becoming suspicious of his frequent trips to the bathroom. (Eventually these came every 30 minutes, often only for passage of mucus.) Finally, he had to be hospitalized and an inoperable rectal carcinoma was found. A colostomy was recommended but the patient resisted because he was afraid it would trigger family abandonment. When the ice was broken between him and his daughters and real communication began, he was relieved of his fears about the consequences of the colostomy. The operation made him comfortable.

Sometimes a previous unfortunate encounter with surgery provokes a family member to discourage an elderly patient from accepting surgery. An elderly man hesitated to go through with aneurysm surgery because his daughter objected. As the daughter recalled it, a surgeon had announced her mother's death with the comment that the operation was a success but the patient died. Fearing a repetition of the scene, the daughter urged her father to live out his days with the aneurysm. It took patience to explain that the expanding aneurysm presented a remediable threat to life. The daughter relented and was overjoyed at the excellent result.

These cases illustrate the pressures that may impinge on surgeons and referring physicians when they advocate a course of action. But pressures also arise when families and patients seek unwise inter-

Factors in Preoperative Evaluation

Life Expectancy
Patient Comfort
Patient Motivation
Will to Live
Risk of Nonsurgical Treatment

Natural Course of Disease
Complications
Long-Standing Morbidity
Operative Risk
Risk of Surgical Failure

ventions. Sometimes a patient's terminal condition simply must be accepted and the family advised against heroic measures. They must be told, for example, that the incapacitated stroke patient who develops multiple stress ulcers and gastric hemorrhage may exsanguinate without operation but that an operation just as surely will produce refractory complications. Each operative round will become all the more difficult, the prognosis all the more dire, and the emotional toll on the family all the more exhausting. The death of Spain's Generalissimo Francisco Franco illustrates the futility of heroic measures in certain circumstances.

I am not suggesting avoidance of procedures necessary to survival when the patient has a chance for a reasonably good life. This is an entirely different issue from prolongation of dying. Cardiopulmonary cessation in a patient with reversible illness obviously merits a more energetic attack than in a terminal cancer patient. I ask families to consider what the patient has to look forward to after resuscitation. I ask them to consider dignity in death. Familiar as I am with the magnificent contrivances available to sustain life, I do not wish for myself or my patients the trickling on of life at the end of an assortment of tubes, with no real hope of becoming oneself again. Similarly, my view is that the taking of major risks is an absurdity when the patient is dead as a personality, for example the patient with advanced, well-documented senile dementia. Is there a point to trying to save someone who vegetates in a nursing home and does not know he or she is there? None of this is to argue that a physician should act positively to end such a life. Rather, the issue lies in when to counsel against action to preserve such a life.

No matter what a family may say, the patient has the right to know what is wrong. Dissembling foments mistrust and sets the stage for future problems between the patient and surgeon. The duty of candor often falls to the surgeon. I recall a patient who, not being told the truth about the extent of his cancer, migrated from office to office trying to find out why he was deteriorating. No one told him. Each physician probably felt that if the surgeon had not explained, why should he. The last six months of the patient's life was a vain round of office visits. This situation was caused by a daughter and son who felt their father could not handle the truth. I find most patients develop an inner strength after the initial shock of a poor prognosis and say, in effect, "I've got the damned disease. Now, what do we do about it?" An honest relationship means that the surgeon will

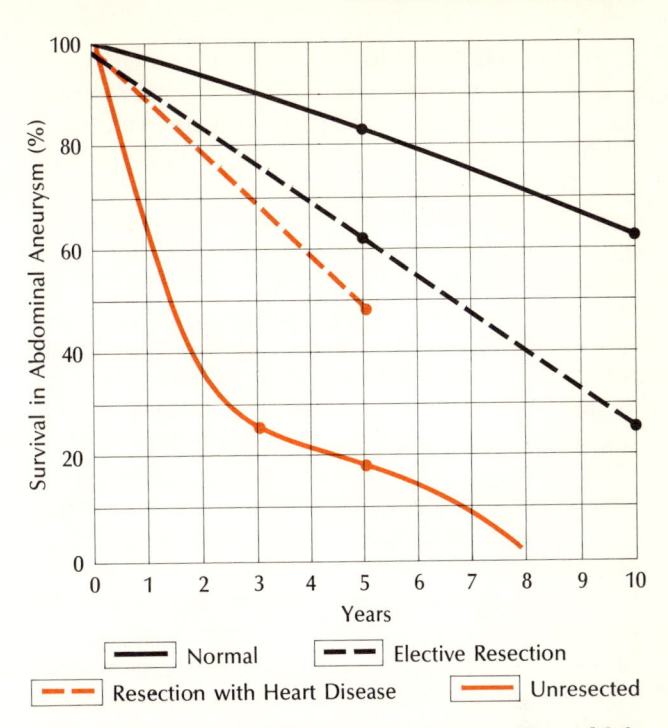

If an abdominal aneurysm is treated electively and life expectancy is good (e.g., no heart disease is present), five-year survival is fairly close to that of general population. But if life expectancy is short, benefit of surgery may be minimal: note that 18% of aneurysm patients live five years without resection. Data, from Baker and Roberts, are adjusted for age and sex.

get cooperation and will not be expected to play God.

In treating the patient as a responsible adult, the surgeon should lay out the diagnosis, prognosis, and treatment options in detail. Length of hospital stay, expected period of recuperation, and outline of activities must be presented – and all questions answered. The patient must know where he or she is in the trajectory of care. A patient must never be allowed to believe that forward motion stops in a nursing home. If, right from the start, the patient knows that the nursing home is not a dead end but part of a plan, there likely will be acceptance. It is cruel to surprise a patient who expects to leave the hospital to go home with the news that he or she must be placed in a nursing home. This happens when relatives suddenly give reasons against taking the patient home. The patient's tendency to feel abandoned and hopeless, as well as other depressive reactions and behavioral problems, will then complicate the prognosis. Worst of all, the patient may feel that professionals have not been truthful about the disease process and that it must be much more serious than portrayed or he has been led to believe.

It may be necessary to go to some lengths to protect the patient's trust. I will inform the patient regarding a colostomy if there is any possibility whatsoever that colostomy may be necessary. I do this so that when the patient awakens after surgery in which a colostomy had to be performed, the chance of acceptance will be good. Likewise, I feel that the patient is entitled to a thorough preoperative depiction of what life will be like after treatment is completed, the disabilities that are likely to remain, and how he or she will or will not be able to manage with respect to everyday activities, hobbies, and other interests.

None of this can be done well without knowing the patient's style of life. Knowing the patient's likes and aspirations may help in breaking bad news. A 73-year-old man with cancer of the breast told me that he liked to go dancing with his wife once or twice a week. Keeping mobile was important. In telling him he had the disease, I could offer assurance that it would not interfere with dancing. I find it important to offer the patient some solace and hope even in the worst circumstances. Elderly patients generally do not expect a totally optimistic picture. They tend to regard each day as a bonus in a long life; they expect major illness that will carry them to their Maker; they tend to be stoic when the news comes. By contrast, younger patients may be far more readily crushed by bad news because they anticipate a long, healthy life. While the young know their age peers will live on, elderly patients have seen many peers die. Sometimes their reason for declining surgery is the belief their time has come, too.

Surgical Approaches

Against this background, let me now turn to some specific surgical approaches. My purpose is not to be encyclopedic but rather to cover enough of the range to give a sense of geriatric strategy. Significant collateral disease obviously complicates the evaluation of geriatric candidates for any surgery; surgical risk is known to rise strikingly with the severity of the collateral disease. Myocardial infarction within the preceding three months brings a mortality of 40% for major procedures; since the risk after three months is much less, surgery should be delayed if possible.

For reasons unknown, preexisting cerebrovascular disease carries less risk of postoperative complication than does preexisting heart disease. However, diminished cerebral blood flow may produce difficulties in the geriatric patient postoperatively, particularly

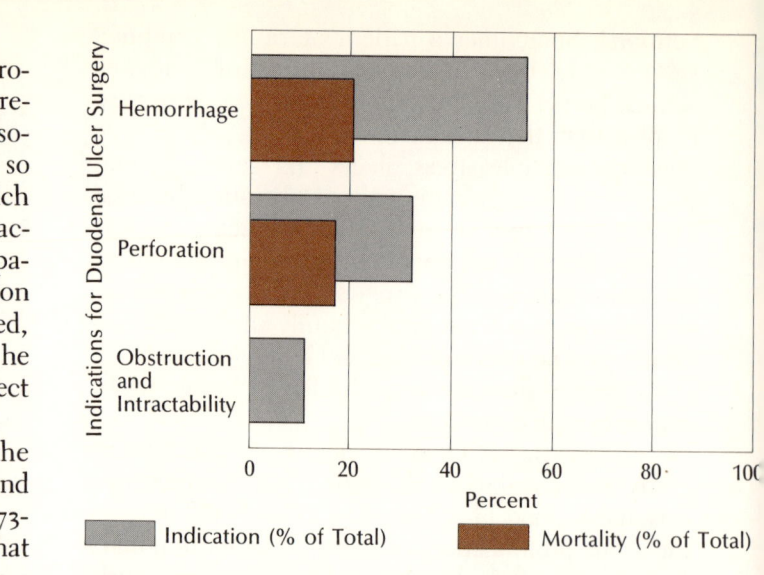

Among patients aged 65 or older, emergency indications for ulcer surgery predominated at Montefiore Hospital (New York) from 1964 to 1968, and mortality in these sit-

when there is even minor body-temperature elevation. Patients may become confused, disoriented, uncooperative, or mentally obtunded when the brain's increased oxygen needs cannot be met by the vascular system. Every effort must be taken to avoid fever or to find and correct its cause quickly. Indeed, geriatric patients generally should be watched postoperatively for mental changes indicative of deterioration in hemodynamics, electrolyte balances, and other factors such as adverse drug reactions.

Diabetes mellitus may alter the patient's tolerance for surgery on several counts: 1) the patient is more prone to have "silent" MI; 2) the infection rate is higher among diabetics, and their ability to overcome infection is lower than that of nondiabetics; and 3) the diabetic is prone to endarterial disease. However, diabetes may provide an urgent indication for surgery, as in patients with acute cholecystitis. The reason here is that diabetics have a much greater tendency to gangrenous cholecystitis and bile peritonitis because of occlusive disease of the cystic artery. Also, their resistance to infection from bile microorganisms is diminished.

Hernioplasty and gastric, intestinal, urologic, and vascular surgery have special indications in relation to the elderly. In general, necessary surgery should be done as simply and quickly as possible, electively if at all possible.

Hernia in the geriatric patient has unusual psychologic impact. It may be taken as evidence of dete-

SURGICAL MANAGEMENT

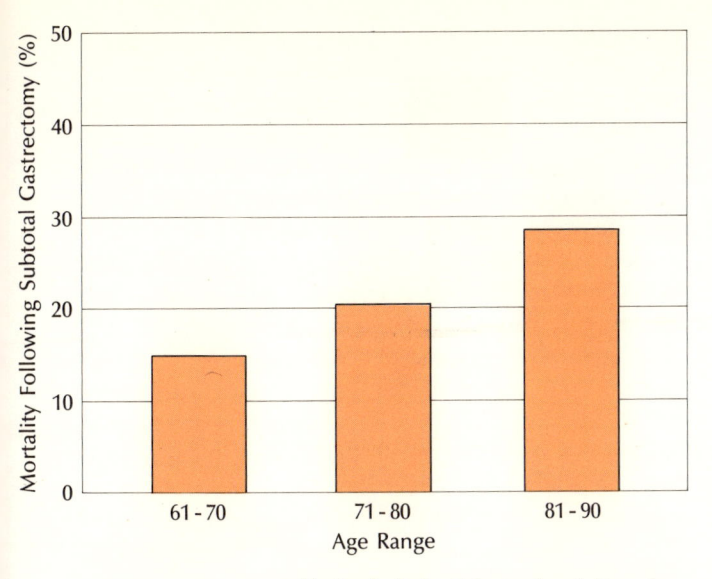

uations was expectably high (left; Schein data). In subtotal gastrectomy, a direct correlation was found by Mitty between advancing age and mortality (right).

rioration that must be hidden from families. Some patients even deny it to themselves. While hernias are not uncommon in the elderly, a bulge in the abdominal wall may indicate an occult neoplasm in the peritoneal cavity; patients often attribute the vague symptoms of an occult neoplasm to an abdominal bulge that has been asymptomatic for years. Vague hypogastric pain, change in bowel habits, or mild cramps – which may cause a patient to believe the hernia is becoming troublesome – actually may indicate colonic neoplasm. My practice is to include proctoscopy and barium enema as preoperative investigations prior to hernioplasty in the elderly.

Progressive enlargement or symptoms proved by exclusion to be related to the hernia are sufficient indication for repair. Even poor-risk patients can undergo herniorrhaphy safely with local anesthesia and intravenous supplementation. Elective surgery almost always is advisable for femoral hernia, especially in the elderly woman. Repair of ventral or umbilical hernias should be performed if they are symptomatic or difficult to reduce. Hiatal hernia repair rarely is necessary in the elderly unless there is obstruction, hemorrhage, or reflux esophagitis refractory to medical therapy. Preoperative endoscopy is mandatory.

While indications for surgical management of peptic ulcer usually are the same for all adult patients, the desirable procedure for the elderly patient with hemorrhage or perforation is not gastrectomy.

Vagotomy, pyloroplasty, and simple plication are preferable because they expose the patient to much less risk. I avoid four- or five-hour operations whenever possible. In an emergency with no time for workup, the safe assumption is that the patient may have collateral disease and the simplest, quickest surgery is best, such as oversewing a perforation (unless there is obstruction and bleeding). Only 15% of patients in whom the perforation is oversewn will need a second operation electively in five years, or 30% in 10 years. If the patient already is 70, the actuarial tables argue against the kind of definitive surgery acceptable in patients with 40 years' life expectancy. In the patient with obstructive complications of peptic ulcer, lower mortality is obtainable with partial gastrectomy rather than vagotomy and drainage. The higher mortality after vagotomy is attributable to "gastric atony" in an already distended, flaccid stomach.

The incidence of gastric ulcer increases with age. In about 10% of patients, lesions thought to be benign will prove malignant. Surgery is recommended when roentgenographic studies after four weeks of medical therapy show failure to heal. The procedure of choice is distal gastrectomy, incorporating the ulcer if possible. When the ulcer is in the juxtacardiac region, wedge excision of the ulcer should be performed, if possible, along with antrectomy. Biopsy should be done for an ulcer left in situ.

In gastric malignancy, exploratory laparotomy should be done with the aim of totally extirpating the lesion. The final choice of procedure depends on operative findings. Palliative resection is recommended to remove the source of bleeding and obstruction in incurable cases. Total or proximal subtotal gastrectomy is not advised for palliation in the elderly because of high morbidity and mortality; only if there is a chance for cure should these procedures be entertained. Gastroenterostomy, gastrostomy, and jejunostomy may be done for symptomatic, unresectable tumors, but they offer little hope of improving the patient's condition.

Treatment for intestinal obstruction must be aggressive in the elderly. Often a barium enema is necessary to establish that the obstruction is in the small intestine and not the colon. Since elderly patients do not tolerate prolonged intubation and nasogastric suction well, early exploration is indicated when intubation alone does not produce a rapid resolution.

Only recently has it been recognized that intestinal infarction, a condition that is almost exclusively confined to geriatric patients, can occur in the

> **Indications for Early Surgery in the Elderly**
>
> **Aneurysms**
> - Aneurysm >7 cm in diameter
> - Evidence of progressive enlargement
> - Hypertension, moderate or severe
> - Calcification, moderate or severe
>
> **Diverticulitis**
> - Recurrent significant hemorrhage
> - Generalized peritonitis
> - Significant urinary tract symptoms
> - Suspicion of coexisting malignancy
> - Failure of medical management
> - Unresolving localized abscess
> - Fistulization to small intestine
>
> **Biliary Disease**
> - Solitary stone, symptomatic
> - Silent solitary stone, diabetes mellitus
> - Symptomatic patient, nonfunctioning gallbladder
> - Recurrent episodes of pancreatitis
> - Obstructive jaundice, even mild or transient

absence of anatomic vascular occlusion, as the result of circulatory inadequacy that produces functional ischemia. Intestinal infarction is far better prevented than treated, since surgery usually consists of resecting nonviable tissue and the residual viable bowel is rarely enough for nutritional integrity. Preventive measures include suspecting ischemia in the elderly patient with typical epigastric postprandial pain and progressive weight loss. Angiography in such a patient may demonstrate a correctable lesion.

Angiography with lateral views is diagnostic and allows surgical intervention with good results in patients whose intestinal angina arises from atherosclerosis of the superior mesenteric artery. Most frequent in men over age 70, intestinal angina usually involves, besides the superior mesenteric artery, either the celiac axis or the inferior mesenteric artery. Unfortunately, medical management of the symptomatic patient with intestinal ischemia usually ends in disaster.

Appendicitis in the elderly may not follow the classic Murphy sequence. The patient may be gravely ill or not sick at all. Some patients may have advanced signs of intestinal obstruction, generalized peritonitis, or intra-abdominal abscess; but others may exhibit only minimal local discomfort, a lax abdominal wall, and little systemic reaction. Roentgenograms to discern any opaque fecaliths are helpful in the elderly. Barium also may be useful if the situation allows, since appendicitis may be the symptomatic presentation of right colon carcinoma. Early surgery with awareness of possible associated disease is indicated; there is little to be gained by observation for suspected acute appendicitis in the aged.

Diagnosis in geriatric patients with colon pathology is complicated by the high frequency of functional constipation and laxative dependency. The diagnostician must maintain a high degree of suspicion. Fortunately, radiologic screening of the colon can be rewarding, because early diagnosis of colon cancer offers an excellent opportunity for cure. In any geriatric patient with unexplained weight loss, anemia, bleeding, hypogastric discomfort, or even trivial changes in bowel habits, sigmoidoscopy and barium enema should be employed.

Diverticular disease is found in about 40% of patients by age 70 and usually can be managed medically, even when hemorrhage is massive. Localized diverticulitis with or without perforation also can be managed medically, provided there is alertness for signs of generalized peritonitis and of any blowout from a localized process. Once inflammation has subsided, a one-stage resection may be carried out safely. In obstruction from acute diverticulitis, much is to be gained by proper bowel preparation followed by elective intervention. There are, of course, instances in which a conservative approach is just not feasible. Indications for early or emergency surgery for diverticular disease include recurrent significant hemorrhage, generalized peritonitis, concomitant significant urinary symptoms, suspicion of coexisting malignancy, failure of medical management, unresolving localized abscess, and fistulization to the small bowel.

Should elective surgery be recommended for the asymptomatic patient when a single gallstone is found on routine abdominal films? One may argue that even the small mortality in such surgery is a contraindication. On the other hand, in patients over age 75, *emergency* cholecystectomy is reported to carry a 14% mortality, as against only 4% for *elective* cholecystectomy and choledochotomy. In elective cholecystectomy alone, mortality is even lower and results from coexisting disease; not the procedure. My suggestion is to perform elective surgery on the asymptomatic geriatric patient with a single stone. If the patient refuses surgery or the procedure is contraindicated electively, cholecystostomy with stone removal may be performed with minimal risk under local anesthesia at the earliest sign of difficulty. Cholecystostomy is clearly indicated for patients with a symptomatic stone; diabetics with a silent stone; patients with multiple stones; asymptomatic patients with a nonfunctional gallbladder; patients with mild or transient obstructive jaundice; and patients with recurrent pancreatitis. In geriatric patients with pancreatic malignancy, attempts at curative resection are so risky that palliative bypass procedures must be preferred.

A ruptured abdominal aneurysm is catastrophic at any age. Only one patient in three escapes serious morbidity or even mortality after resection once rupture has occurred. Some patients never make it to the operating suite. It is of great importance, therefore, to manage aneurysms electively when rupture impends. The key signs are aneurysmic diameter of 7 cm or more, progressive enlargement, moderate or severe hypertension, and moderate or severe calcification on x-ray.

The predominant reason for urologic surgery in elderly men is prostatism. The threat obstructive uropathy poses to the kidneys can be relieved by transurethral resection, which is generally well tolerated. However, if renal failure is present, surgery should be preceded by catheterization and fluid therapy for several days to return blood urea nitrogen values to as close to normal as possible.

Cystectomy for carcinoma of the bladder makes little sense in most geriatric cases, especially when collateral diseases carry a poor prognosis. Periodic cystoscopy and fulguration of the tumor seem far more reasonable: patients usually live for several years, during which they pass their urine normally and avoid the discomfort of a urinary diversion.

The rule of doing the least procedure that will relieve symptoms and reduce threat to life or limb holds for vascular problems. Even angiography should be avoided, if possible, because of its invasive nature. Despite the potential of gangrenous changes, intermittent claudication may be considered a blessing in disguise for the patient with angina pectoris: the claudication keeps physical activity within the range of coronary sufficiency. Bypass surgery to improve leg circulation should be reserved for patients with unmanageable distress or those in whom amputation otherwise would be unavoidable.

To conclude this perspective on geriatric surgery, I offer a case history that demonstrates the need to look ahead before taking definitive action. Doing so may make possible a comprehensive surgical strategy that results in more function on the part of the patient than would occur otherwise. A diabetic patient presented demarcating skin below the right knee and with gangrenous changes in the distal half of the right foot. Above-knee amputation was an obvious choice, but clinically the patient's left leg, though alive and free of pain, was not much behind the right in arterial insufficiency. Therefore arteriograms were obtained of both legs and showed that vascular repair would be much more difficult in the left should it become necessary. If gangrenous changes were to occur in the left leg after above-knee amputation of the right, a second above-knee procedure would be obligatory. Two above-knee amputations make the nursing problem tremendously more difficult, since most patients cannot even turn over in bed without help. Preservation of even one knee enables one to do so without assistance.

Accordingly, the decision was to place a femoral popliteal bypass graft in the right leg, which changed the level of amputation from above the knee to the arch of the right foot. In the event an above-knee procedure became necessary in the left leg, the patient would at least have retained the right heel and knee. The ability to ambulate would be preserved. The ability to turn over in bed would be assured, too, in the event of further circulatory deterioration. Thus the toll disease might take on the quality of this patient's life was minimized.

That goal, I believe, is what geriatric surgery is all about.

21

Dental Problems

HOWARD H. CHAUNCEY and JAMES E. HOUSE
Harvard School of Dental Medicine

Preceding chapters in this book dealing with the medical care of the elderly have voiced several common themes: 1) these patients usually have multiple problems, which, singly or together, may compromise functional independence and the quality of life; 2) attempts to alleviate these problems, even when relatively minor, can frequently result in a marked improvement in quality of life; and 3) the primary care physician often is the individual most suited to assist and/or organize the variety of efforts necessary to meet the multiple needs of the patient.

These themes are also germane to the dental requirements of the geriatric patient. Dentists share this desire to promote the life satisfactions of the elderly, and since medical and dental problems are frequently intertwined their collaboration is requisite. Various systemic diseases, nutritional deficiencies, and psychosocial and socioeconomic problems can affect oral health. Conversely, the condition of the oral cavity can have a pronounced influence on these factors.

Awareness of oral problems by the physician plays an essential role in providing comprehensive care for the elderly. It has been documented that the average individual 65 years or older visits the physician at least six times a year, but is seen by a dentist about once a year. Given his more frequent contacts, the physician has a greater opportunity to identify the major dental needs of his geriatric patient.

One reason that elderly patients seek dental treatment so infrequently is that private insurance plans, Medicare, and Medicaid have severe restrictions regarding provision of dental care. The elderly are frequently unable to pay for their dental needs without outside financial assistance. Less than 32% of all persons, including the elderly, who have an annual family income of less than $5,000 visit their dentist in the course of a year.

In contrast, approximately 32% of family members with an annual income of $15,000 or more visit their dentist between two and three times a year. Persons over 65 years of age spend more than $1,100 annually for all health services but only $105 is used for dental care. Public programs generally expend about 7% of their monies for dental problems. Thus, during the prolonged time interval between dental visits serious problems can develop and go undetected in low-income elderly persons.

The National Health Survey conducted in 1971 indicated that approximately 50.8% of all persons 65 years of age and above had lost all their teeth, both upper and lower arches. A considerably higher proportion (approximately 65%) had lost all teeth in at least one arch. More than 22 million persons in this country were completely edentulous. Six percent of all persons over 65 years needed but did not have dentures, while almost 4% had incomplete sets of dentures. Perhaps the most important observation is that 30% of all denture wearers reported that their prostheses needed refitting or replacement.

Information gathered in a survey of problems encountered by persons who wear full dentures indicated that 38% had worn the prostheses for more than 11 years without professional reevaluation. Retrogressive oral changes associated with the use of ill-fitting dentures are accentuated in older persons. Angular cheilitis as well as various undesirable changes in facial appearance or muscular imbalance can occur in edentulous persons who do not wear dentures and in patients who continue to use dentures that lack retention, stability, or proper occlusion. Similar alterations can occur in older people with excessively abraded natural teeth. Unfortunately, the geriatric denture wearer usually seeks professional assistance only when extreme discomfort occurs or a dental crisis arises.

This information acquires great importance when we recognize that an ever-increasing proportion of our population is 60 years of age or older. The Veterans Administration has indicated that 13%, or four million, of the 29.6 million veterans in the country were 60 years of age or older in 1975. This proportion is expected to rise, so that by 1985 nine million, or 31%, of the 28 million living veterans will be 60 years old or older.

Fortunately, the American Dental Association, as well as a number of public and private institutions, has initiated a variety of efforts designed to increase public awareness of the need to maintain good oral health. These have been launched simultaneously with preventive dentistry programs, by dental practitioners, and may be in part responsible for the improving current oral health picture. Between 1972 and 1975 there has been a steady rise, from 47.3% to 50.3%, in the number of persons who had a dental visit during the previous 12-month period. Similarly, in the period from 1958 to 1971 the percentage of edentulous persons in the age category 65 to 74 years dropped from 55.4% to 45.2%. Thus, more and more individuals over 60 are retaining some natural teeth. In turn, an increasing number of people are seeking fixed or removable partial prostheses.

Two factors that have an impact on oral health and whose constant change results in an increase in the demand for treatment are income and education. The interaction of these psychosocial and socioeconomic factors is changing the face of dentistry. As people become more health conscious, their pattern of oral care maintenance will change. Health-conscious individuals maintain better oral hygiene and seek treatment more frequently.

One of man's most complicated biologic activities is eating. To date, a valid assessment of the interrelationship of masticatory impairment, nutritional intake, and psychologic gratification derived from eating has not been obtained. In theory, the absence or elimination of masticatory deficiencies should promote a selection of food items that provide a nutritionally balanced diet. However, individuals with removable partial and/or full dentures show a marked diminution in their ability to chew. Many other factors contribute to the reduction in chewing ability noted in old age. These include diminished sensory perception, lowered motor ability, and bone resorption. There is a dynamic interplay between bone resorption and chewing ability in denture wearers. As the bone in the dental ridge resorbs with age, the biting force of the prosthesis in the molar region diminishes. In turn, this has been associated with changes in the textural preference in relation to foods. Low biting force and a preference for softer foods by the patient can increase the probability of inadequate nutrition. In the older person, lowered motor and sensory responses may reduce chewing ability even further and amplify this effect. Diminished flavor perception after the insertion of a maxillary denture can adversely affect the appetite.

It has been stated that the dietary preferences of the elderly change with their progressively decreas-

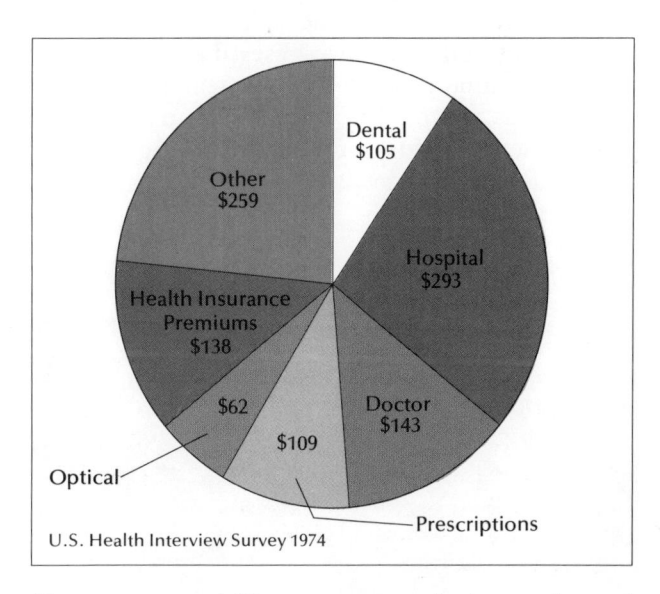

For persons aged 65 years or more who incurred out-of-pocket expenses in the health-care categories shown above, average outlay for dental care was relatively low.

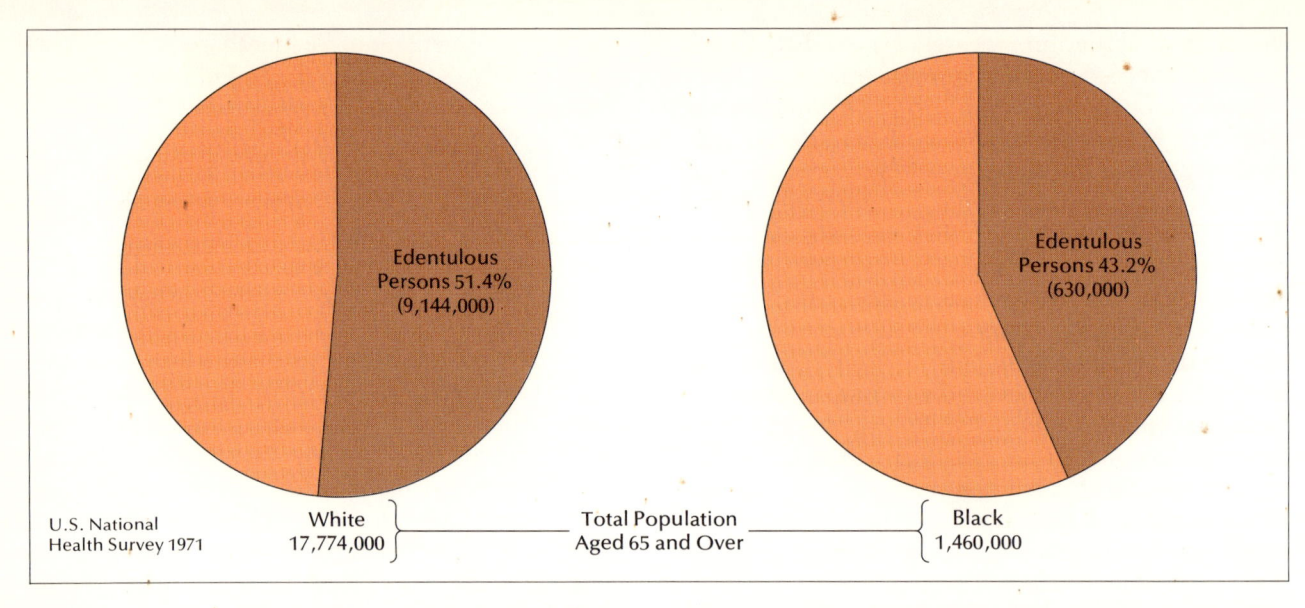

CHAPTER 21: CHAUNCEY AND HOUSE

Disparity between elderly whites and blacks in edentulousness is due in part to higher percentage of whites in older age groups. Nonetheless, rates for black males (but not black females) are genuinely lower than for whites.

ing masticatory ability and that patients over the age of 70 have a consistently inadequate nutritional intake. The type, maintenance, and extent of prosthetic replacement can produce marked changes in food selection. There may be a shift to more easily chewed foods. Avoidance of certain foods may occur because they do not "taste right," since the smell-feel component, believed to affect flavor, is diminished. The individual may seek oral gratification from foods that are easier to chew. In the patient who has visual, hearing, and other sensory losses the reduction in oral gratification may intensify the search for "satisfying" foods, often salty or sweet. This may prompt some patients, against the advice of their physician, to shift to more salty foods. Thus, it is of great importance to have valid information regarding the effect that changes in dietary habits, arising from lowered masticatory ability as well as other factors, may have on the health status of the individual. Current information gathered from the Veterans Administration Normative Aging Study is expected to assist in clarifying the relationship between reduced chewing ability in denture wearers and their food selection and/or preference.

The potential impact and interaction of these multiple factors may emerge from the information contained in the U.S. Public Health Service Health Statistics Series and other surveys. In addition, a number of investigations have been established to ascertain the interrelationship between the incidence of

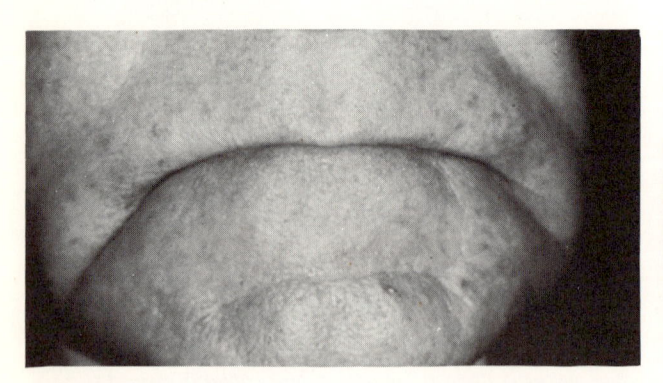

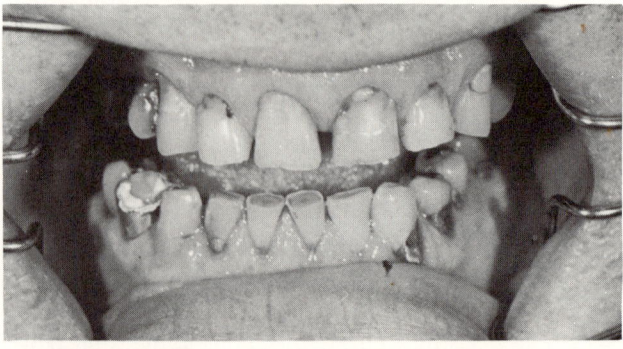

An illustration of the type of change in facial appearance that can occur in an edentulous person who does not wear a denture is shown at left. Excessive abrasion of natural teeth is also a common phenomenon in the elderly (right).

disease and various socioeconomic factors. These health status studies have provided excellent cross-sectional data on a variety of populations. There are no comprehensive longitudinal health studies that encompass an evaluation of oral status, other than the Veterans Administration Normative Aging Study, which is collecting longitudinal data from multiple medical, socioeconomic, and psychologic evaluations. When initiated in 1963, the Normative Aging Study contained more than 2,000 healthy males ranging in age between 25 and 75 years. The participants were selected because they met specific health criteria, represented a broad range of socioeconomic statuses, and exhibited geographic stability. Their age distribution was quite similar to the general veteran population. Oral health status was not a consideration in their selection. In 1970, slightly more than 1,200 of these subjects volunteered to also participate in a dental (orofacial) longitudinal study.

The dental longitudinal study consists of several series of examinations or procedures. These are: 1) an interim dental health history; 2) a comprehensive orofacial examination; 3) masticatory function tests and a survey of dietary habits; 4) biochemical analyses of stimulated whole and parotid saliva; and 5) various general procedures, including intraoral and panographic radiographs, lateral and frontal cephalometric radiographs, study casts, and oral cytologic smears.

Although the number of participants with dentures in one or both jaws increases with age in this health-conscious group of volunteers, only 55 of 785 subjects over 45 years old (7%) are edentulous in both jaws. This is a substantially lower rate of edentulousness than the national average of 31.5% for this age group of males.

Masticatory performance can be accurately assessed using a standard test food. In the dental longitudinal study, the 1,200 participants were classified into three major dentition groups: 1) a complete removable denture in one or both jaws; 2) a removable partial denture in one or both jaws; and 3) no removable replacements, even if indicated. Chewing performance on the right side and on the left side and the performance needed to prepare the test food for swallowing, as well as the number of strokes used to reach the swallowing point (threshold), were different for the three groups. These differences were statistically significant. Subjects with natural dentition not only reduced the test food to a finer size, but applied less effort, in terms of chewing strokes.

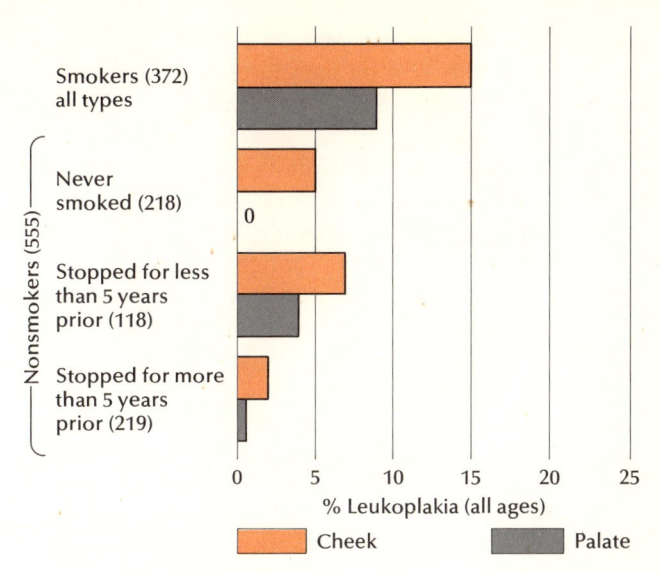

As shown in the graph above, marked association exists between tobacco smoking and the incidence of leukoplakia in participants in dental longitudinal study.

When the right side masticatory performance for the three dentition groups was recalculated, with a statistical adjustment for age, it was found that age had no discernible effect. This indicates that chewing ability, which is markedly reduced with the loss of the natural dentition, can be only partially restored by a prosthesis. Studies now being conducted to determine the effect of this diminished masticatory performance on food selection have indicated that certain foods, especially apples, carrots, and celery, are avoided as more teeth are lost and the extent of prosthetic replacement is increased.

Tobacco smoking is a major public health problem. The dental longitudinal study has provided information confirming the increased frequency of leukoplakia in smokers, specifically concerning the location and prevalence of this lesion in 372 current smokers and 555 nonsmokers who do not wear a full upper denture. The nonsmoker group includes 219 former smokers who had stopped smoking more than five years prior to examination. The most common sites were the cheek and palate. Leukoplakia was observed on the cheeks in only 10 of the 218 subjects who reported no previous history of smoking. For smokers, the prevalence rate on the cheek was more than three times greater than for the nonsmokers, while the risk of developing leukoplakia on the palate was infinitely greater in smokers than in nonsmokers. (Of 145 persons wearing full upper dentures, only three exhibited leukoplakic lesions of the palate.)

CHAPTER 21: CHAUNCEY AND HOUSE

Many pathologists consider that leukoplakia is a premalignant lesion and frequently recommend that a biopsy be done to determine whether a malignant change has occurred.

The incidence of oral tumors increases with age from 22.8/100,000 population at age 50 to 54 and twice that by age 80. Malignant tumors are frequently located on the side of the tongue and the floor of the mouth but can occur in any area. Primary oral malignancies have been noted to develop more frequently in persons who use excessive amounts of alcohol and tobacco. These persons usually exhibit a low level of oral care.

In a recent study of 1,200 healthy adult males, the incidence of coronal caries was related to age. The men were between 25 and 74 years of age and primary caries, restorations with secondary caries, and restorations without caries were noted. The findings indicated that, contrary to common belief, there is a significant increase in caries incidence associated with aging, mostly secondary caries.

The foregoing information clearly indicates that physicians must reevaluate their responsibility in maintaining the oral health of their elderly patients. The most expeditious procedure is to conduct a brief survey for gross problems during office visits, preferably semiannually. This survey should include a comprehensive examination of all oral tissues. Patients with dentures should remove them so that the tissue beneath can be examined. The patient, a nurse, or an aide can assist by reflecting the cheeks when the mouth is opened. The physician then grasps the tongue and extrudes it, using a 2 x 2 gauze, for careful inspection. The tongue, floor of the mouth, palate, cheeks, and tonsillar area are examined for tumors and other lesions.

The physician should specifically inquire if the patient has a chewing problem or denture-related soreness. These may require a dental referral. While physicians are not expected to be aware of all the nuances concerning denture fit and condition, they can examine the denture and determine if a fracture exists or there has been a "home repair." The patient should be informed that self-repair of dentures not only can cause serious harm to the tissues but can damage the denture beyond repair. Most dentists are willing to provide repair service for a minimal fee.

Monilial infections are common in the elderly and can contribute to the development of denture stomatitis or angular cheilitis. This can be diagnosed and treated, either by the physician or by the dentist, with nystatin preparations (oral rinses). Stomatitis is characterized by erythema of the tissue under the denture. Cheilitis is recognized by the cracked corners of the lips.

Among the drugs that affect oral tissues, diphenylhydantoin is most often cited. It causes a marked proliferation of the gingival tissue around the crown of the tooth. In patients receiving this medication, the teeth must be professionally cleaned at frequent intervals and the patient must maintain good oral hygiene. Tranquilizers especially reduce the rate of saliva production and lower its pH and buffering capacity. The change in pH and subsequent alterations in the oral microflora balance may cause a generalized stomatitis or angular cheilitis. Broad-spectrum antibiotics can also alter the microbial balance so that an overgrowth by *Candida albicans* develops. Ny-

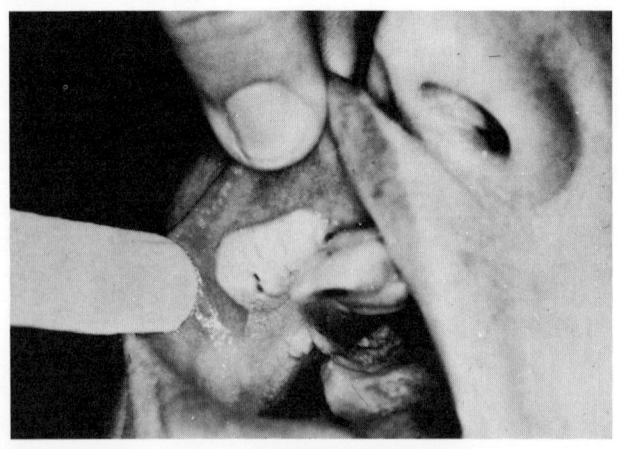

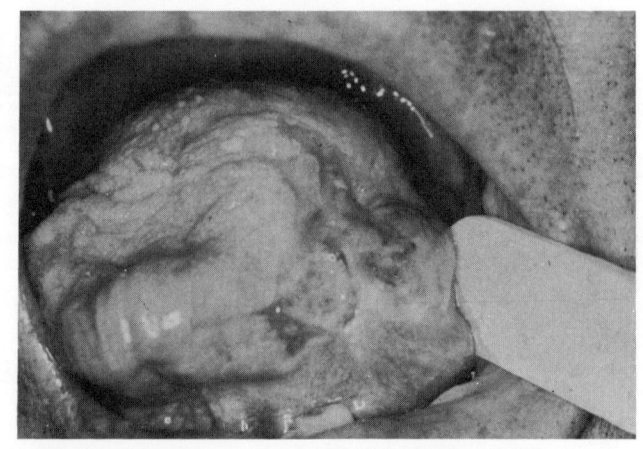

Leukoplakia on the cheek (left) is often considered a premalignant lesion that calls for biopsy. Incidence of oral tumors doubles between ages 55 and 80; a carcinoma of the tongue is seen in an elderly man (right).

statin therapy is usually indicated for these patients.

In addition to the patient who can be seen in the physician's office, the homebound and institutionalized patient has dental problems that often are ignored and become acute. In the individual with hand and/or arm function compromised by arthritis, stroke, or other disability, good oral hygiene should be maintained with the assistance of another person, using an electric toothbrush or various special implements such as toothbrushes with extenders and/or flushing devices. The dentures of chronically ill or bedridden patients must be regularly cleaned and checked for alignment and fit by the physician, nurse, or a family member.

Similarly, the physician must not assume that dental care is routinely given in nursing homes or chronic-care hospitals. Nursing aides often are reluctant to inspect or clean dentures, unless explicit orders are given. Nor should the physician assume that nurses instruct their patients regarding the need for good oral hygiene. Moreover, dentures occasionally are mixed up, misplaced, or lost. An elderly patient receiving dentures that belong to another individual can experience great distress when he or she attempts to use the prosthesis. This can be prevented by having the dentures labeled. The patient's name can be inserted by a dentist or dental laboratory technician within 20 to 30 minutes. Labeling kits for use in a hospital ward can be obtained from medical or dental supply houses.

Access to dental treatment – involving barriers of both cost and practitioner availability – must be resolved for the elderly. How costly are these services and what is the most efficacious procedure for providing them? This question is under study in the various Triage programs.

Comprehensive assessment of patient needs, by Triage, includes requisite dental treatment. A dental survey is conducted by a nurse-clinician, and the patient is referred to his or her own dentist or allowed a choice of available dentists. Triage pays for the treatment according to a fixed fee schedule. If the fee for treatment exceeds the schedule, the dentist is notified, and he determines whether he is able to reduce the fee to the allowed fee limit. The patient is duly informed and can reject the care or pay the difference between the allowed amount and the fee requested by the dentist. Triage provides transportation when necessary. Homebound and institutionalized patients are visited by the dentist.

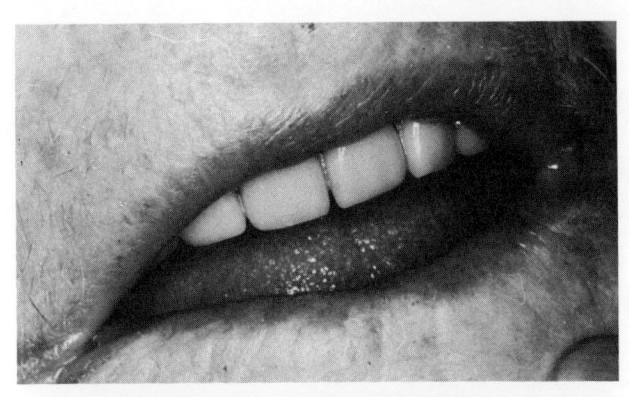

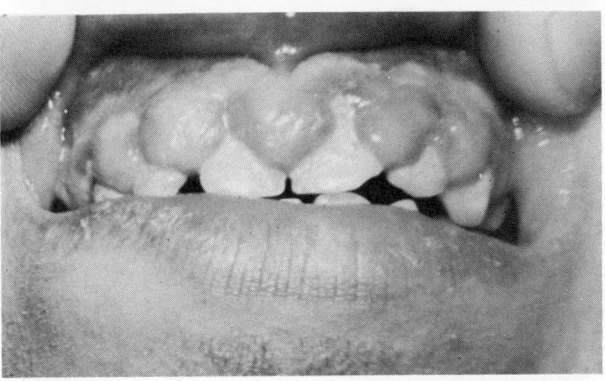

Monilial infection may cause cheilitis (top), producing cracked corners of lips. Diphenylhydantoin treatment may lead to gingival tissue proliferation (bottom).

Preliminary findings from the Triage programs indicate that the increase in the public funding necessary to provide dental treatment for the elderly is not as great as anticipated. Thirty-one percent of these treatments were prosthodontic procedures. Prosthodontics accounted for almost 77% of the total monies used for dental care, and was only 1.2% of all Triage funds expended. The mean dental expenditure per patient was $252.

Current circumstances dictate that the physician must actively participate in any initiative directed toward improving oral health in the elderly. Physicians who view dental treatment as an integral part of total health care perform an inestimable service for their elderly patients. The time when the physician viewed his jurisdiction as beginning beyond the tonsils while the dentist focused his attention on the region anterior to this area should be long past.

22

Rehabilitation of the Elderly

T. E. HUNT
University of Saskatchewan

There is no reason why the family physician cannot prescribe for the bulk of elderly patients in need of straightforward rehabilitative services. While it is helpful to have guidance available from specialists in geriatrics and rehabilitation medicine, the special geriatric considerations and rehabilitative principles can be mastered. In complex cases, especially those refractory to treatment or complicated by collateral disease, consultations or referral probably will be necessary. By and large, the family physician is well situated to assess rehabilitative needs and manage the case in the environment most comfortable for the patient. Even without an elaborate team, the family physician can do a great deal for the patient simply with the aid of a well-oriented nurse and a physical therapist.

Medical management of incapacitation encompasses four activities: control of the underlying disease; prevention of secondary disabilities (i.e., bedsores, contractures); restoration of functional ability; and adaptation of and for the patient (to maximize residual functional capacities and psychosocial adjustment, and to modify the environment).

To these general considerations, special features of geriatric rehabilitation can be added. These include the difficulty of controlling illness of multifactorial nature, confusion related to abnormal presentations of disease, and the impact on recovery potential of collateral diseases. Dementia, depression, withdrawal, and other psychosocial problems give disability in the aged population a dimension disproportionate to that found among the young.

A treatment program for a geriatric patient must be shaped to such realities. The susceptibility of elderly patients to secondary disabilities makes imperative the rapid initiation of rehabilitative measures in the hope of maximizing function. Paradoxically, the chances of unpredictable improvement may be greater than in the young, therefore enhancing the value in persisting with treatment of the geriatric patient over an unusually long period of time.

There are reasons why physicians underachieve in geriatric rehabilitation, or give up on it. I will discuss a few of the main pitfalls, because they are avoidable. The setting of unrealistic goals – or goals more appropriate to an earlier stage of the life cycle – is one. In young patients, with fewer collateral diseases and an essentially upbeat outlook on life, achievement can be measured by successful return to gainful employment. For the elderly, the goal may not be the full restoration implied by gainful employment. Rather, the goal may be return to the previous degree of independence in such activities of daily living as grooming, walking, kitchen work, and hobbies. To strive for "cure" is to invite defeat, frustration, and abandonment. I recall an elderly woman whose arthritis was untreated for 30 years. Her physician, a surgically oriented general practitioner, did nothing for her because "you can't cure arthritis." She was never referred to a rehabilitation or rheumatic disease unit where the disease might have been controlled and where she certainly would have achieved greater functional independence. This was not misdiagnosis but mismanagement – nihilism engendered by the physician's orientation toward "cure."

Of course, the reverse attitude often prevails as well – that is that the restorative potential is assumed to be nonexistent or much less than is actually the case because the patient is old. In the past many elderly disabled have been denied perfectly feasible rehabilitation services because of their advanced age. The aged amputee is an example. Fifteen or so years ago many persons over the age of 65 years were rejected for prosthetic fitting and training "because they were too old to learn or to handle a prosthesis." Today most rehabilitation centers are successfully training persons of 80 to 90 years or even older to use artificial limbs.

Nonrecognition of dehydration and hyperthermia is another barrier to rehabilitation. Older persons tend to drink insufficient amounts of fluid on their own initiative because they do not feel thirst as keenly as younger persons. Dehydration can result rapidly with even the slight additional fluid loss through respiration (as well as perspiration) where the respiration becomes increased with infections, dyspnea due to other disease, or rehabilitative exercises. Older persons, especially women, sweat less than do younger persons and do not start to sweat until higher body temperatures are reached. Heat applications, particularly those to extensive body areas, may then provoke hyperthermia. Dehydration and hyperthermia may result in acute but reversible organic brain syndrome with confusion and other behavioral changes, such as irascibility, aggression, and occasional violence. Precautions to assure sufficient fluid intake and to prevent excess heating are necessary steps to take in geriatric rehabilitation.

Poor analysis of pain also may hinder rehabilitation in the elderly. Older persons tend to have abnormal presentations and sensitivities to pain. Acute pain does not seem to be as sharply perceived or reacted to as it is in the young. But chronic, niggling pain seems to be worse. Diffuse, persistent pain may indicate a variety of physical and mental problems, ranging from depression and anxiety to osteoporosis, cited here because it is one of the most common causes of diffuse pain of the back and the pelvis in elderly women.

Pain perception and recognition by geriatric patients may be strikingly abnormal in a crisis. For example, up to half of acute myocardial infarctions (MI) in the elderly occur without pain. The only symptom of a painless MI – or, for that matter, an inflamed, thrombosed external hemorrhoid – may be the sudden onset of noisy, agitated behavior or confusion. For rehabilitation and other purposes, the physician's interpretation of geriatric pain is crucial.

Abnormality of clinical presentation of pain in the elderly has been illustrated well by the geriatrician

Prognostic Indicators in Stroke Patients

Clinical Features	Good Prognosis	Poor Prognosis
Conscious level	No loss or rapid return	Delayed return
Mental status	Alert, responsive, and orientated to time and place	Continuing dementia
Emotions	Normal for individual	Inappropriate crying or increased lability
Psychologic state	Normal progression of reaction to severe disability	Undue depression or apathy
Motor function (including bowel and bladder)	Early return	Delayed return, especially continuing flaccidity
Sensation	No loss or early return	Delayed and lack of proprioception
Perception (especially left hemiplegia)	No loss or rapid return	Continuing loss after first month
Language	Isolated problem of expressive dysphasia; rapid return of single appropriate words	Global dysphasia Jargon Perseveration
Concurrent disease	Absent or insignificant	Incapacitation by severe concurrent illness
Age	Usually younger	Very aged, especially with previous strokes or other vascular disease

CHAPTER 22: HUNT

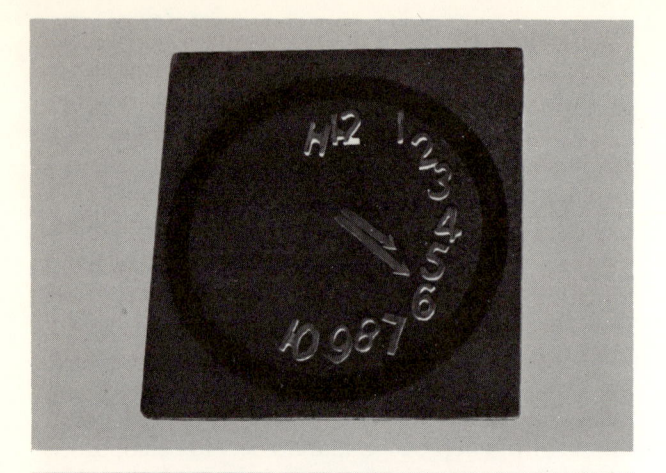

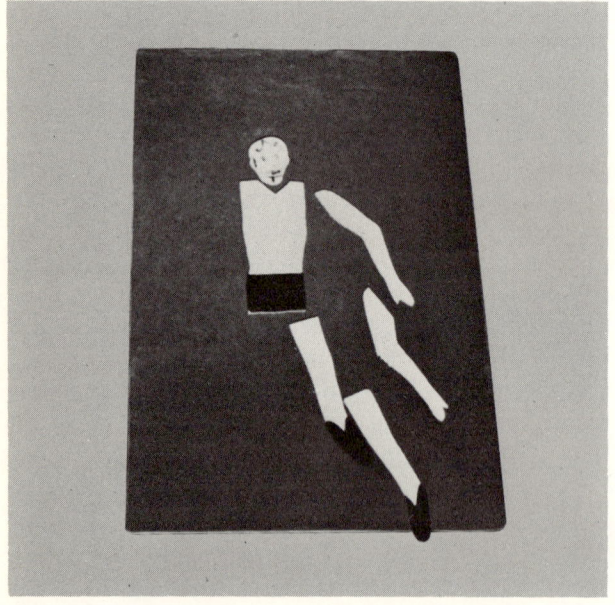

Test of perceptual loss assesses patient's ability to place numerals on imitation clock and to position parts of body. Left hemiplegic might perform as shown.

Sir Ferguson Anderson of Glasgow. In referring an elderly woman to him, a physician wrote, "She has a pain in her neck and is one in mine." Indeed, her neck pain was serious. But it was not intractable: it disappeared when thorough investigation revealed, and treatment alleviated, a stomach ulcer. The point, of course, is that in the elderly, pain from internal organs often is referred to locomotor regions. Referred pain appears to dominate pain of local origin. A complaint of arthritis in a knee may be the only symptom of a hip lesion. Painful shoulder syndromes often represent pain referred from the cervical spine, where the most common etiology is cervical spondylosis.

Back pain may indicate metastatic carcinoma, even when the spinal roentgenogram is negative. Traumatic lesions often are unsuspected causes of chronic pain. The aged patient may recall no traumatic episode and may even have persisting, though limited, joint functions that disguise the trauma, such as the "arthritis" that actually represents an impacted femoral neck fracture. Minor or forgotten accidents may produce pathologic crush fractures of osteoporotic vertebrae, a cause of pain that is often missed.

With pain properly assessed and managed, the chances are enhanced for rapid mobilization of the elderly patient. Rapid mobilization is a high priority for many reasons. Prolonged disuse of a joint or muscle tends to promote deformity, contractures, and other handicaps. It should surprise no one if a fractured or dislocated shoulder never moves again after being held in an immobilizing sling for six months. Yet, mobilization must not be pursued too rapidly. A course must be charted between the risks of immobilization and the need of the elderly person for more time to heal. Not only do bony and soft tissues in the elderly heal more slowly than in the young, but the healing often is less complete. A fracture site may still be visible on x-ray film in an aged person's hip a year after pinning.

Therapists may have to be warned to avoid overstretching soft tissues in attempts to maintain range of motion of joints, because the patient may be insensitive to pain.

For this reason, the patient's temperature sensation should be tested prior to giving heat treatments. Deep heat by ultrasound, shortwave, or microthermy must be used cautiously in the elderly. They tend not to realize they are burning, especially in the legs. Intense heat may also be detrimental because it can enhance muscle metabolism; if the circulation is poor, gangrene may result. These hazards suggest that, where thermal therapy is indicated, low-intensity heat from a warm bath or moist pack is often the modality of choice.

The choice of surgical procedure should be made with rehabilitation goals in mind. Pinning a fractured femur may seem the procedure of choice. And it actually may be, because of collateral illness that forecloses complex surgery. However, the more risky operation, total hip replacement, may be better for the hemiplegic patient because remobilization is possible the first day after operation, and the patient may experience less disability in the long run. Considerations of rapid mobilization may have priority for the elderly candidate for amputation when vascular disease, cancer, or some other disease severely limits life expectancy. A wise surgeon will choose an operation that immobilizes the patient for the least amount of time, such as a through-the-knee procedure. This area with a good blood supply heals easily, and the patient can be walking with a prosthesis relatively quickly.

I would like to turn from pitfalls in geriatric rehabilitation to a discussion of case management. In Chapter 8, "Stroke in the Geriatric Patient," Dr. Solomon Robbins has reviewed the principles of diagnosis and management of acute stroke. Let us pick up the story of the patient with a completed stroke and take it into the rehabilitation phase. I will try to dramatize the principles of geriatric rehabilitation, including diagnosis of functional defect as a basis for a treatment plan and functional prognosis.

Let us postulate an 82-year-old widow who has had a stroke while visiting her 60-year-old daughter's family. Under the care of the daughter's family physician, the mother has been admitted to a 200-bed community hospital. It is three days after the stroke and she has just regained full consciousness. The physician is about to make rehabilitative plans. He must complete his assessment of brain damage. This will allow a tentative estimate of functional loss and potential for functional recovery. He knows that nothing can be done to increase the rate of tissue recovery in the brain. But he also knows that by recognizing physiologic improvement early, he can help speed functional recovery with the aid of nurses and physical, occupational, and speech therapists.

Upon examining the patient, the physician finds she has expressive dysphasia. She is able to understand. She can say "yes" and "no" appropriately, sig-

Stages in the Management and Rehabilitation of the Stroke Patient

Time or Stage	Guide to Ability	Details of Management
Admission	Unconscious patient	Life support measures through medical assessment; control of concurrent significant disease; frequent changes of position in bed; correct postures; bladder and bowel management
Day 1 – day 3	Consciousness regained	Start multidisciplinary assessment of disability; add passive mobility to extremities; start sitting on edge of bed or in chair
Day 3 – day 7	Alert, fully orientated; moving contralateral extremities adequately	Start standing-up exercises, language retraining; try independent bowel and bladder function; self-feeding (may need some devices)
Reassess Progress and General Condition		
Second week	Return of some movement on affected side; understands simple conversations; appropriate "yes, no" answers; appears aware of own body and environment	Now in Rehabilitation Department for walking reeducation; training in activities of daily living; speech training if needed; social planning NOTE: frequent rest periods; assure adequate fluids
Third week	Increasing functional return	Increased practice and training in ambulation, activities of daily living, and speech
Third – fourth week	Partial independence	Thorough reassessment; plan for discharge; arrange home care
Fourth – sixth week	Continuing functional improvement	Continue home care until able to come in as outpatient or go to hospital
Sixth week plus	Physiologic return usually complete; may yet improve functionally and psychologically	Thorough reassessment; continuing home or outpatient program to assist possible further adaptation; reevaluate frequently; day hospital to alleviate family care

CHAPTER 22: HUNT

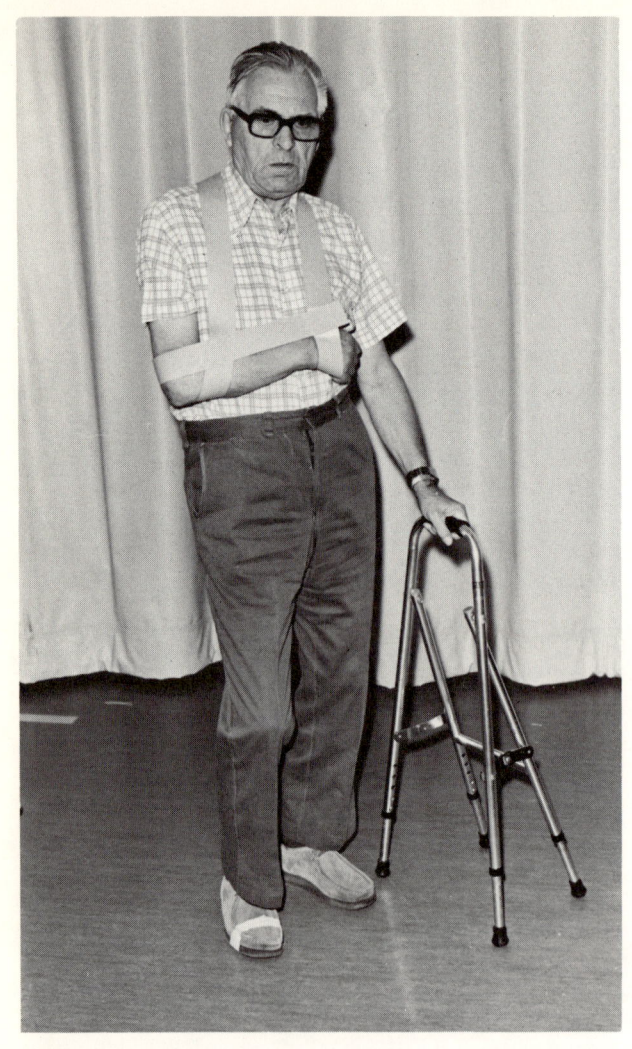

Man with right hemiplegia starts to ambulate with a quadriped walking aid, which greatly improves balance. Sling supports paralyzed arm with minimal drag on neck.

nifying a fairly good prognosis for speech recovery. He asks her to lift her right arm, but she does not. She does lift her left arm when asked. To test ability to perform a complex act, he asks her to touch her nose with her left hand, and she does. He discovers that while she cannot move her right hand or arm, she shows good right-leg motion.

With these results, the prognosis is not bleak. Indications of the most severe brain damage are largely missing. Though there is right hemiplegia, there is no clouding of consciousness, homonymous hemianopsia, or inappropriate crying or laughing. On the first hospital day, semicomatose, she had to be catheterized. Because she is fully conscious and is recovering voluntary movement, she is probably regaining continence. The physician may expect the nurses to remove in a day or so the catheter that had been placed when she was admitted.

According to the daughter, the patient had a heart attack at age 65 but has not recently shown chest pain or shortness of breath. She had received digoxin and, because of edema of the feet and ankles in the last few years, a diuretic. Currently, there is no evidence of cardiac failure. ECG abnormalities are consistent with an old myocardial infarction. The physician concludes from all the evidence that the heart disease is well controlled and is no bar to stroke rehabilitation, though she will not be pushed to maximum effort.

A noteworthy finding is a poststroke blood-sugar value of 180 mg/100 ml, but this is not unexpected after brain damage. If it persists for more than a week, the significance of hyperglycemia will be reevaluated; but at this point, the hope is to avoid prescribing insulin or oral hypoglycemic drugs because these can create a risk of hypoglycemia during exercise.

For years, the patient had had osteoarthritis in her right knee and had been walking with a cane. The osteoarthritis does not appear to require major restriction on therapy in the long run, though weight bearing in the immediate recovery period will have to be limited.

After making his own examination, the physician asks for the appraisal of a physical therapist for strength and range of motion, of a speech therapist for language abilities, and of an occupational therapist for evaluation of expectation with regard to dressing, washing, and other activities of daily living. In addition, the occupational therapist can test perceptual abilities. The appraisals can be made within a few days.

Experience tells the physician that the woman probably will have a cycle of emotional reactions to her disability: a period of unreality ("This can't happen to me; I'm walking out of the hospital in a week."); then depression, upon realizing that disabilities will not suddenly clear ("Why did this happen to me? I'm no good any more."). This despairing attitude is particularly common among individuals who had been managing independently but now fear dependency upon family or society. As time passes, the elderly tend to become apathetic, which means a reduced motivation to pursue rehabilitation; this contrasts with the tendency of younger patients to become hostile.

The physician, the nurses, and the therapists will

REHABILITATION

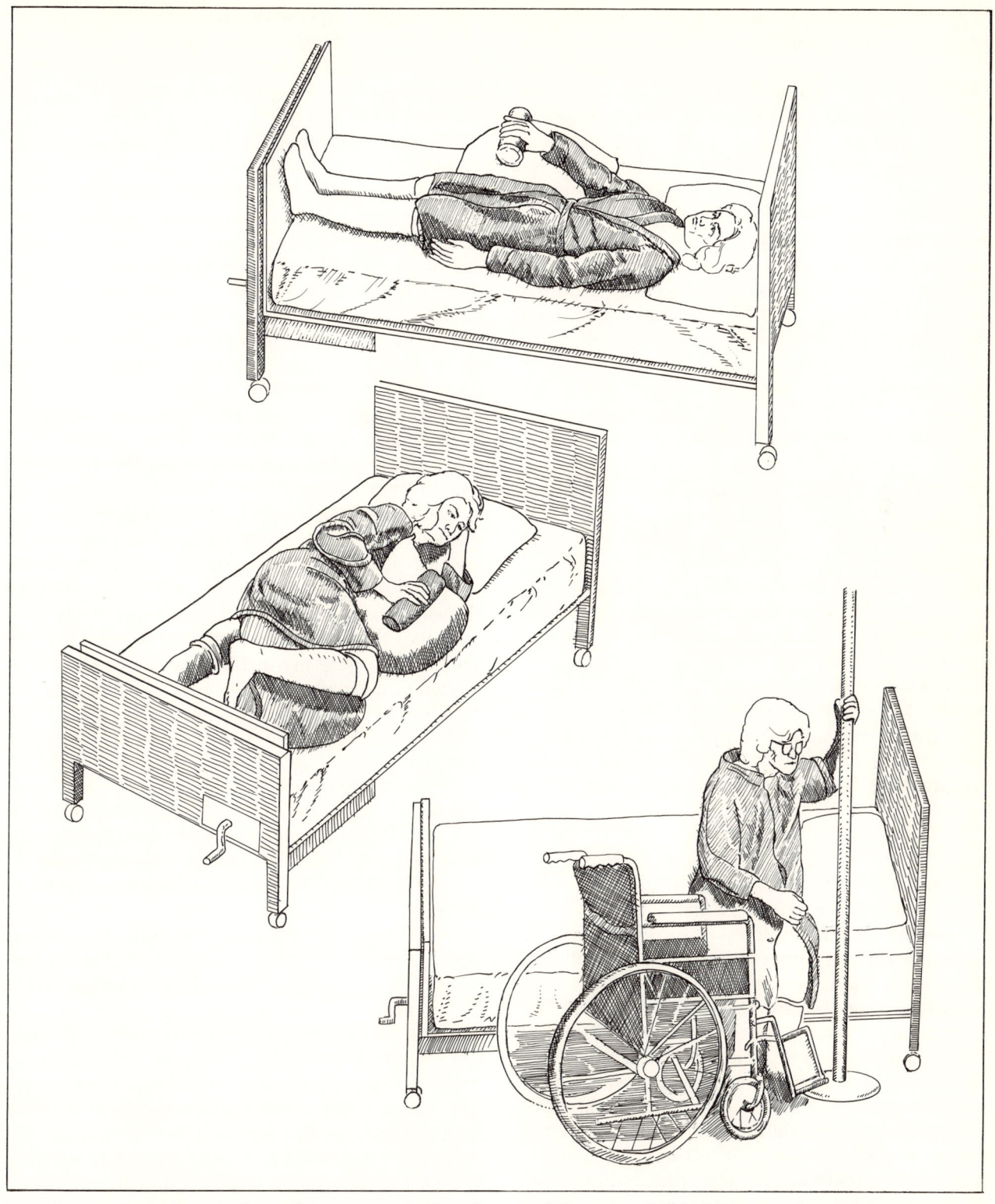

Female patient with right hemiplegia is postured and supported in supine position (top), body and legs fully extended and feet held at right angles by footboard. Paralyzed arm is abducted and flexed, supported on pillow, and fingers curled lightly around a rolled facecloth. In left lateral position (middle) pillow is between knees, and paralyzed arm still supported. About day 7, she uses a "Saskapole" (bottom) to transfer to wheelchair.

177

have to vary their approaches according to the patient's reactions. From the outset, the patient needs as accurate an explanation of medical status as possible. Later, in the depressed stage, the need is to convey that recovery potentials exist. When physical condition permits, the woman will be invited to meet other patients who can demonstrate what stroke rehabilitation can accomplish and how adjustments can be made. This often encourages accommodation to disability.

Family support also is taken into account by the physician. A patient tends to do better if the spouse is alive, if the family gives good emotional support, and if residence is among neighbors with positive attitudes toward aging and chronic handicaps. A patient who has lived in a community lacking facilities for the disabled tends to be more apathetic than one who has seen other disabled persons functioning, and who is aware that society has taken measures to ease the pain of the handicapped by providing such devices as wheelchair ramps at public buildings.

In the case we are describing, the patient has no spouse, but she does have the devoted concern of her daughter and the daughter's family. Whether the home and neighborhood environments are favorable will be determined in part by a social assessment that has been started as a basis for discharge planning.

The comprehensive plan emerges at the end of the first week of treatment. Based on the consensus prevailing in a conference with nurses and therapists, the physician tells the patient and her daughter that the prognosis is good and that over the next four to six weeks the patient will probably attain considerable, though not full, independence. The doctor explains what the therapists will do and the patient's part in the plan. He holds out the hope that she can return home by the end of the third or fourth week. (Under the Canadian medical care system, there are no major barriers to her staying in the hospital for this length of time.)

Basic rehabilitation has already been initiated. The nurses have assured proper changes of position and posturing to prevent decubiti and contractures from developing. The speech therapist has already commenced language reeducation at the bedside. For brief periods on the third and succeeding days, the patient has been placed in a wheelchair by the nurses and, with provision for rest periods, gradually allowed to start standing up with support. The foot of the bed may be used for this. In our hospital, a portable pole (the "Saskapole") can be wedged at the bedside between the floor and the ceiling. Convenient to the patient's good side, the pole is used for support in standing up, both as an exercise and in transferring between bed and wheelchair. In this early stage, the physical therapy objective is to maintain mobility of the extremities and to encourage the patient to move limbs more and more as physiologic improvement occurs. The urgency of preventing secondary disabilities is well understood by the multidisciplinary team. Contractures, pressure sores, disuse weakness, atelectasis, thrombosis, osteoporosis, and other sequelae of immobility can delay or impede therapies at critical times when the patient is most ready for functional gains.

The physical therapist and nurse see to it that the patient is properly positioned at all times, in and out of bed. The occupational therapist provides temporary splinting for the leg, ankle, and foot, so they are positioned to avoid dropped foot or other contracture. An arm splint is prepared to hold the hand with no wrist flexion and a slight flexion of the fingers. If one wanted a power grip, the wrist would be held extended (in an aged person, the need is not for power but for holding utensils). The desired position is a neutral or slight wrist flexion with fingers slightly curled. The occupational therapist also provides a board for the wheelchair to support the affected arm and hold the wrist in the desired position. An unsupported or dangling arm will cause shoulder subluxation in a hemiplegic patient, producing pain and instability. When walking, the patient may need a hemiplegic sling.

Let us say that, during the first week, contractures, depression, apathy, and other impediments have been prevented, and some early mobilization has been realized on the right side. The therapist now increases the use of assisted exercises of the right leg. Since no recovery in the right arm has occurred, a passive range of motion is employed: the limb is moved, and the patient is encouraged to try to feel and to will the motion. The therapist tries to sense the moment the muscles respond volitionally, indicating further physiologic recovery of brain tissue.

In addition, the occupational therapist has been teaching the right-handed patient to work with her left hand, so that if no right-arm recovery ever occurs, she will be able to brush her teeth, wash her face, apply makeup, dress, and perform other activities of daily living. The woman is taught how to use big buttons, special holders to pull stockings, and other adaptive devices. Thus, the processes of restoration and adaptation go together, with the emphasis shifting to adaptation when it becomes clear that fur-

Potential Care Resources for the Aged

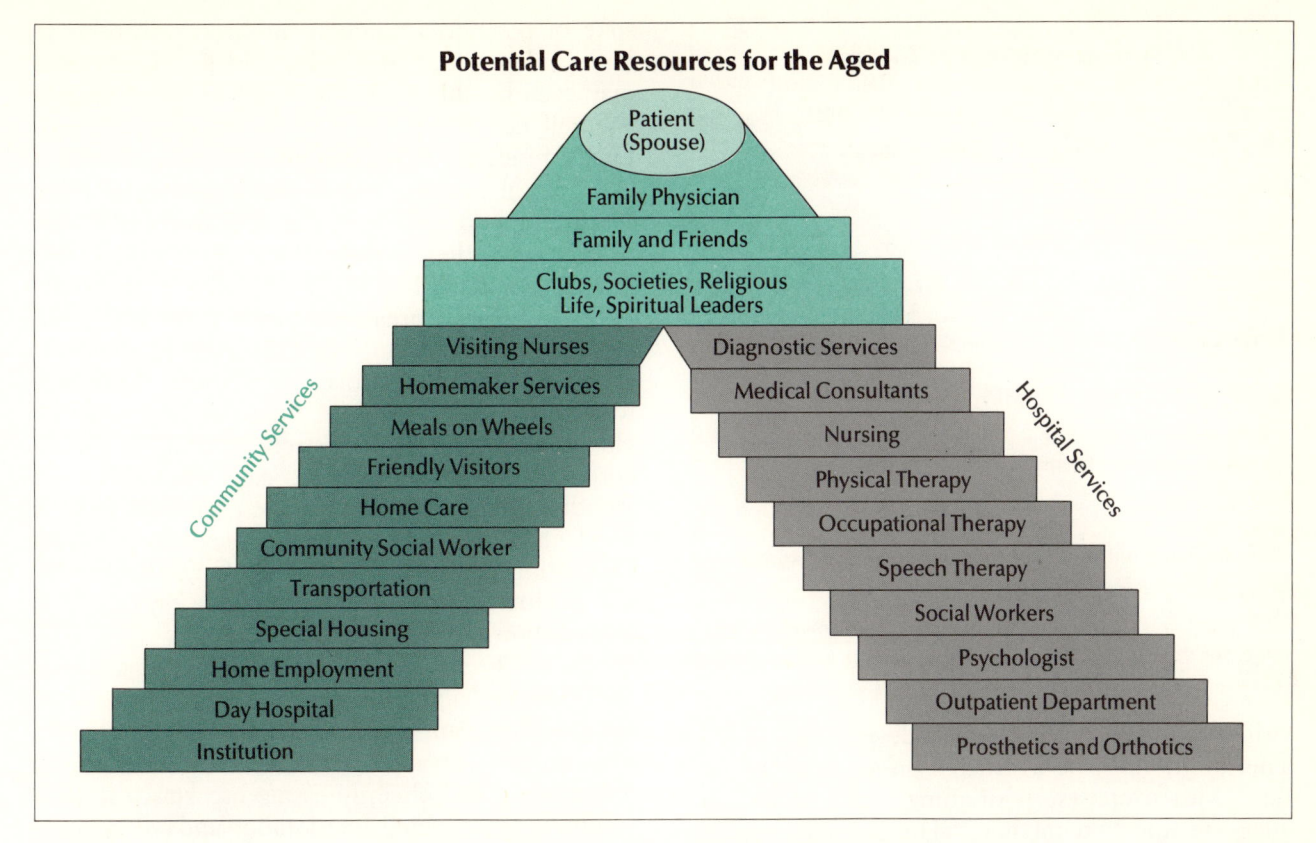

Patient (Spouse)
Family Physician
Family and Friends
Clubs, Societies, Religious Life, Spiritual Leaders

Community Services:
- Visiting Nurses
- Homemaker Services
- Meals on Wheels
- Friendly Visitors
- Home Care
- Community Social Worker
- Transportation
- Special Housing
- Home Employment
- Day Hospital
- Institution

Hospital Services:
- Diagnostic Services
- Medical Consultants
- Nursing
- Physical Therapy
- Occupational Therapy
- Speech Therapy
- Social Workers
- Psychologist
- Outpatient Department
- Prosthetics and Orthotics

ther functional restoration is not likely or delayed.

By the end of the second week, the patient may be walking between parallel bars with assistance. At this stage, she will probably need some type of foot-drop support. This can be simply a rubber tube stretched between a calf band situated below the knee and a D-ring fastened by adhesive tape to the anterior instep area of the shoe. (Later, if there is insufficient return of controlled movement of the foot and ankle, she will probably require a permanent short-leg brace, i.e., below the knee. In this instance, a consultation with the specialist is certainly indicated.)

Considerable recovery has occurred thus far, but the patient is not yet a candidate for home care. During the third week, good progress might involve improvement in right-leg function, with the patient still lacking fine movements but able to transfer from bed to wheelchair with practically no assistance. She can also balance, without aid, between the parallel bars and take a few solo steps. At this stage, the professional staff will encourage the woman to try to dress herself and to manage well in a small kitchen designed for rehabilitation patients.

Let us also say that, most encouragingly, the right arm has begun to show gross movement. It can now be used to hold a sheet of paper on a tabletop while writing with the left hand. At the same time, the patient's spoken vocabulary has expanded so that she can utter a few simple words, such as "bedpan."

On the more conventionally medical side of the picture, one can also postulate that cardiovascular status is stable, and fasting blood sugar has declined, indicating that diabetes mellitus is not likely. Blood pressure may be stable at 180/90 mm Hg, up from 130/80 upon hospitalization. This rise probably does not warrant prescribing antihypertensive drugs, which may carry the risk of hypotension and syncope in exercise.

The individual who has come back this far is now a feasible home-care candidate. A decision for home care depends not only on recovery but also on the ability of the household involved to help in care, the availability of home-care services, and the interpersonal relationships between the patient and members of the household. An alternative might be *temporary, restorative* care in a skilled nursing facility.

If the patient is discharged to "go home," the physician requests the hospital's home-care department to make necessary arrangements. He provides orders for treatment and medication. The planning of visits by a nurse and a therapist is done by the home-care department. The occupational therapist may also

> **Summary of Aims of Therapy**
>
> Control of underlying disability-producing illness
>
> Control of other significant concurrent disease
>
> Intensive supportive critical care
>
> Relief of pain
>
> Prevention of additional superimposed disability due to increased weakness, contractures, decubiti, urinary infection resulting from enforced bed rest
>
> Avoidance of pitfalls introduced because of aging changes
>
> Early restoration of mobility, ambulation, and functions of self-care, including control of bladder and bowels
>
> Early restoration of communication and social interaction
>
> Use of community resources for supportive and restorative care following hospital discharge
>
> Frequent reassessment, reevaluation, and revision of therapy throughout the course of disability

visit occasionally to see if helping devices are needed. The family must be instructed on assisting the patient with exercises, positioning, and simple language reeducation methods. The home-care team will report to the physician at intervals. Any complications – especially dizziness, shortness of breath, or headache – must be reported at once.

I will close the story at the sixth week. Reexamination shows only a gross grip in the right hand. Further progression of return in the arm is problematic. Conventional wisdom is that by this time virtually all physiologic recovery has occurred, but this may be less true for the elderly than for the young patient. An unresponsive elderly patient sometimes improves because of motivational – if not physical – change, especially over a period of time at home. If secondary disabilities have not been prevented, functional recovery at this point would be foreclosed.

In this case, the prognosis is that the patient, in spite of poor arm function, probably will become fairly independent in walking and in self-care and may even be able to do some housework. Probably she will not be able to live entirely alone. If prolonged residence in her daughter's home is not possible, special housing nearby, with additional community support, will be essential. If she is otherwise well, either of these is preferable to institutional care.

The case described here, involving a stroke patient, embodies principles of assessment and management applicable in other diseases. However, it should be noted that stroke differs in that the underlying disease process is not amenable to control. A clinical strategy for arthritis rehabilitation would incorporate control measures, e.g., chemotherapy. Another difference is that in the arthritides there is no place for passive exercise because of the potential for tearing intra-articular tissues. Guided, assisted, and graduated active exercises are the key to restoring function and relieving arthritic pain.

The ability of elderly persons to survive depends on a delicate balance of weaknesses and strengths. I am sure that many physicians have observed that an older person who appeared to be at death's door one day was up and cheerily eating breakfast the next morning. Unexpected deterioration and recovery are common in the elderly as delicate balances are tipped one way or the other, sometimes by minor illnesses and other times without any apparent cause.

What must be emphasized, in conclusion, is the tremendously increased vulnerability of the patient if restorative measures are delayed. A physician can add a substantial load of permanent disability by taking too long to investigate the geriatric patient and by ignoring the need for concurrent rehabilitative therapy. Hospitalization for the elderly should be short and restorative. This thinking at our hospital is leading us to a strategy of more home care and less hospitalization, even to the extent of managing some stroke patients entirely in the home by bringing the hospital team there.

23

When To Institutionalize the Elderly

JACK KLEH
George Washington University

While one in 20 persons aged 65 or older is in an institution (principally nursing homes and homes for the aged) at any single point in time, perhaps one in four will be in a nursing home at the time of his or her death. The elderly population, now 22 million, will reach 30 million in the year 2010 and 50 million in 2030. The segment that is the greatest user of nursing homes, the elderly aged 75 or more, is growing faster than the elderly population as a whole. Thus, both the immediate and long-term prospects are that more and more patients and families will depend on physician understanding and recommendations for long-term care, especially use of nursing homes, when the individual can no longer function independently in the community.

Hospital utilization-review (UR) systems, a response to public demand to hold down on health care spending, bring pressure on physicians to consider nursing home and home health services in another context as well, the convalescent/rehabilitation phase of care. The lengths of stay of the elderly, who occupy one third or more of the nation's hospital beds at any given time, are of obvious concern to UR committees. The elderly have an average hospital stay of 11 days, as against six for the rest of the adult population. Review systems are cutting those stays in some hospitals by a day or more, on the average. For patients who need additional but nonhospital care, it can be given in a skilled nursing facility or through a home care program at an average cost of one third of hospital care, according to the American Hospital Association, which reports that nearly 2,000 hospitals have a discharge planning program to screen patients for home care or skilled care.

At the same time, many physicians are not confident about the quality of care a nursing home can give. A recent survey by *American Medical News* of several geriatrics-oriented physicians showed that 25% rated the care in nursing homes they visited as fair or poor, 33% excellent, and 43% good. A major criticism was lack of medical personnel or supervision. The same survey showed that 50% of the respondents thought physicians generally shunned their responsibilities to nursing home patients.

The purpose of this chapter is to help the family physician assess the need for institutional, especially nursing home, care and guide the patient and family in making a decision. To do this, the physician must understand the diagnostic workup of the chronically ill aged patient, the need for continuing comprehensive treatment, including meeting his or her psychosocial needs, and the goals and organization of the nursing home as one of several vehicles of long-term care. As compared with our conceptions concerning use of the hospital, our employment of long-term care services must be acknowledged to be disorganized and primitive. (Chapter 24, "Options for Care of the Aged Sick," discusses use of modalities not requiring the institutionalization of the patient.)

A first lack in the long-term care field is an appropriate scheme for classifying patients in terms of service needs. Some who are nursing home candidates are bedridden, some ambulatory, and some are

CHAPTER 23: KLEH

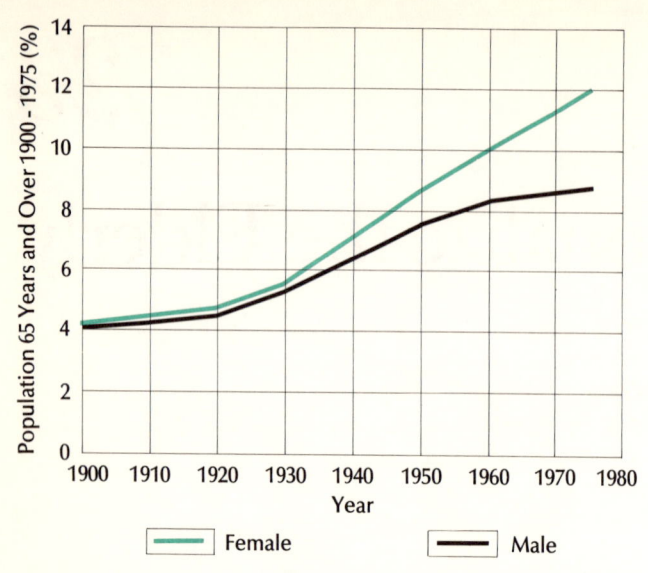

Rising proportion of aged in U.S. population is shown by Census Bureau data. Between 1900 and 1975, proportion of women 65 or over nearly tripled (from 4.1% to 12.1%), that of men more than doubled (from 4.0% to 8.8%).

both at different times. Yet all may have the same disease. Physicians are taught triage on a disease basis, but this orientation may not work in long-term care. A disease may be a precipitating factor in the institutionalization, but the significant consideration is how well the patient can function in the context not only of this disease or diseases but in terms of all factors that contribute to his disability including psychosocial circumstances.

Thus, an important statement for long-term care purposes would be *not* that the patient has a stroke producing right-sided hemiplegia but that he or she cannot use the right arm and leg and, lacking assistance at home or motivation to learn compensatory motions, cannot bathe, feed, move, take medication, or otherwise rely on himself or herself for activities of daily living or even survival. In some instances, two patients may have the same physical capacity for independent living but one is a definite nursing home candidate because of anxieties and personality factors that require a highly structured and secure environment beyond what the family may be reasonably expected to provide at home.

Functional and psychosocial assessments are central to the placement decision. The former covers ability to carry out activities of daily living, such as feeding, toileting, dressing, grooming, and bathing. The latter deals with ability to relate to and work with others, and both are concerned with ability to function in his or her environment. A patient with good interactions with family members, peers, professional caretakers, and other persons will be able to mitigate the effects of his or her disabilities.

In stressing these evaluations, I by no means dismiss categorical evaluations: medical, neurologic, psychologic, and socioeconomic. Any or all may be needed to define the patient's problems so that the most effective treatment plan may be devised. The problem list may include diagnoses of disease states, undiagnosed but significant symptoms, inadequacies in interpersonal relationships, economic limitations, and environmental impediments. The plan that evolves from the problem list will change as specific problems are resolved or, perhaps, new ones are added. For example, family members bring a disoriented aged patient to the physician and request nursing home placement. The patient is obviously "senile" and the family has no way to care for the patient at home. The physician finds that the patient has an acute brain syndrome caused by infection and dehydration. With medical treatment, the syndrome clears. But, since the physician has done a thorough appraisal, the problem list also shows a hitherto undetected hearing and vision loss, contributing to a depression that originated when the wife died a few years before. Add the fact that the patient has not been taking medication for angina pectoris and because of pain on climbing stairs has not been leaving a walk-up apartment to shop or meet friends. Meals have been skipped. Thus, even after the medical crisis is resolved, the patient remains at risk of another functional breakdown.

Is the answer a nursing home? It depends on the interventions attempted (hearing aid, spectacles, friendly visitors, meals on wheels, medications, counseling) and his response to them. Will the family agree to visit more often, to provide transportation so the patient can go out, to cook occasionally for him? Counseling may help the family understand that the patient's fear of dependence may underlie his hostility. Environmental changes may make institutionalizing unnecessary – such as eliminating stair-climbing or moving to a residential facility with services for the elderly. The patient may need help in qualifying for welfare grants and food stamps.

While there is obviously no formula for determining when nursing home placement is indicated, decisional inputs can and should be developed systematically. This may only amount to a systematic review of already available information if patients and their circumstances are well known to the family physician. Indeed, the physician may have discerned a trajectory of needs and implications for kinds of service at different stages and may have already prepared the patient and family. Case management then becomes relatively straightforward.

Often, however, the physician confronts an unknown patient or a complex situation with unknown or ambiguous elements. Aid in specific assessments can then be sought from consultants; the medical, rehabilitation, nursing, or social service departments of hospitals; and such other sources as county health departments and welfare agencies. The family physician's role becomes that of coordinator and counselor in making analyses and recommendations to patient and family.

A new organizational vehicle in long-term care is available in some localities: the geriatric evaluation unit. It studies the patient and produces multidisciplinary diagnoses and treatment recommendations, providing comprehensive workups not otherwise available to the family physician.

One such unit, of which I am clinical director, is the Gerontological Treatment Center, a division of the Psychiatric Institute of Washington, D.C. In addition to workup and management, the center serves a purpose for which neither hospitals nor nursing homes are well suited: the short-term evaluation and treatment of the disturbed elderly patient in a "non-institutional" environment, that is, one that enhances the patient's self-image. Housed in the top floor of a downtown hotel, the center has 16 semiprivate beds. Staff members wear street dress and join the patients and their families in a dining area.

Most patients are referred by family physicians for evaluation and management of behavioral changes. To determine the extent of these changes, the basis, if possible, and the likelihood of reversibility, each patient receives an initial comprehensive evaluation by an internist, neurologist, psychiatrist, and social worker and a functional appraisal in a therapeutic milieu. Additionally, where dementia exists, feasibil-

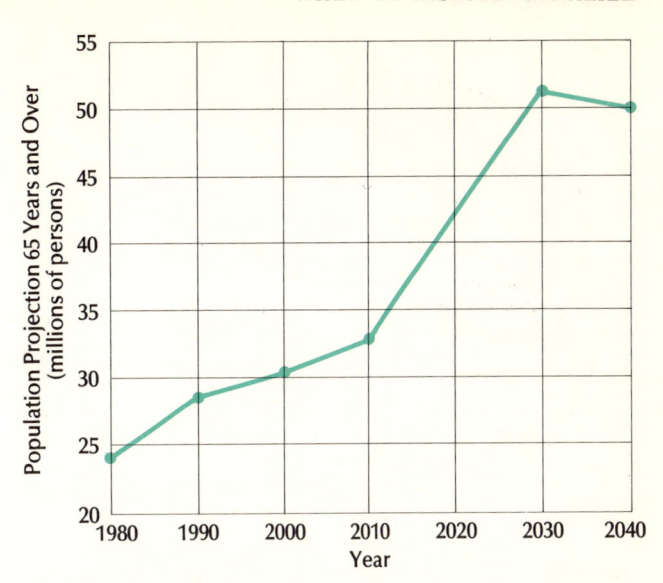

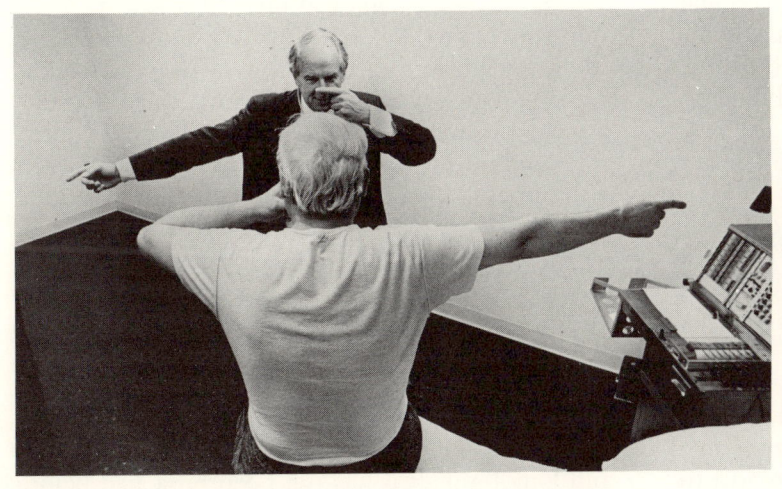

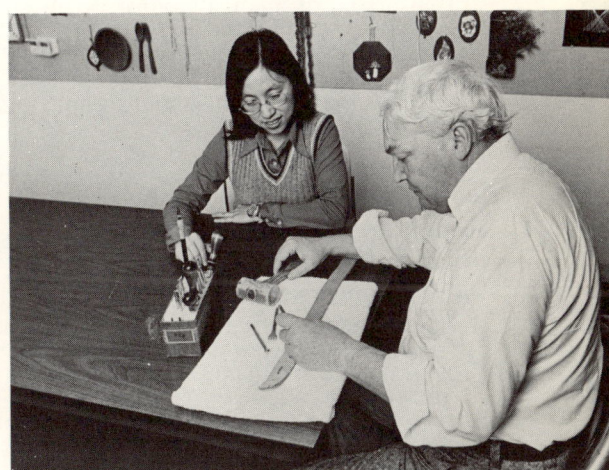

Effects of post-World War II "baby boom" are projected by Census Bureau as sharp increase in over-65 population from year 2010 to 2030. Downward trend thereafter reflects drop in birth rates that began in 1965.

Neurologic testing is part of routine evaluation of every patient (simulated here) at Gerontological Treatment Center, Washington (left). Occupational therapist (right) assists in evaluation, observing patient's ability to follow verbal and demonstrated instructions for leatherwork and expressions of emotions such as hostility.

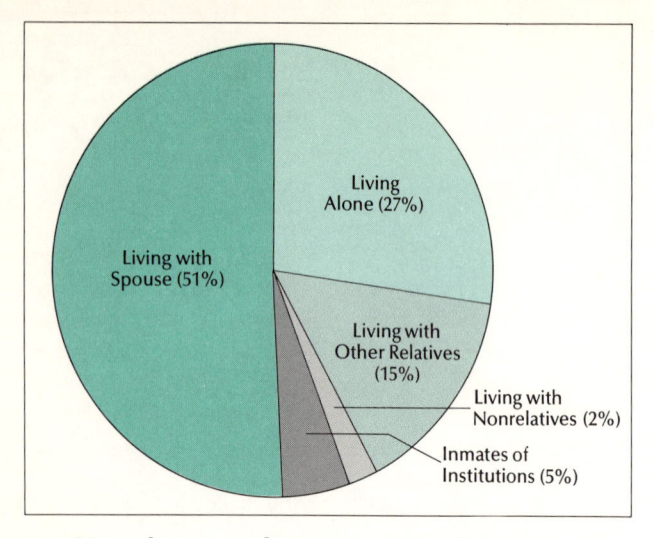

In 1975, only one aged person in 20, or about 1.1 million, lived in institutions, Census Bureau found. Proportion of women is higher than of men in homes for aged; reverse is true in chronic disease and mental hospitals.

ity for reality orientation is included. The key assessments of functional ability and social interaction are made through direct observation of the patient as he or she lives in the center and during excursions, to see how the patient behaves in stores, on the street, and at home. Family relationships and socioeconomic circumstances also are examined.

Evaluations are made on entry and during or after short-term treatment, with a variety of therapeutic modalities, including milieu therapy, group or individual therapy, psychotherapeutic drugs and so on, so that a trial of medical and/or psychosocial measures can be taken into account in diagnosis and placement recommendations. Review of the problem list, proposed management plan, and a placement recommendation are developed at a discharge conference. The family physician, who may or may not have been involved during this period, is given an extensive report at the time of discharge. Family members have opportunities to discuss the results with the center's staff, particularly in terms of understanding the patient's illness, care needs, ongoing living arrangements, and their own role.

Almost 80% of patients are recommended for a return to community living. Generally, elderly persons can manage with assistance and/or environmental change, since few are completely in need of institutionalization. The staff tends to recommend it only when there are compelling reasons, such as safety of the patient and those around him or her. The availa-

bility of home care and other outreach services also figures in placement recommendations. When referring physicians decide against continuing primary treatment themselves, the center arranges for follow-up care. The breadth and complexity of the problems may prove too much for physicians in certain types of practice.

Comprehensive evaluations of this type help correct medical misconceptions about the elderly that promote premature or unnecessary institutionalization. This has been demonstrated not only at our center but also through the experience of the Evaluation-Placement Unit of Monroe Community Hospital in Rochester, N.Y. Dr. T. Franklin Williams and associates reported in 1973 that most of 332 patients examined by this unit were originally considered ill or disabled enough to be nursing home candidates. More than half lacked a personal physician whom they saw regularly. No placement decisions were attempted until efforts were made to resolve depression, anxiety, urinary tract infections, uncontrolled diabetes, anemia, liver dysfunction, previously undiagnosed cancer, and malnutrition.

Ultimately, only one third of the candidates were recommended for nursing homes. Of the rest, many were able to remain at home with assistance, such as home health services. Some were advised to use a supervised boarding home. For a few, psychiatric hospitalization was advised. The validity of the recommendations was checked independently six weeks after placement. The degree of appropriateness was judged appreciably higher than in previous placement studies: patients were properly placed 80% to 90% of the time, an improvement of 20% to 30%.

In concluding that many nursing home candidates could remain in the community with proper assessment and planning, Dr. Williams warned against placements based solely on written data from physicians and nurses; these are likely to be inadequate for a sound clinical recommendation most of the time. Gratifyingly, personal physicians of the Rochester patients were reported to be happy to have the unit's evaluation. This has been the experience of our Washington center, too.

After the appraisals have been obtained, the family physician or the evaluation unit staff is prepared to counsel the patient and family, separately and together, about the findings and options for the short and long term. If it has not been broached before, this is the time to begin the adjustment of patient and family members to the realities of disability. Unless there is a crisis, there is no need to be abrupt. Chronic illness generally allows time for adjustment, and people need time to work through the implications. Pushing a subject when the patient is unreceptive may provoke resentment, mistrust, overreaction. I find that patients in a hospital or specialty facility tend to adjust in a week; outpatients take longer.

As noted earlier, the family physician who has been seeing the patient regularly over the years has ample opportunity to prepare the adjustment. I recall an 80-year-old spinster who had a variety of ailments: cardiovascular, hepatic, osteoarthritic. She was living alone and doing well until an arrhythmia, paroxysmal atrial fibrillation, produced syncope. She was admitted to the hospital, converted spontaneously, and was able to return home still mentally sharp and socially adept. Subsequently, however, she had syncopal episodes that were believed to be transient ischemic attacks, and her arthritic symptoms worsened, threatening her independence. She responded by taking in a medical student as a boarder. I then began talking with her about moving into an apartment complex in which meals, maid, and other services would be available. This time she responded by acquiring a live-in companion (on the third try). Further physical difficulties occurred, and the possibility of admission to a nursing home has had to be broached despite a reasonably satisfactory arrangement. Gently and repeatedly it is being pointed out to her that she is having more and more problems of coping with independent living and that there are limits to what she can do at home. Because she has come to recognize the progression of her needs, I believe she will make the adjustment if placement in a nursing home becomes necessary.

When patients and families absolutely refuse to consider a nursing home, such denial of the reality of disability may produce behavioral problems, not the least of which may be hostility toward those who wish to help and unsafe attempts to continue in old routines. (The physician too may become an "enemy.") Sometimes family members have an erroneous view of the patient's restorative potential; belief that intensive rehabilitation will work may prompt shopping for a "more realistic" physician or institution. The result may be a program the patient cannot handle, engendering more frustration and depression. In these cases, I find myself forced to confront relatives with the harm they are inflicting on the patient by holding out false hopes. Most do stop when they realize what they are doing.

The education of patients and families in the evaluative and planning stage should not stop with a review of disability and need for supportive services. Negative and positive attitudes toward nursing homes should be probed for, so that they may be discussed or built upon. Sometimes, hostility to nursing home placement reflects fear of professional abandonment; the positive response is to assure the patient and family that the physician intends to continue the care or will remain associated with it through a colleague, preferably someone the patient and family already know and like. From newspaper and legis-

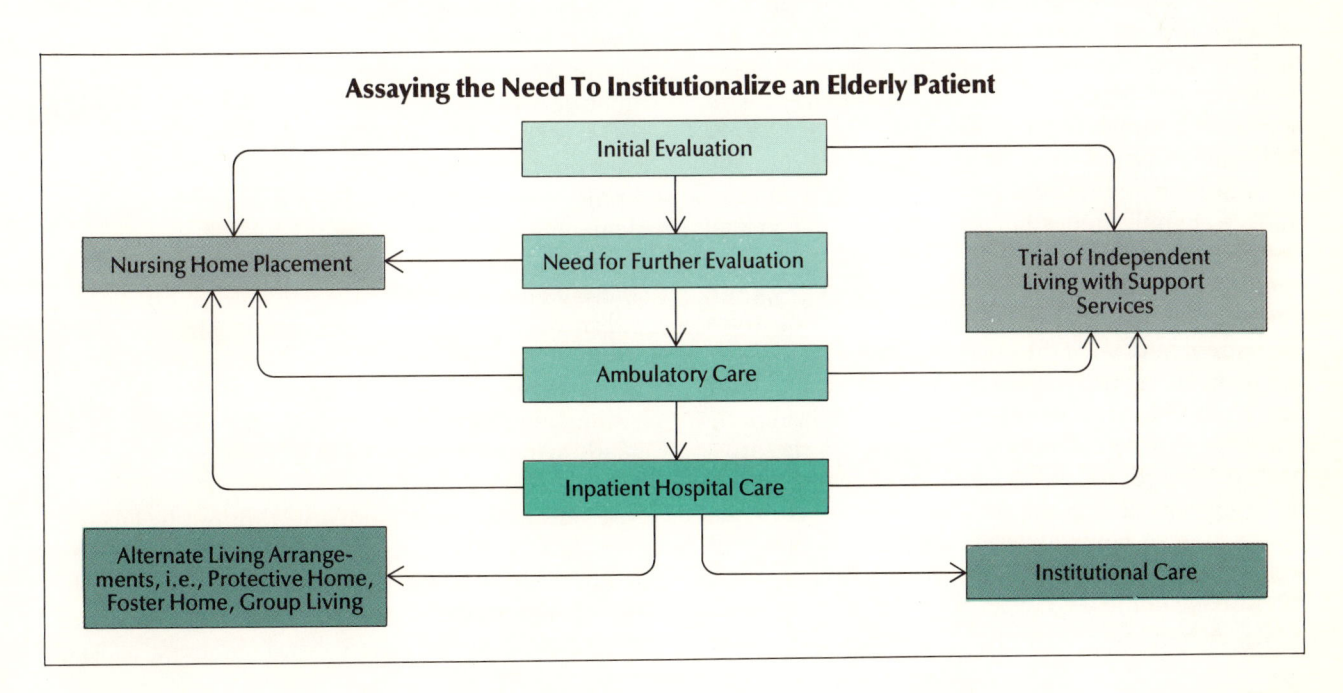

Assaying the Need To Institutionalize an Elderly Patient

Initial Evaluation → Need for Further Evaluation → Ambulatory Care → Inpatient Hospital Care

Outcomes: Nursing Home Placement; Trial of Independent Living with Support Services; Alternate Living Arrangements, i.e., Protective Home, Foster Home, Group Living; Institutional Care

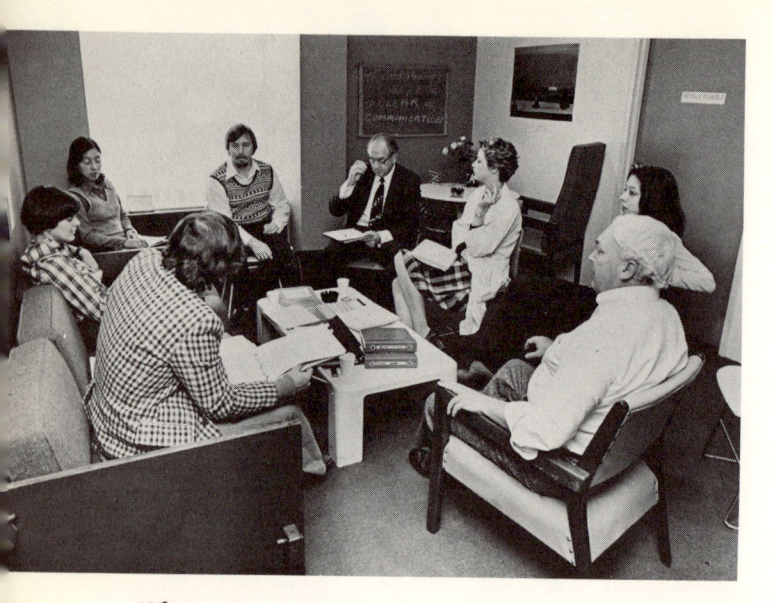

When appropriate, patient may attend conference at Washington center in which psychiatrist, medical director, social worker, and others discuss his progress.

lative investigations, patient and family may have the notion that all nursing homes are pesthouses. To meet these feelings, I find it helpful to have the family and patient visit one or more of the nursing homes I recommend; it tends to relieve much of their fears.

Another source of resistance is the patient's fear of loss of control over his or her life. The nursing home then looms as a stigmatizing defeat. Here, the positive approach may lie in emphasizing how the new setting provides opportunities for care, activities, and relationships the patient has missed and how its safety may confer peace of mind. I find that family members will become supportive when they recognize that other options have been considered and the nursing home is the best option under the circumstances. Family understanding and consent are all the more important when the patient is unable to conduct his or her affairs or where a healthy spouse needs to be accommodated in the separation from the patient bound for the nursing home.

The breaking up of aged couples because one partner needs to be in a nursing home may be traumatic but often can be cushioned. Resistance to the prospect of separation can be overcome in many cases if the well spouse can be located near the nursing home or in a complex that includes residences as well as nursing facilities. Sometimes, both may need the nursing home. I recall an aged man and wife who managed together in their own household. The husband compensated for the wife's beginning dementia and other disabilities by shopping and cooking, by reminding her when to take medications, and by arranging for visits to the doctor. When the husband developed prostatic cancer and had to be institutionalized, it was clear that the wife too would have to be institutionalized. The physician, with a son from a distant city, worked out a plan by which both the wife and husband were admitted to a nursing home near the son.

Having developed a comprehensive evaluation and plan and having found the family and patient agreeing to nursing home placement, the physician now must deal with recommending a specific institution. There are a number of considerations:

1) Which facility best meets the patient's medical, nursing, and psychosocial needs?

Again, there are no automatic answers. A "level of care" classification set up primarily for reimbursement purposes can be helpful but must be used cautiously, since facilities at the same "level" may vary considerably in ability to manage different patient needs. The best match for a patient with heavy medical and nursing requirements may well be a facility at the "skilled" level, in which patients receive professional nurse supervision around the clock. There is a high ratio of RNs to other personnel, and the facility tends to be better equipped for rehabilitation therapy. The "intermediate" level may be the best fit for a patient whose chief requirements are assistance in activities of daily living and only occasional care by a professional nurse. The intermediate care facility may offer restorative, recreational, and reality-orientation programs, but the intensity probably will be much less than in the skilled facility. The "residential" level is represented by facilities that chiefly offer room and board plus some supportive services and arrangements to help the individual obtain occasional nursing and restorative care when needed.

Some patients experience changes in functional ability, being ambulatory at one time and bedridden and in need of continuing nursing care at another. Fortunately, some institutions offer more than one level of care, a capability that may be valuable in minimizing "transfer shock" (the untoward reactions elderly patients tend to have in relocating from one institution to another).

Besides differences among institutions by levels of care, there are the differences at the same level alluded to earlier. Some nursing homes are excellent for stroke patients; their staffs have developed an expertise in managing the physical and emotional aspects.

Others may be especially adept at caring for the disoriented patient. Such special capacities probably are known to hospital social service departments, county health departments, and county medical societies, among other sources available to the physician and his office staff. Again, parallels with hospital types of organization and service are seldom helpful. The nursing home is unlikely to have the well-developed medical/surgical staff or substantial laboratory that one takes into account in selecting a hospital for an acute problem. The nursing home's objective is to help a disabled patient make the most of functional capacity over the long run; it is a residence, while the hospital is not. Thus, psychosocial needs and a staff oriented accordingly have a much higher priority in nursing home than in hospital selection.

2) Is the facility acceptable to patient and family?

The considerations range from the amenities offered to religious or other social preference to convenience for the family. The impressions made by the home may be major factors. For patients paying their own way, cost also is a major factor, since charges may exceed $10,000 a year. Many aged patients have to apply for Medicaid coverage for the first time in their lives.

3) Is the facility acceptable to the physician? The issues here are quality of care, the institution's general policies, and efficient use of physician time.

A nursing home's acceptability depends very heavily on its nursing staff, since there will be long periods of time without direct physician supervision. In the stable case, the physician may see the patient once every month or two. While retaining overall responsibility for the patient's care, the physician must rely on the staff to communicate changes of status or treatment potential and make timely suggestions on modifying the regimen.

In appraising the staff, one should be concerned about those who will interact most with the patient. In addition to the nurses, the nurses' aides have a significant role. A hostile or poorly oriented aide, by ignoring the patient, or conversely overprotecting him, can engender or intensify physical and behavioral problems. Besides looking at the qualifications of the director of nursing, charge nurses, and therapists, I talk to the aides and observe them. The inservice training a facility gives its aides and nurses becomes especially important where there is a large turnover in personnel.

The physician should observe the staff in operation, if at all possible. The nurse or aide who quickly fetches a vase for the flowers brought by a visitor makes one feel more confident that the nursing home's emotional environment is good. Absence of bedsores, institutional cleanliness, attempts to ambulate patients, efforts to converse with them rather than to leave them in silence at the television set are other indications of good care. Naturally the observations of patients, families, colleagues, and others all have a bearing.

The institution's accreditations and certifications, including the details of inspections or surveys, should be available for the physician's appraisal. A facility's recordkeeping procedures may be evidence of quality of care. It is a plus if the home maintains problem-oriented records and nursing-evaluation forms, structures nursing care plans, and follows up-to-date policies on emergencies and basic patient care developed with the aid of a medical director. It is a minus if a facility offers no reality-orientation or recreational programs or if it has no active medical direction.

Accessibility of the nursing home to the physician is a consideration; if patients are placed in a few nursing homes rather than many, the physician can not only conserve his precious time, he can also get to know the homes better. If the most appropriate placement for a patient is inconvenient for the physician, the possibility of referring the patient to a colleague should be discussed with the patient and family. This is often preferable to allowing rapport with the patient and family to disintegrate through inadequate supervision.

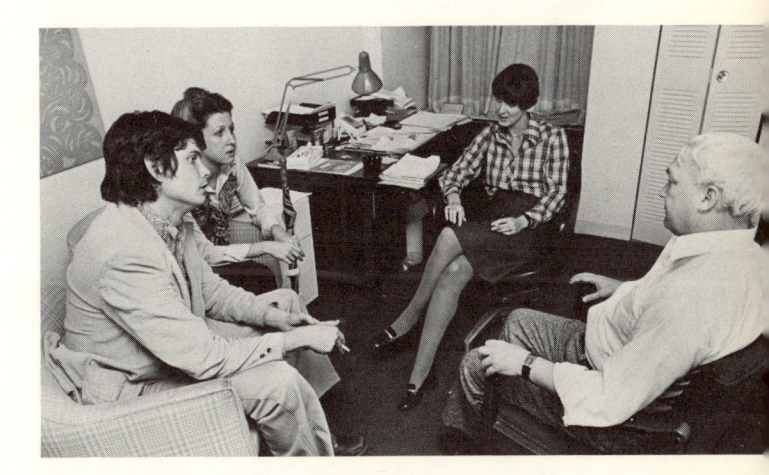

Recommendation for patient's return to community living includes social worker's evaluation of family's willingness to help, as well as of possible environmental changes and outreach services needed.

4) Is the patient acceptable to the facility? Is there a waiting list, and is the waiting time too long?

Some nursing homes have policies against accepting patients who have severe behavioral problems, who are Medicaid recipients, or who are not members of a facility's sponsoring religious group. The physician who lacks information on such practices and limitations may turn to medical colleagues, social workers, nurses, other professional persons, clergymen who visit congregants in various facilities, and nursing home associations.

Let us assume that a nursing home has been chosen. The physician now provides a treatment plan and discusses it with the facility's staff to assure that it is understood and to determine whether modifications are necessary to capitalize on or compensate for in-house capabilities. Besides medications, diet, and physical therapy, the plan should cover instructions on activities of daily living, special nursing needs, and application of socialization, reality orientation, recreational and other programs. Arrangements should be made for any therapies needed from outside sources, such as hospital visits for irradiation treatments. In monthly or bimonthly visits, the physician should review the patient's progress with the director of nursing to determine if changes in the treatment plan or its execution are needed. The practice of some physicians of reviewing only the chart is unacceptable; the visit to the facility is an occasion to continue a rapport patients value as indicating they have not been abandoned. Moreover, the chart may not tell the physician all he or she needs to know.

Some of the interplay of medical and other factors in the decision to admit to a nursing home and its sequelae is illustrated by the following "true story." Over a 12-year period after her husband died, an 84-year-old childless woman showed increasing depression, enhanced by marked deafness and social isolation. On physical examination she was found to have significant hypertension and a urinary tract infection. Her deafness proved not correctable, and efforts to treat her depression as an outpatient with a tricyclic antidepressant produced syncopal episodes. She refused hospitalization at that time.

Subsequently, however, and despite discontinuance of the apparently responsible medication, she sustained a prolonged period of unconsciousness and was hospitalized. A computed tomography scan showed a brain infarct. Although it left almost no motor residua, she began showing dementia. Since it was clear she could no longer live independently, the physician contacted the nearest relative, a nephew, as part of discharge planning. The nephew agreed that placement in a nursing home was the only feasible option. However, despite the physician's advice that it was medically unsuitable, the nephew chose a nursing home convenient to his residence. Several weeks later, the nephew reported that the patient was confused, disoriented, paranoid, and hallucinating. At the physician's suggestion, the widow was transferred to a short-term treatment facility for acute care, where she improved on antipsychotic and antidepressant drugs.

A new nursing home was chosen on the physician's recommendation. It offered a good socialization program, but deafness and inability to cope with a hearing aid were found to limit the patient's participation. At the same time, the patient experienced side reactions to the psychotropic drugs. Reduction of the dosages brought a good response. A companion was hired by the nephew and given instructions for a program of activities that would not overwhelm the patient. She began showing marked improvement in physical, neurologic, and social status. The dementia and depression were, and continue to be, well controlled in the nursing home.

In summary, the decision to admit to a nursing home requires a judicious balancing of functional, medical, and psychosocial considerations. The decision cannot be taken casually. Rather, it should arise from a comprehensive evaluation, followed by the preparation of a treatment plan and counseling of patient and family. Approached systematically, the question of when and where to institutionalize the chronically ill aged patient can be answered expertly and sympathetically.

24

Options for Care of the Aged Sick

ISADORE ROSSMAN
Albert Einstein College of Medicine

An alternative title for this discussion might well be "When *Not* To Institutionalize" the elderly person with a significant medical problem (or problems). The physician should not fear to treat at least some geriatric patients suffering from coronaries, strokes, and other major illnesses at home rather than in the hospital or nursing home. Yet the possibility of employing home care in acute geriatric illness is often overlooked. One reason may be that physicians and other professionals mistakenly regard the home as invariably too primitive an environment for delivery of adequate care. For some geriatric patients at least, it may be the therapeutic locale of least risk.

In general, we physicians tend to accept the hospital without question as a convenient, beneficial, and necessary milieu for acute care. Similarly, we are likely to think of a *good* nursing home as a benign, or at worst neutral, environment. In making these casual judgments, we tend to underestimate the trauma, iatrogenic morbidity and mortality, the deterioration in coping ability, or the outright confusion that may be produced when a frail, elderly person – in equilibrium with a known environment – is transferred to a strange one.

There are specific reasons why the hospital and nursing home are risky for the geriatric patient. These institutions may be perceived ominously by the patient made anxious by new symptoms or progressive weakness. Institutionalization often connotes abandonment or impending death to the aged.

Also it invariably produces a destruction of defined roles in the family or community that have given the elderly individual a sense of identity and security. Physicians caring for geriatric patients, especially males, should keep in mind that they have the highest suicide rates, even without associated chronic illness. They can take for granted that distress or depression will be intensified when admission to a hospital or nursing home is proposed. The reaction is thus far different than that of younger adults, who generally look forward to restoration of function and lifestyle.

Besides major psychologic decompensation, the risks of the hospital environment to the elderly include nosocomial infections, medical or nursing errors, adverse reactions to medications and procedures, and accidents and trauma. These risks were documented in a study of 500 elderly patients carried out a decade ago by Dr. William Reichel (see Chapter 3, "Multiple Problems in the Elderly"). He found that 146 patients experienced 193 untoward reactions as a result of hospitalization. Falls from bed or chair accounted for 42 episodes of trauma; other accidents, 19; reactions to medications, 54; serious reactions to procedures, 31; hospital-induced major psychologic decompensation, 19; hospital-acquired infections, 17; and medical and nursing errors, including errors of omission, 11 episodes.

Thus hospitalization may be counterproductive in terms of caring for the whole person. The point I would stress is not that geriatric patients do not need the resources of the hospital or nursing home. Rather, it is that institutions, like drugs, must be employed with awareness of the individual risk/benefit ratio. My experience suggests that both hospital and nursing home are overutilized in dealing with elderly patients, often to their detriment. Stereotyped thinking, insurance and welfare benefit structures, and lack of (or indifference to) options in outpatient care are all contributory factors. Stereotyped thinking refers to the tendency to institutionalize aged patients almost automatically – whether they have a few nursing needs or advanced cancer, for wandering or episodic nocturnal confusion, as well as gross organic mental syndromes – without considering the negative effects. Incentives to hospital and nursing home placement are built into insurance and welfare programs; examples of rubber-stamp transfer of Medicaid patients from hospital to nursing home are legion. Conversely, out-of-hospital benefits are scarce or grudgingly allowed, or have been up to now. These aspects of the subject will be discussed more fully later on.

Sometimes the use of institutions may be attractive principally to relieve a practitioner's diagnostic or therapeutic anxieties in confronting the multiply burdened elderly patient. Another contributory factor may be the predominance of specialists with hospital-based work patterns, in contradistinction to home-oriented primary care physicians. The lack of community organizations with a strong financial interest in home services is yet another reason for the shortage of health and social service programs to support the elderly patient. Thus, in discussing alternatives to the use of hospitals and nursing homes, one must necessarily be concerned with the structure in this country of medical care, related services, and their financing. The virtual disappearance of the house call, which in other countries is a mainstay of geriatric care, reflects our country's heavy focus on institutions.

Admittedly, because of inadequate noninstitutional options in many communities, the question of "when not to institutionalize" often cannot be answered simply in terms of medical advantages and disadvantages to the patient. But unless we examine the question critically, too many of the aged will continue to be served inappropriately if not counterproductively. Accordingly, in this chapter I will explore first the negative aspects of hospital and nursing home settings and some means of mitigation; and second, the options of home care, "after care," and day care with which I have had practical experience.

When the elderly are taken from their homes to a hospital or nursing home, depression, disorientation, agitation, and anxiety are likely to be accentuated. Hospital routines tend to intensify feelings of helplessness. The very intensity of a workup may convince elderly patients they are mortally ill.

Adding to anxiety and confusion, especially in patients with some degree of brain syndrome, are the surrealism of blaring page systems, early morning awakenings for taking temperatures and receiving pills, groans and screams of nearby patients, and the inexplicable appearance and disappearance of silent nurses, attendants, and other functionaries. If hospital admission is taken to confirm approaching death or descent to a new level of weakness, it can hardly be accepted cheerfully. The patient who has had progressive disease or a traumatic procedure like mastectomy or colostomy may be described, with some justification, as having been negatively conditioned to readmission.

What is routine to the hospital staff may be terrifying to elderly patients. Anxiety and confusion may be aggravated by diagnostic and operative procedures or their prospect. Yet, in my experience, hospital staffs are either unaware of or unable to deal adequately with this or with the fragility of the aged. Thus, the elderly are susceptible to shock-like reactions when given cool enemas. Intravenous pyelograms are particularly difficult for older persons with unstable blood pressure regulation. Standing and holding the breath for a chest film also may be trying for an older person even when he is in good health; if weak and feverish, an older person may collapse or feel like collapsing. Few hospital staffs are made aware of these problems or are taught the necessity of pa-

Disorders Developing at Home and Managed by Montefiore Home Care

Pneumonitis
Pyelonephritis
Cellulitis
Thrombophlebitis
Phlebothrombosis
Abscesses (incision and drainage)
Exfoliative dermatitis
Dermatitis herpetiformis
Ischemic gangrene
Minor cerebrovascular accidents
Transient ischemic attacks
Acute congestive heart failure
Myocardial infarction
Osteoporotic fractures
Uremia
Obstructive lung disease, asthma
Paroxysmal arrhythmias
Systemic lupus erythematosus
Multiple myeloma, leukemia, other cancers (including chemotherapy)

tience and the need to be supportive of the elderly.

Because of the risks of hospitalization and hospital procedures to the elderly, it becomes all the more important to weigh the necessity for using them. What is the point of an elaborate, trying hospital workup to confirm a suspicion of cancer when the patient is not an acceptable candidate for surgery or chemotherapy? In such patients, is it not more humane to wait and let time reveal the diagnosis? I would choose to do so and let the patient stay at home.

Often a painful workup is undeviatingly carried through to its conclusion by "formula," even though no practical outcome can be expected. A value prized in the teaching hospital – detailed perfection in the workup – may be at odds with good geriatric practice. Time and again, workups are continued while the elderly patients complain that the x-ray table is too hard, that they cannot retain a barium enema, and that procedures are so debilitating that they cannot cooperate any further. The procedure may be suspended for the time being, but the patient is subsequently sent back so that the workup can be finished, obviously a distressful experience. How often do we stop to ask, "If with a good deal of trauma we confirm that there are multiple diverticula or diverticulitis with narrowing, can we really do anything about them in this patient?"

Sometimes unnecessary workups are initiated because the specific nature of geriatric problems is not understood. Because of diminished testosterone titers, the red blood cell mass of aging males may drop to female levels. Poor dietary patterns may make a further contribution. I have seen elaborate workups ordered routinely for mild anemias, including bone marrow studies and examinations for possible gastrointestinal malignancy, when such anemias are typically nutritional – as a good history would indicate. A trial with dietary supplements may well tell the story without subjecting the patient to the uncomfortable workup. True, at the present time, fears of malpractice litigation may be a factor, and there is no absolute protection against such litigation. But the likelihood can be diminished if the physician develops a good rapport with patient and family and explains the reasons for his decisions.

Let us assume that hospitalization is required and turn to ways to mitigate its negative potential. One way is to prepare the patient and family by explaining the need for the admission, the procedures likely to be applied and the reasons for their use, the benefits expected from the stay, and its probable length.

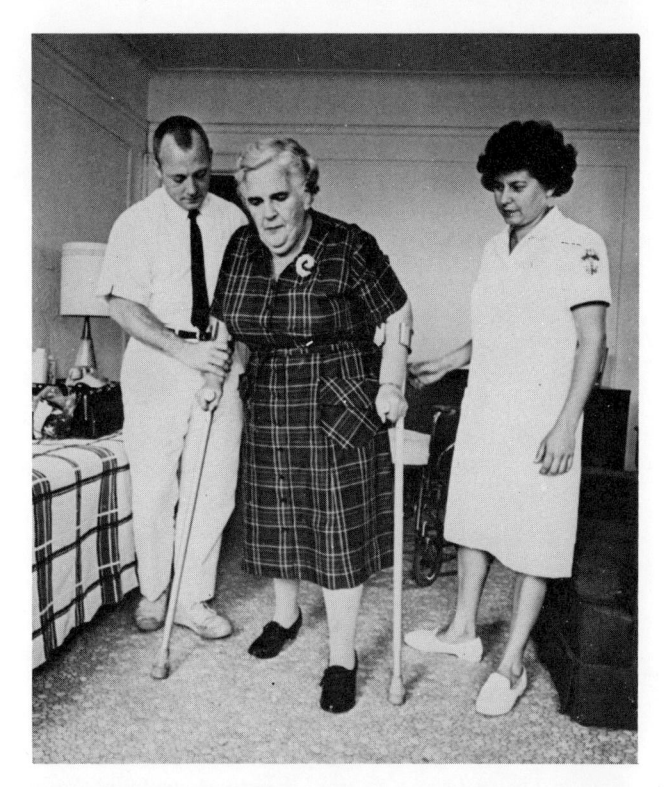

Despite bilateral (below-knee) amputations, patient above was restored to full ambulation on home care, got typing job. Multiple sclerosis patient (below) refused to enter nursing home, was managed at home for several years despite progressive neurologic deterioration.

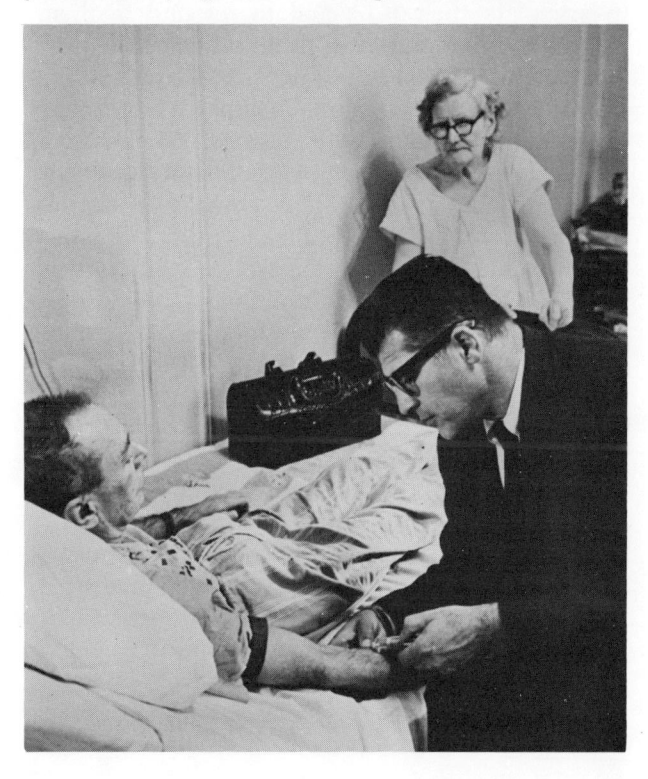

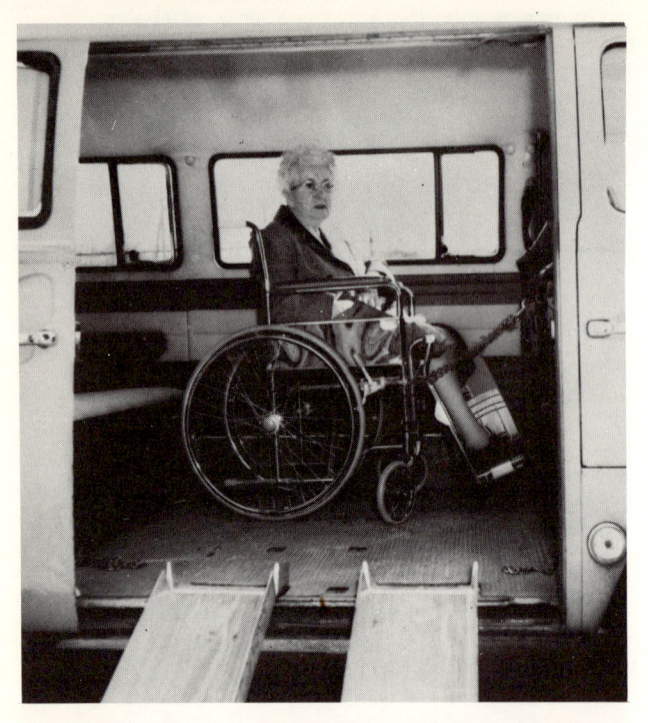

For after care program, van especially adapted to wheelchair transport brings groups of patients to Montefiore for treatment by physicians, nurses, and therapists.

Another way is to encourage the patient and family to articulate their fears and to respond to them. Many patients fear unrealistically that facts are being withheld and that they will never come home again or will lose major functional abilities. One value of eliciting the fears or anxieties is that these may incorporate a realistic perception of difficulty in coping with a new environment. The physician can probe the specifics of this perception and assure the patient that he and the hospital staff will be ready to help. Perhaps nothing is more calming to an anxious patient than to present hospitalization as one step in a positive plan that contemplates an outpatient stage. One cannot overemphasize the uplift given the patient by initiating discharge planning on or before the day of admission.

One of the most demoralizing aspects of hospitalization is lack of sympathetic attention during treatment intervals. Elderly patients often are alarmed or perturbed when left in bed for two or three hours with no human interaction. Professionals do not seem to realize how anxiety-reducing it is to elderly patients when they are visited, addressed by name, and touched. At the early stages, particularly, frequent visits by the physician, who may be the only familiar professional in a strange environment, are enormously supportive. Depersonalization has a greater depressive effect on the elderly than on the younger patient, a point that nurses and aides should remember. The professional tendency to respond to anxiety and depression only with psychotropic drugs is unfortunate; although tranquilizers may be necessary in some cases, they have such side effects as dizziness, with its potential for producing falls.

Besides sympathy, the elderly patient needs explanations – including many repetitions thereof – about what is happening and why. Patients generally are poorly oriented as to what goes on during the hospital day and why routines of blood taking, temperature readings, roentgenography, and other maneuvers are in their interest. Some elderly patients attach traumatic symbols to such procedures; vacupuncturing tubes of blood, for example, may signify "they are taking my life's blood away and I am getting weaker." Some patients believe they are viewed as so depersonalized that the hospital is subjecting them to "experiments" that would not be done on important human beings.

I am indebted to a nurse for an example of how hospital personnel can improve their concern for the elderly through very simple changes in routine. "When I make night rounds to check on patients and the flashlight wakes them up, I immediately shine the light on *my* face. I don't leave it on theirs. They can see it's me and what I'm up to. Keeping the light on their face confuses them," she explained. If the awakened older patient was hard of hearing, she would put her stethoscope to the patient's ear and speak into the diaphragm, amplifying her voice so the patient would appreciate that there was nothing to be alarmed about. The same kind of concern should motivate other adaptations of hospital routines: an enema should be kept warm, a portable x-ray machine at the bedside may substitute for a standing admission film, the patient's propensity to allergic reactions should be reviewed before an intravenous pyelogram is done, and drugs should be initiated in low dosages and reactions carefully monitored. Before giving drugs that may aggravate postural hypotension, the patient's blood pressure should be checked not only in a sitting position but also while standing and after standing for a minute. The use of firmly anchored floor mats and stanchions in the rooms of geriatric patients would help guard against falls and fractures.

The nursing home may be an even more powerful symbol of disaster than the hospital. It may signify family abandonment and, since physicians tend to make infrequent visits, professional abandonment, too. The fact that abysmal conditions exist in many nursing homes often signifies to the elderly that society is shunning them as well. More precisely, I should say *our* society. In Europe, the elderly respond differently because society there conveys different values about aging. These values are reflected in a higher caliber of nursing homes, home care services, and congregate living facilities. In Amsterdam, I observed a nursing home that had elaborate therapy rooms. All patients were dressed as for normal life. Lying in bed or sitting in a wheelchair in nightclothes was not permitted. Rather, every patient was gotten up in the morning and helped to get dressed, a tremendous morale builder. Many different safety devices were commonplace. The normalcy of such an environment had an enormously positive effect.

In our society, the nursing home is perceived so negatively that it is not unusual to encounter patients who are adamant against placement. I recall a multiple sclerosis patient who was deteriorating at home and placing increasing burdens on the home care team and a family member. He was taken to visit an exemplary nursing home and introduced to a congenial staff in preparation for subsequent placement. The next day, he was found unconscious from an overdose of sleeping pills. The man survived. Despite progressive severe neurologic impairments, he was maintained on our home care program for five more years, lest another suicide attempt be precipitated by forced institutionalization. A reaction pattern consisting of depression, anorexia, and general decline upon institutionalization has been dubbed the "transplantation reaction."

Having outlined the risks inherent in institutionalization, at least for some geriatric patients, I will turn to outpatient options and criteria for their use. In contrast to the strong professional orientation toward the institution, there is growing lay support for outpatient alternatives. Hearings recently conducted by the U.S. Department of Health, Education, and Welfare showed that laymen strongly favor expansion of home care. New York State's recent Moreland Commission, of which I was a member, found in investigating nursing home scandals that older patients quite uniformly want to stay at home and receive services there. I believe this is a medically feasible option in many instances. An analysis of a nursing home waiting list some years ago showed that one quarter of the patients could remain at home if they had homemaker and other supportive services. With-

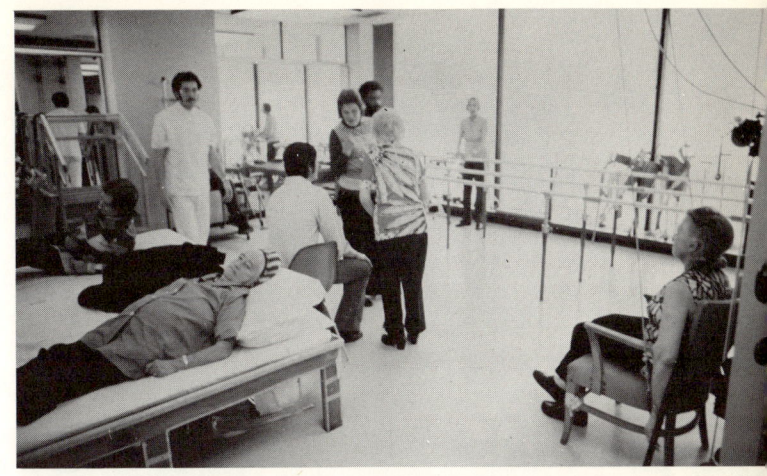

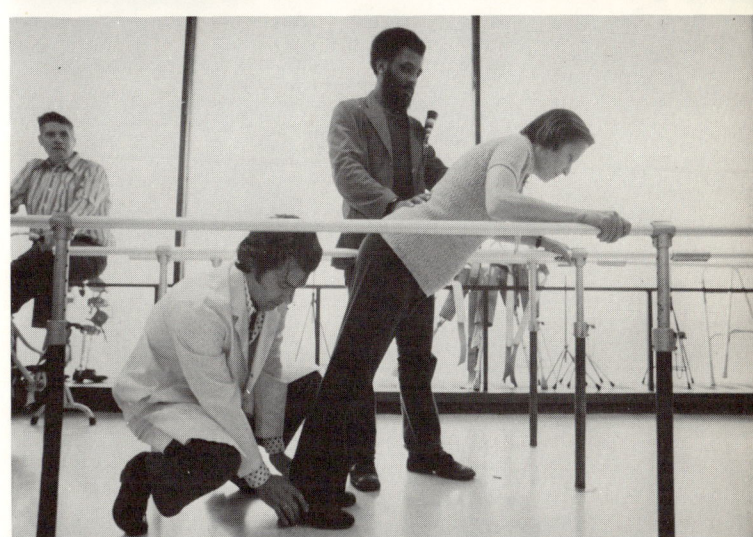

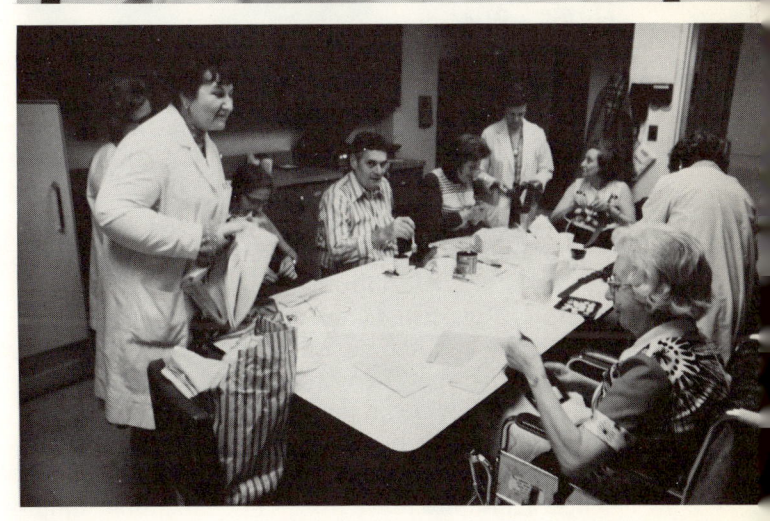

In Montefiore physical therapy department (top and center), one therapist can treat six after care patients in an hour, as many as in full day of home visits. Program also offers recreational therapy and socialization (bottom).

CHAPTER 24: ROSSMAN

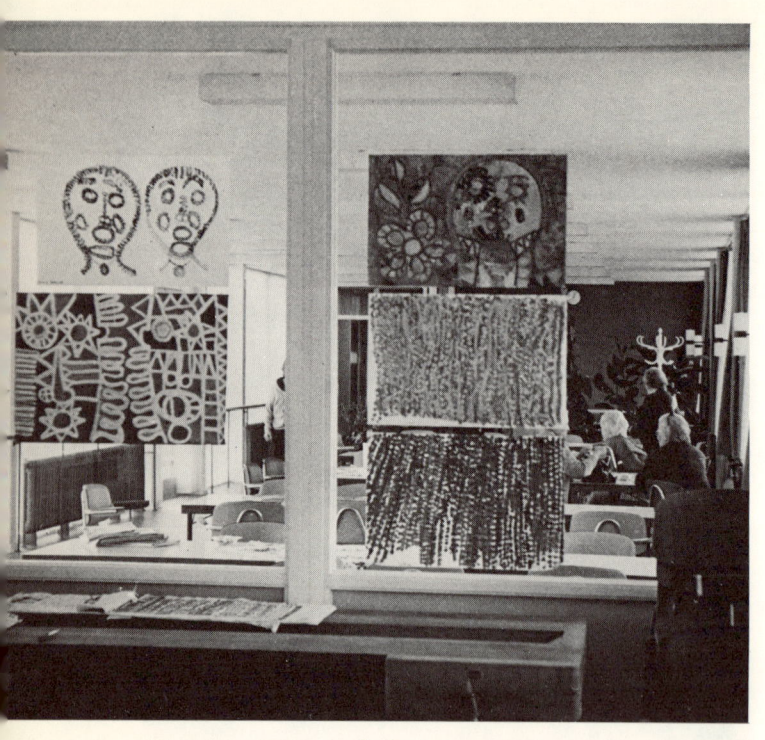

Paintings were made by severely impaired patients with organic brain syndrome in Amsterdam nursing home, which allots much space to recreational therapy.

out a doubt, patients equally as sick and incapacitated as many in skilled nursing facilities and chronic disease hospitals can be cared for at home.

Home Care

A prototype hospital-based program of home care was inaugurated in 1947 by Montefiore Hospital in New York City to demonstrate the foregoing point. Essentially, the therapeutic team in the hospital – with a core of doctor, nurse, and social worker – was adapted for patient care in the home. In my view the program has in many cases prevented deteriorations that lead to rehospitalization for such conditions as chronic congestive failure and other cardiac disorders, stroke and hypertension, rheumatoid arthritis, and even cancer. From both professional and other viewpoints, home care has often been found preferable to extended hospitalization. However, experience indicates that if the patient requires frequent or almost daily physician visits, close laboratory monitoring, or intravenous therapy, then it is usually too taxing to manage him at home – though all this can and has been done.

The belief that patients with major acute illness will fare worse at home than in the hospital is by no means always true. For example, there is evidence that an elderly coronary patient may fare as well if not better at home than in the hospital. A recent British study showed that randomly chosen home care male MI patients had a mortality rate of 12% at 28 days, as compared with 14% for those chosen for hospital care. At 330 days, the home care mortality rate was 20%, that for hospital care, 27%. An intriguing question is why coronary care units in the British study did not produce a record far superior to that of home care. Pending further studies, I offer the speculation that two subpopulations are involved: one comprising patients for whom anxieties and procedures associated with the hospital and the CCU environment are detrimental; the other comprising patients for whom the ability to treat rapidly (e.g., when cardiac arrest occurs) is essential to survival. The negative effects on the first group may have cancelled out the benefits that accrued to the second. I believe that many geriatric patients in whom a coronary attack is documented but does not produce major cardiovascular changes would fall into the former group. In contrast, the patient experiencing tachycardia or shock does need prompt hospitalization. (An accompanying table lists other major illnesses for which diagnosis and treatment may be accomplished in the elderly without hospitalization, although hospital back-up facilities may be necessary for workup.)

The Montefiore program has a census of 80 homebound patients. The initial evaluation of a candidate for home care is done by a team consisting of a physician, a nurse, and a social worker. From the physician's viewpoint, a patient is acceptable if he or she has an illness requiring 1) services of a physician weekly or biweekly, occasionally less often, and 2) services of a nurse with the same frequency. Periodic visits by a physical or other therapist and homemaker may be required also. On occasions when an elderly patient has needed but has refused hospitalization, we have reluctantly continued home care rather than withdraw services. We continue to be surprised over how long many of these patients – often frail, weak, dizzy, ataxic, and episodically confused – can be maintained at home. Despite early forebodings, on home care we rarely encounter drug overdoses, and no one has gotten into difficulties using oxygen or IPPB at home.

From the viewpoint of the social worker, a patient is acceptable if there is a reliable, caring person to give assistance in the home. An unwilling or indifferent family is a strong contraindication to home care. However, family resistance may represent ambivalence and is seldom an absolute: one basis for it may be a fear of being unable to cope with the patient, a fear often dispelled by an offer of professional help. On the other hand, there are instances when long-standing family conflicts make home care inadvisable even though a willingness to assist the elderly relative is expressed. To evaluate the realities here is the task of both the physician and the social worker, who also assess the physical environment. Unless there are gross overcrowding and poverty, most homes are found physically suitable for home care.

The use of home care for a typical "nursing home" type of patient is illustrated by a recent case of a 73-year-old man, victim of two strokes. He had spastic lower extremities, contractures, a mild organic brain syndrome, and stasis dermatitis. Admitted after hospitalization to the Montefiore home care program in February 1975, he required physical therapy, assistance with activities of daily living, and training in ambulation.

The patient, who lived with his wife in a tiny, cluttured apartment, was visited once every 10 days by a physician, weekly by a nurse, and biweekly by a physical therapist who treated the contractures and provided training in ambulation and activities of daily living. A physiatrist made a recheck house call soon after the patient came home from the hospital. The nurse saw to it that pressure areas on the legs were allowed to heal. The wife was trained to handle some of the basic nursing and physical therapy. A month after returning home, the man not only was out of bed and in a wheelchair but also – thanks to the wife – was able to leave the apartment house during the day in his wheelchair. Subsequently limited ambulation became possible.

In September, a fever refractory to antibiotics produced a seizure, and the man was hospitalized. A chest film showed right lower lobe infiltration. He died in the hospital of pneumonia and cardiac complications. Home care can be said to have given the patient and his wife seven months of home life instead of institutionalization.

We find that the doctor-patient relationship, or the team-patient relationship, tends to be much better in the home than in the hospital. The same functionaries and procedures that elicit suspicion in the hospital are readily accepted in the home. This improved trusting relationship almost inevitably leads home care patients to become more dependent emotionally than hospital patients on their care givers. I have known patients to decline better housing outside the Montefiore service area because of fear they would lose touch with the home care team.

The Montefiore demonstration cannot be said to have inspired a mass movement into home care among hospitals. Only 450 of the nation's 6,000 hospitals sponsor home care programs; these usually offer services of a physician, a visiting nurse, home health aides, and physical, speech, and occupational therapists. (Podiatrist, practical nurse, and other services also may be offered.) Some programs are primitive, and the total number of home care programs for Medicare and Medicaid purposes recognized by the federal government now stands at 2,000.

Hospital home care programs thus are available in only a fraction of the nation's communities. Considering that there may be almost five million elderly persons with significant physical restrictions, many homebound, absence of home care means that there often is little choice other than to use the hospital or nursing home when a major illness occurs. The homebound patient has less of a chance today to obtain a physician's house call than a few decades ago. The chances of admission to the hospital or nursing home are correspondingly greater, even though the house call might produce enough information to make hospitalization unnecessary. In the usual course of events, the patient meets the physician at

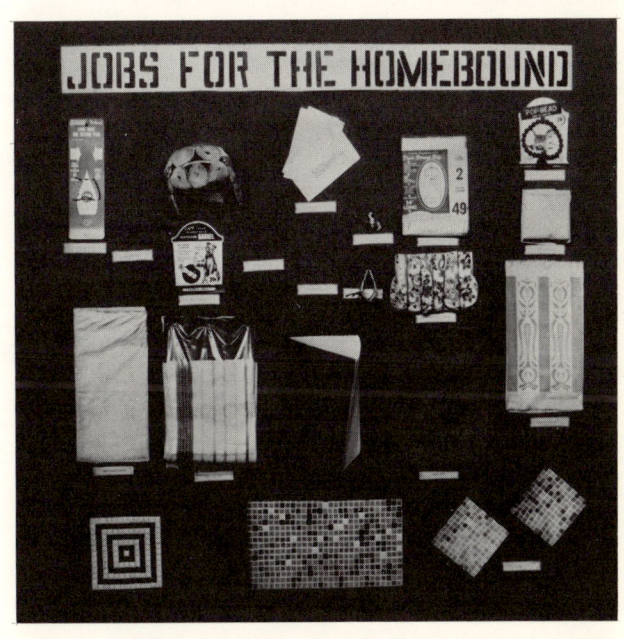

Montefiore bulletin board displays examples of simple packaging, mosaics, and other sorts of handicrafts done under commercial contract by home care patients.

CHAPTER 24: ROSSMAN

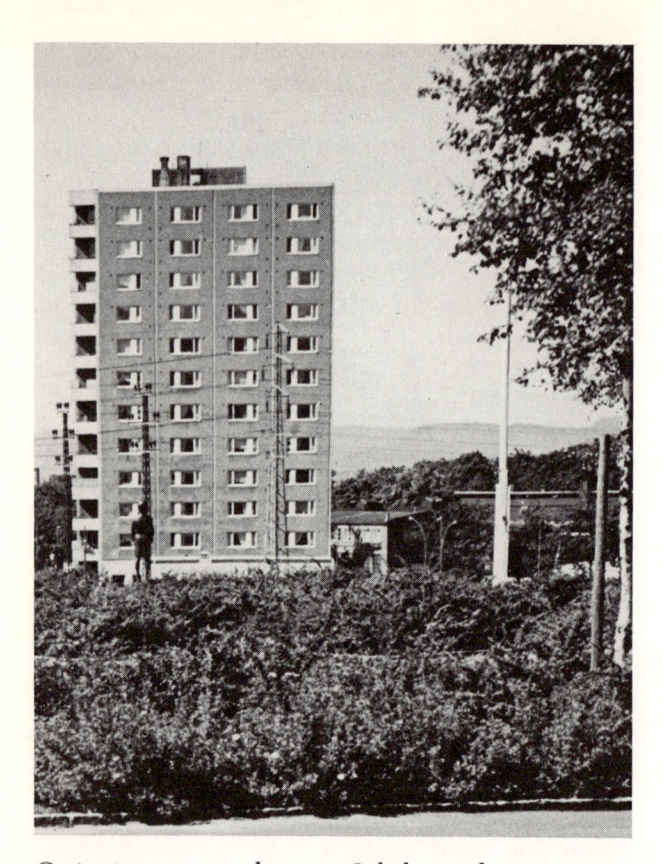

Geriatric apartment house in Oslo has such conveniences as ground-level stores, compact apartments, and supervised rooms where residents take showers sitting in plastic chairs, thus avoiding risk of falls and burns.

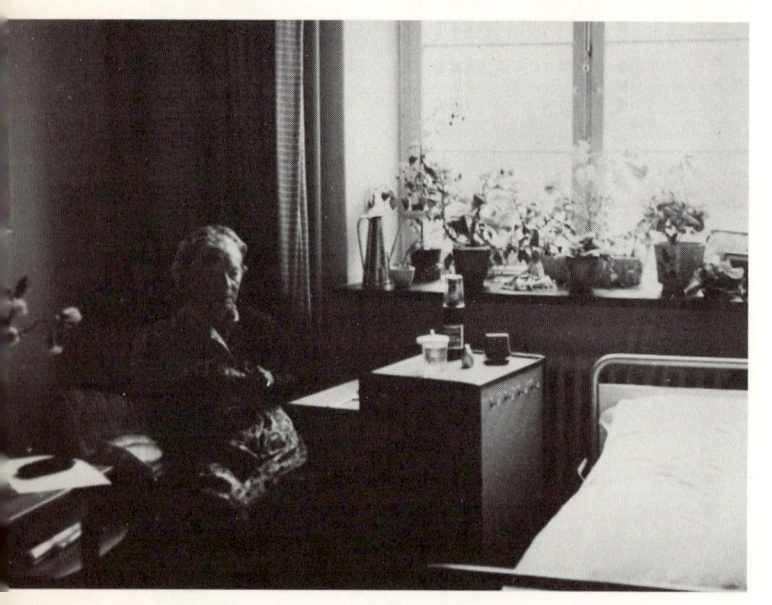

In Copenhagen's De Gamles By (old people's town) residents have single rooms (with baths) where they enjoy privacy and pursue hobbies such as raising plants.

the hospital and, because he or she actually appears sick, is admitted.

After Care

An alternative to home care that may be more acceptable within the traditional framework of hospital activity is "after care." The term is short for services to homebound patients after hospitalization, although there is no reason why offering the services must be conditioned on prior hospitalization.

For four years, Montefiore has offered an after care program as an alternative or adjunct to home care. Services are provided in the hospital setting to patients who, although homebound, are well enough to be moved by van to the hospital in groups of six to eight. A driver and attendant bring the patients from their apartments to the van, which is equipped to carry wheelchairs safely.

Each afternoon, a different group is brought to the hospital for a three-hour period to receive care, as needed, from physicians, nurses, social workers, and therapists. Laboratory and other hospital services are available. A group social hour has been innovated for these patients, most of whom are lonely and isolated. The capacity of the van for wheelchair patients is one reason why the patients are grouped into modular units of six to eight. Another reason is that this number can be comfortably supervised by a physical therapist or aide.

Economical use of professional time is a major advantage of after care. In home care, a physical therapist can visit six patients in a working day; in after care, six patients can be treated in an hour in the physical therapy department. (Another advantage to professional personnel is that it resolves the problem of their anxiety about visiting patients in certain high-crime neighborhoods.)

The program is under the immediate direction of a registered nurse who has a home care background. She evaluates patients' progress, refers to physicians when indicated, and confers with consultants, especially the physiatrist. The nurse checks medications, maintains contact with families, and provides liaison with ancillary personnel. The home care social worker is involved routinely in developing a program of care for the patient. When after care is inadvisable because the patient has deteriorated, classical home care becomes the back-up program.

Patients generally prefer after care despite the inconvenience of being in the van for a half hour or more while other patients are picked up or returned home. They do not object to dressing and leaving home. In fact, they prefer after care because it does get them outside the home and links them with a patient group. Friendships often develop.

Day Care

Some elderly patients find it difficult or impossible to be alone at home because of physical or mental impairments and the absence of a supportive family member. These often are patients with hemiplegia, arthritis, amputation, arteriosclerotic heart disease, hypertension, visual difficulty, and chronic brain syndromes. They are mobile but unable to deal with the needs of daily living. The concept of a "day hospital" was developed in England for such patients, who can be described as being on the verge of institutionalization. The prevention of minor as well as major medical or social decompensations thus becomes a key issue for these "frail ambulants." Some may be primarily in need of supervision and social services rather than medical care and rehabilitation. Some may be in posthospital convalescence, and others may have been disabled in many activities of daily living for years. Transportation from home to day hospital is provided by a fleet of taxis and ambulettes.

A companion to the day hospital is the geriatric day care center. Centers sometimes are defined as serving patients who are not primarily in need of medical services, but this is not a hard-and-fast distinction. The services found in day hospitals and day centers may be the same. British day hospitals, for example, serve recent stroke patients who need therapy, as well as patients with old strokes who, although able to perform activities of daily living, are unable to be left at home safely when the family is at work. Another source of confusion comes from drawing parallels between geriatric and child day care centers. A major difference is that patients in the geriatric center participate in their own care programs as adults who make up their own minds.

In day care hospitals and centers, patients are fed, cared for, and given recreational and diversional activities during the nine-to-five day for several days a week. Many patients are medically indistinguishable from patients admitted to nursing homes and homes for the aging. An English study comparing patients in a day hospital with a matched group of nonattenders estimated that the day care group had 8% fewer hospital admissions and that almost 12% of those who did have to be hospitalized were able to be discharged earlier. For almost 7% of the day care group, hospitalization occurred later in the course of deterioration than it did with nonattenders.

A day care movement seems at hand in the United States. There were 15 centers counted a few years ago, and there probably are more today. They may be freestanding or under auspices of a hospital, county health department, nursing home, or geriatric center. The average daily patient census in 10 centers varies from 11 to 115. The Day Center for the Elderly, affiliated with Montefiore Hospital, has a total of 92 patients, of whom 25 to 35 come in each day; 13% have had strokes. More than half of our participants live alone; 80% are women, and 20% are over 85. The staff consists of two social workers, two nurses, one occupational therapist, and one recreational specialist. Patients are handled in groups.

One of the centers having the greatest range of services is San Francisco's On Lok Senior Health Services Center, which serves 47 patients daily. The center offers initial assessment and periodic evaluation, physical examination, physiotherapy, occupational therapy, podiatric and dental services, health education, meals, reality therapy, grooming and bathing assistance, laundry, and recreation. Social work, nursing, and personal services are given at

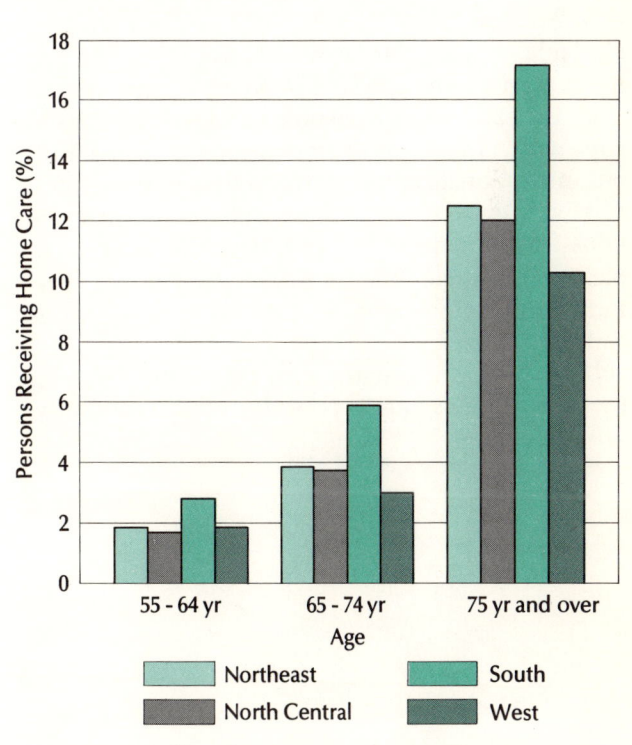

Most recent data from National Health Survey (published in 1972) show 1,747,000 persons 55 and over received personal care at home each year in 1966-68.

home as well as at the center. On Lok is unaffiliated.

Another facility is the Adult Day Treatment Center of Baltimore's Levindale Hebrew Geriatric Center and Hospital. The 57 participants, transported to and from home during the work week, are required to have a private physician and a family member or other person to assume responsibility after day care hours. Each participant is given a treatment plan devised by an interdisciplinary professional group and acceptable to the participant. Almost half the participants are severely or totally disabled. One in four has a severe mental impairment. A comparison of attendees and a three-segment (institution-, community-, and apartment-living) control group was made in terms of ability to perform activities of daily living and other parameters. The attendees showed improvement or maintenance of status 94% of the time as against 32%, 63%, and 52%, respectively, of the three groups of control subjects.

Specialized Housing

A relatively unexploited solution to many sociomedical problems of the elderly is specialized or congregate housing. Such housing can offer compact apartments, dining facilities, and cleaning services. Medical, nursing, and social work services are available on a regular or consultative basis. Most of these services are provided in Ketay House in New York City and make it possible for elderly persons to cope with minor or temporary health problems without institutionalization. Europe offers housing projects with even greater refinements in accommodations for the elderly. A Copenhagen housing complex, for example, offers a full range of health services – from ambulatory to hospital care – on one campus.

If we take as a geriatric goal the maintenance of the patient for as long as possible in the community, the need for restructuring our institutionally biased systems for delivering care will be apparent. Since the passage of Medicare and Medicaid legislation 12 years ago, our country has focused disproportionately on a bricks-and-mortar approach to health care. It is biased toward premature admission of elderly patients to hospitals and nursing homes.

The impact of this bias is perhaps most clearly seen when an elderly person or couple, marginally surviving independently in the community, has a temporary exacerbation of a chronic illness or the superimposition of an acute illness upon their frailties. With temporary assistance, the intermittent crises could be met without removal from home and community. As matters now stand, the crisis probably would mean an end to independent living.

It has become clearer than ever with passage of time that many institutionalized patients could have fared just as well at home with supportive medical and social services that utilize family and community relationships. This is another way of saying that we have lacked a system for treating patients in the locales most suited to their medical and psychosocial needs. Such a system could be organized in various ways. One certainly would be a hospital-based system in which institutional/noninstitutional services were blended as each geriatric case required. The benefits of such a system would not only be improved patient morale but greater cost-effectiveness. For example, in contrast to the costs of a skilled nursing facility (about $45 a day in New York City), home care at Montefiore averages $12 to $14 a day. Day care may average $23 to $25 a day, about the cost of an intermediate care facility. From the viewpoint of patient, family, and taxpayer, there seems to be good reason for encouraging mechanisms to provide care in or close to home.

When not to institutionalize? When a rational alternative is available.

25

The Doctor and the Aged Patient

ROBERT N. BUTLER
National Institute on Aging

The subject of the doctor–aged patient relationship is most apt at the conclusion of this book. Unless the patient and the physician have a good relationship, the many approaches discussed in the preceding chapters will not be fully or effectively utilized. The chances of accurate diagnosis diminish when the physician is "turned off," while the chances of patient cooperation in adjusting to acute or chronic diseases are diminished in the context of unresolved or suppressed resentment.

Sometimes the patient and the physician have hang-ups about aging, disability, disfigurement, and death that prevent rapport and good communication. As a practicing psychiatrist before becoming Director of the National Institute on Aging, I have had opportunities to observe good and bad doctor-patient relationships. For the lonely and worried patient, I have no doubt that simply being seen and heard by a trusted physician has a therapeutic effect; the patient may still have heart disease or cancer, but his or her morale is uplifted and the encounter promotes ability to function. When trust and respect are lacking on either side of the consulting desk, the results can be disastrous: instead of making the most of the patient's abilities, the relationship becomes an obstacle to effective clinical strategy.

The fact that many physicians and their elderly patients do get along well must be considered a testimonial to the personal resources they bring to one another. Much in our society works to denigrate the aged. "Ageism" – prejudice against the elderly as being unworthy of investment of time and effort – causes many physicians and patients to trivialize or deny needs for care. When they bring to their encounters a belief that nothing much can or should be done for the "inevitable" consequences of so-called aging, the stage is set for frustration, hostility, paranoia, depression, abandonment, and indifference. The stereotype of the cantankerous, sullen, apathetic, or unresponsive older person becomes much more likely to materialize. In short, a relationship infected with "ageism" contributes to fulfilling the expectation that older patients are "crocks" and promotes resort to the "senile write-off."

I hope preceding chapters have shown that much of what is called aging is disease that is treatable, if only recognized in time as such. Effective medicine is impossible without the physician's seeing past the stereotypes, without viewing patients objectively. The reality is that there is as much, if not more, diversity among older adults in terms of physical and mental status, socioeconomic circumstance, personality, and, of course, experience in meeting stress as there is among younger adults. This diversity makes diagnosis and care much more of an intellectual feat and challenge. Consider, too, that virtually any disease with a classic complex of signs and symptoms is likely to present atypically in the elderly. This holds for diseases as varied as appendicitis, myocardial infarction, hyperthyroidism, and pulmonary embolism. Moreover, the symptoms of these diseases may seem nonspecific and be attributed carelessly to senility. Yet we have seen in this book that dementia or confusion frequently is reversible when recognized as a treatable symptom of infection, drug toxicity, dehydration, or congestive heart failure, among many conditions.

Physicians are coming to recognize that the proper diagnosis and care of the elderly patient are indeed worthy challenges. A 1976 survey by an American Medical Association publication showed that three fourths of physician respondents agreed with the statement that doctors need special training in geriatrics. This recognition reflects the fact that geriatric patients not only have different disease presentations from other classes of patients and have multiple conditions at the same time but also that they form a large and growing medical clientele. Half the nation's disease load is chronic disease, much of it borne, of course, in later life. Half the nation's annual spending for personal health services – now at the rate of $160 billion or more a year – is attributable to chronic disease.

Geriatrics seems destined to be even more important in tomorrow's medical practice. The growth of the population aged 65 or older has been more rapid than the growth of the U.S. population generally. Constituting 4% in 1900 and 10% currently, the elderly will compose 12% of the general population by the year 2000 and 17% by 2030, according to some demographic projections. Not only will physicians be seeing more geriatric patients, they will be seeing them far more often than they see younger patients. One has only to cite some of the common geriatric ailments that require repeated attention: cardiovascular and cerebrovascular diseases, cancer, osteoporosis, diabetes mellitus, and rheumatoid arthritis. No wonder that an estimated 40% or more of physician office time and 33% of hospital time are devoted now to older patients; in 40 years, the elderly may account for as much as 75% of the total time physicians spend with patients.

Clinical strategy becomes complex and prolonged for elderly patients with multiple conditions. The physician seems constantly to be balancing priorities. A choice of courses of action is all the more challenging in the context of life-style adaptations required by chronic diseases and the socioeconomic resources available to the patient. The physician aware of the patient's disabilities and diseases must consider preventive and health-maintenance tactics to forestall further complications. The physician must truly be a "doctor" – the word means "teacher" – helping the patient learn new ways to maintain his or her independence and self-respect. He must undertake to counsel on diet, exercise, and emotional adjustment as well as on how to make use of rehabilitative modalities. Clinical strategy also may involve the physician in making referrals of the patient and family for social services.

Geriatrics is thus very much in tune with the person-orientation of family practice, as distinguished from the disease-orientation of specialism. While all physicians are concerned with the doctor-patient relationship, perhaps family physicians feel most keenly the long-term responsibilities of relating well to the patient, especially the aged patient. In the absence of scientific examination of these relationships this chapter will present what is perforce a personal view of how to establish a good relationship with older patients. I will discuss the expectations and resources the patient brings to the relationship, what the physician brings to it, and the elements I think help build a good relationship.

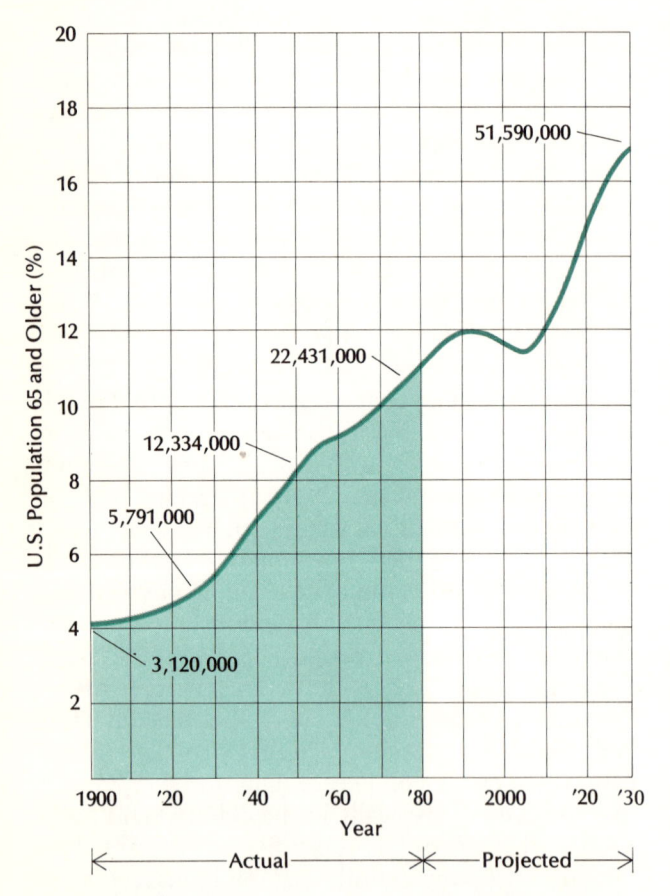

Currently about 10%, the proportion of persons aged 65 or over in U.S. population is expected to rise to 17% by the year 2030. Projections are by U.S. Census Bureau.

What the Patient Brings

As already noted, the aged are a diverse group. In classifying as elderly anyone over age 65, we assemble a population that spans 30 years or more. Some observers quite imprecisely divide the elderly into the young-old and the old-old, those over age 80. The latter tend to have the more serious deficits and poorer prognoses and may warrant more intensive claims on medical and social supports. Besides these diversities, the elderly must be recognized as composing peer groups who have had distinctive social experiences in terms of wars, economic depression, mores, and immigration. Tomorrow's aged surely will be different in these respects. As professional views of the elderly change, the self-image of the elderly will change, and the interaction of patient and physician is bound to be different.

All of which is to say that my generalizations about elderly patients must be qualified. While many of the elderly have an admirable optimism about themselves and old age, others are intensely negative. Given this spectrum, we must recognize that many patients share, in one degree or another, a negative view of old age. They tend to accept deterioration fatalistically. A patient may be reluctant to see a physician because he fears confirmation of "bad news" or is reluctant to seem unrealistic about seeking help for something irreversible. I find many patients bring to the relationship a tendency to underreport or make light of symptoms they fear indicate dread diseases.

At the same time many cherish the hope that the physician, who is generally held in high esteem, can do something. This combination of fear and hope may make them highly vulnerable to intimations of rejection and sensitive to sympathy. They tend to accept the doctor's judgment that something is wrong but nothing can be done. But they can become covertly or openly hostile if patronized by being told not to worry when they know that pain or some other symptom is worsening.

Elderly patients often bring a desire for human contact and attention. About one in every four of the nation's elderly lives alone. Many have experienced losses of spouse, friends, and work role, as well as inability to cope with idleness and financial insecurity. As with younger patients, somatic symptoms may reflect psychogenic problems. But being old, the elderly react to illness as a sign of approaching death, dependency, abandonment, and loss of self-esteem and the respect of others. The life-styles they want to continue seem in jeopardy, and they dread recommendations for institutionalization. When these fears are intense and no rapport with the physician exists, some elderly persons will readily believe that the physician is an ally of relatives who insist on admission to a nursing home.

What the Physician Brings

Like patients, physicians may have hang-ups about death and dying and what their own old age will be. Negative expectations are incorporated in such expressions as "crock." What I have had to say about mental health professionals may be relevant generally to physicians in explanation of negative attitudes toward the elderly:

• The aged stimulate the therapist's fears about his own old age.

• The aged arouse the therapist's conflicts about relationships with parental figures.

• The therapist believes he has nothing useful to offer old people because he believes that they cannot change their behavior or that their problems are all due to untreatable organic brain disease.

• The therapist believes that his psychodynamic skills will be wasted if he works with the aged because they are near death and not really deserving of attention (similar to military triage in which the sickest get the least attention because they are least likely to recover).

• The patient might die in treatment, which could challenge the therapist's sense of importance.

• The therapist's colleagues may be contemptuous of his efforts on behalf of aged patients, e.g., attributing to him a suspicious, morbid preoccupation with death.

To this list one might add that the older patient with chronic disease is hardly attractive to the physician imbued since medical school with cure as the criterion of therapeutic success. There is a tendency to dismiss the patient as soon as the disease is recognized as beyond benefit of treatment. Moreover, professional "ageism" surfaces sometimes as a hostility toward the handicapped elderly as "defective" or "crippled." Patients may be seen as demanding something the physician cannot provide, adding to the physician's frustration and incipient hostility.

I believe there are reasons for these negative attitudes. Some of those who become doctors choose medicine because of unresolved conflicts about death. I do not know of any medical school with a program to assist the medical student in working out his or her emotional reactions to patients with dis-

CHAPTER 25: BUTLER

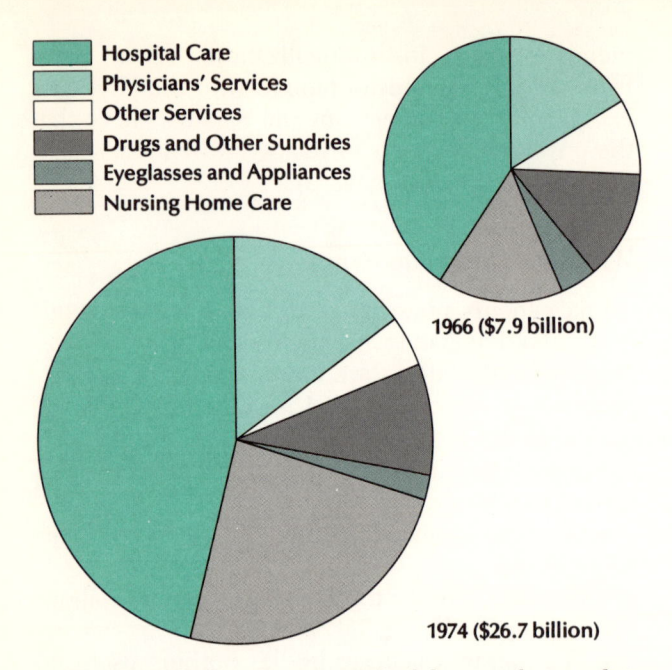

Legend (pie charts):
- Hospital Care
- Physicians' Services
- Other Services
- Drugs and Other Sundries
- Eyeglasses and Appliances
- Nursing Home Care

1966 ($7.9 billion)

1974 ($26.7 billion)

While the elderly represent 10% of the population, their health care costs account for about 30% of nation's spending for health services. Between 1966 and 1974, health care spending for the elderly more than tripled (graph above), with a high proportion of the costs in the latter year coming from public funds (graph below). Data are from National Center for Health Statistics.

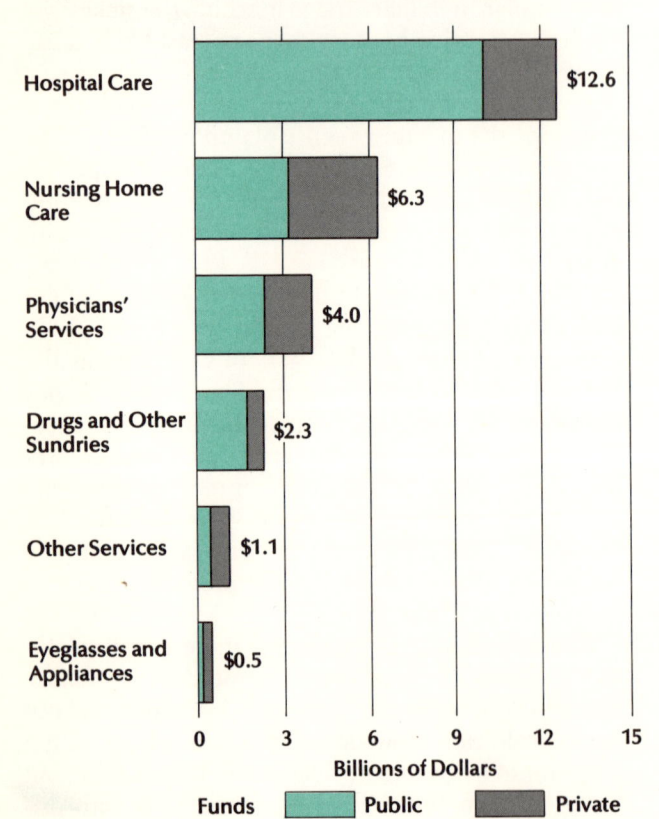

Bar chart (Billions of Dollars):
- Hospital Care: $12.6
- Nursing Home Care: $6.3
- Physicians' Services: $4.0
- Drugs and Other Sundries: $2.3
- Other Services: $1.1
- Eyeglasses and Appliances: $0.5

Funds: Public | Private

---

ability, disfigurement, and pain and to patient and family reactions to death and dying. It might be extraordinarily helpful if the medical school designated a mentor to work informally with students on these personal matters.

The older people emphasized in medical training include those institutionalized for chronic disease and cadavers on the dissection table. These encounters produce an image of the aged, even though they occur in relation to only a tiny proportion of the aged population. At any given time, actually, 95% of the nation's elderly are living outside of institutions. The segment seen becomes an illustration of therapeutic futility and nihilism in geriatrics. Medical students are not exposed to healthy older people; no medical school rotates students through community senior centers, for example. One might expect the same negative outlooks to occur in pediatrics if students saw only youngsters with fatal diseases.

A study of University of California medical students in 1968 showed that their attitude toward old people actually deteriorated during four years in medical school. In general, student experience with the aged tends to reinforce deep fears about mortality and disability, with the predictable result that the more such fears are suppressed, the greater the likelihood of corrosive relationships with aged patients. The so-called senile write-off is an easy, genteel maneuver to adopt: to interpret the patient's ailments as trivial, requiring no serious treatment, and dismiss the patient with a drug prescription or patronizing advice. Moreover, I have known physicians to resist evidence that conditions traditionally considered part of aging are, in fact, disease states. Arteriosclerosis, for example, is not an invariable geriatric concomitant. Years ago, I participated in a National Institute of Mental Health study aimed at differentiating aging from disease. We studied two groups of old men. Those in one group had only minimal evidence of major disease and were, by any traditional criterion, healthy. Those in the other group were free of even minimal evidence of major disease. As we followed these men over the years, we found that it was the appearance of major disease, or its intensification, that produced the physical and behavioral changes typically ascribed to aging. The very behavioral symptoms that feed into the senile write-off often proved to be premonitory of disease and death.

Another aspect of professional negativism is inadequacy in dealing with problems involving family, environment, and need for supportive services. Physicians are not prepared by conventional training to deal with these problems, but they do often recognize that their solution would facilitate the patient's recovery or attainment of maximal feasible function.

Building a Sound Relationship

There are institutional and personal approaches to building sound doctor-patient relationships. An essential institutional step lies in recognizing the validity of geriatrics and gerontology in the competition for research and training resources. Whatever priority is assigned to geriatrics and gerontology represents a clear message in our research-oriented medical world. The National Institute on Aging, the newest of the National Institutes of Health, is an encouraging message of this type. The National Institute of Mental Health's new Center for Studies of the Mental Health of the Aging and the Geriatrics Research and Educational Clinical Centers of the Veterans Administration are other influential commitments. Our institute's research-support activities are also directed toward issues of practical interest, such as studies of drug metabolism in old age. We can support postdoctoral research training in geriatrics and textbook revisions to emphasize geriatrics.

Let us cross over to personal approaches by discussing physician motivation to acquire and share geriatric knowledge, and to examine attitudes and emotional needs as they relate to older patients. To Socrates' injunction to "know thyself," one may add St. Luke's to "heal thyself." The modalities for dealing with emotional and practical problems are fairly obvious, including discussion with colleagues.

What must not be omitted are opportunities to learn from the elderly themselves. Getting to know the elderly patient has been valuable to me as a person and physician. If you want to learn how to survive, they are the tutors. Professionally, knowledge of the patient's personality, history, mental status, and typical responses to stress can provide the necessary context for assessment of symptoms.

Unfortunately, office examinations rarely go comprehensively into such matters. The lack of a careful mental status examination is particularly regrettable in geriatrics, given the need to assess the performance of the central nervous system and its relevance to information processing, subjective experience, behavior, and adaptation.

The usual history taken by the physician covers the systems of the body and present and past illness. It is minimal on personal and social history. Often amazingly little is elicited concerning the patient as a

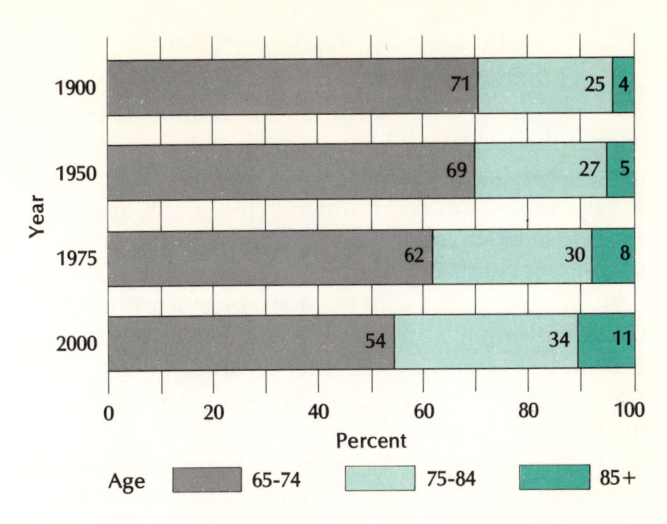

Longer survival (an increasing "old-old" population) is another trend that may be expected to increase the number of elderly persons requiring physician services.

person. What is needed is a "life history," another element in comprehensive assessment of the patient. A life history concentrates on such personal and social aspects as the conflicts a patient has or has had, their resolution, relationships with surviving family members and those deceased, patient acceptance of current place in life (especially in regard to dependency), and indications of how the patient is likely to come to terms with aging, illness, and death.

How one comes to terms with death depends on how one views one's life, not just material success but performance in such roles as parenting. I find many patients have a sense of failure about their children. Yet, as they give a life history, many resolve these feelings (by recognizing first that failures were not entirely so and second that they were not the sole influences on their children) and feel relieved. Thus the life history can be beneficial by allowing the elderly to expiate a sense of guilt. The history-taker must not discount this experience by making such statements as, "Oh, now, you shouldn't feel guilty about that." It is important to say, "Well, you do feel guilty about that; let me hear more about your guilt." The patient is helped to unwind and discuss grief, anger, envy of a sibling, and so on.

Such a life history is not likely to be completed in a single session. It is a process. The patient at first may not reveal much. But he or she will in time, if openness and interest are indicated. It is important that the family physician show concern with the process. The message this effort conveys is critical to the relationship: it makes it clear that the physician wants to get to know the person in depth.

The life history takes time to document, and I am not suggesting that the physician cannot delegate part of the process. There are printed forms for the patient to complete alone, which include basic personal, family, and environmental questions, such as the financial, work, housing, transportation, marriage, recreational, and community situations. Other parts are completed with the assistance of a nurse or paraprofessional. (An example of a life history form is found in *Aging and Mental Health*, pp 165-186. See Selected References.) Physician and patient then review the history together, the physician eliciting further information as necessary and making observations. Do the patient's patterns of coping with stress have noteworthy features? Does the patient tend to become angry and paranoid or to withdraw in a feeling of helplessness?

Whenever possible, a physician should spend an hour or so on a life history at the beginning of a relationship. Besides the bond it can help create, it is cost-effective. An hour spent carefully on life history and mental-status examination can save many hours later. I have met internists and family practitioners who would no more examine a patient without a life history and mental-status examination than a cardiologist would close an examination of a patient without having had the shirt removed. I am convinced that the care of the older patient – who may be making major life-style changes because of chronic illness or situational developments – will be ineffective without these tools. They help the physician formulate treatment strategies that will work because they are based on the patient's mental capacity, circumstances, and moral values. Listening to the patient against the background of the life history, the physician can pick up clues to transient ischemic attacks, anemia, aphasic changes, or mood trends indicating growing depression. Even the sound of the person's voice and a change in the way information is processed can be indicative of cognitive and personality changes. These clues tell the physician to investigate not only for mentation but also for physical illness.

I have mentioned one benefit the patient may receive from a life review – emotional release. In giving the history, patients may have the feeling of receiving a total hearing in which the physician has played a focal role. Because they have had this experience, I find that many patients do not resent it if the doctor, on one or another occasion, is rushed; they remain secure that he understands. Moreover, the life history helps the physician judge more perceptively when the patient needs more or less time during a visit. To those who may worry that a life history will invite habitual exploitation of the physician's time, I can only share my experience that few patients are inclined to do so. If anything, most older patients bend over backwards to be undemanding.

Candor is a hallmark of a sound relationship. The physician is free to give advice and the patient is free to reject it, without risk of sarcasm, rebuff, or isolation. The physician is free to acknowledge that some social and family problems are beyond him or her. But they can be acknowledged and appropriate medical advice given. Let me illustrate: the physician is speaking to an old woman. "I don't know how to help you in your housing problem. But I do appreciate that, with your shortness of breath, it's hell to go up two flights of stairs. Don't be embarrassed that you have trouble. Carry a newspaper. When you need to, stop at the top of the first flight, sit on the step, and read awhile before going on." Such an approach is far better for patient morale than pretense, based on fear of involvement, that the problem does not exist. While it might be helpful too, for the physician to refer the woman to a housing or social-service agency, the most significant gesture has been the showing of sympathy. I recognize that little is taught in medical school about how an office practitioner can draw on community social services. I have learned much from the way shrewd family members discover and use local resources for the elderly, such as Area Agencies on Aging, senior citizen centers, welfare departments, homemaker groups, and philanthropic and church agencies. But some families are adrift and could use advice, if the physician feels competent to give it.

Respect for the patient is another major element of rapport. It not only allows but requires unpleasant issues to be raised. Aware of rapid deterioration of a patient who lives alone or with a family unable to provide more care at home, the physician may have to broach the issue of the nursing home. It is respectful to raise the issue and give reasons for and against admission to the nursing home. I never say that the only choice for the patient is of timing – to go now rather than wait. In a free society, the patient has a right to decide to die in his or her own home. Even if there were incontinence and other complications, even if I disagreed with the decision, I would assist in meeting the patient's wishes. Forcing patients into institutions "for their own good" is antithetical to a sound relationship and to maintaining the patient's self-respect. Rather than to tell the patient, "You're foolish for not following good medical advice," the physician is better advised to take the tack, "I think it makes more sense at this time for you to go into the nursing home." This approach reinforces recognition that the patient is in control of his or her own life, and it serves to counter a sense of helplessness and the hostility or depression that may follow.

Nor does a sound relationship require the physician blindly to accept the patient's word about dependency and illness. If a patient reports a heart attack but there is no electrocardiographic evidence or clinical sign, the patient should be told. The problem may be depression because of an unresolved emotional conflict. A patient once complained to me of heart pains that made him unable to take walks, but he was in obviously good physical condition, and a

---

Examples of the 'Senile Write-Off'

Case A

A vigorous 72-year-old man has fibrosis of the penis, Peyronie's disease. Although worried about sexual function, he is too embarrassed to ask his internist about it during a physical examination. The internist focuses on possible hernia as the cause of nonspecific physical complaints and anxiety. No hernia is found. The internist refers the patient for a psychiatric evaluation. The psychiatrist finds the fibrosis and telephones the internist for a medical history. The internist gives it, with no mention of the fibrosis. What about it? "Oh, that," says the internist. "Well, that would hardly matter at his age."

COMMENT: *Evidently, the internist's indifference or embarrassment about sex and especially sexual function in old age was the basis for trivializing or missing the obvious disease. The patient was entitled to a frank diagnosis and treatment or advice on how to achieve sexual satisfaction without intercourse if treatment was unavailing. The internist needed to resolve his embarrassment and to try to open the subject of sexual desire in old age for the patient. A clinician's willingness to listen sympathetically to the older patient with sexual impotence may, in itself, permit resumption of satisfactory sexual relationships.*

Case B

An older woman becomes anxious about a scheduled operation for cataract lens extraction and is given a tranquilizer. Postoperatively, she is confused; more tranquilizer is prescribed by the ophthalmologist in the hospital. The dose is increased when the anxiety persists, despite evidence that the operation has been successful. Finally, the specialist – the patient has no regular physician – recommends placement in a nursing home, which is done. At this point, the woman appears senile – confused, with poor memory, and anxious. In the home, a new physician takes her completely off medication. He learns that she was apprehensive about the operation and remained so postoperatively because of the "fractured glass" vision. She is counseled that this is an expected, normal result of a successful operation and vision will improve. The anxiety subsides and she is discharged home.

COMMENT: *The specialist substituted the senile write-off, with drug prescription, for active listening and counseling. His evident predominant concern was with the operation, not the patient. A second senile write-off was recommendation of nursing home placement.*

Case C

During an unusually busy day for the physician, a garrulous elderly woman comes in for examination, complaining of "not feeling well." She seems to want the doctor's sympathy. The physician finds nothing wrong in a cursory examination and tells her so but prescribes a tranquilizer, with advice to take three a day or some more if she feels the need. "Don't worry," he says. In a few days, the woman is drowsy, dizzy, and confused much of the time, appearing senile to family members. She later reports increasing pain in the upper right shoulder and general abdominal discomfort, actually the unexpressed reason for visiting the physician. It is now a month after the first visit. She returns to the doctor and gallstones are diagnosed.

COMMENT: *The physician attributed the first visit to hypochondriasis, not realizing that this may be an early symptom of disease. Had he taken time for questioning (rather than dismissing the patient as another "crock"), he might have elicited the referred right shoulder pain, a tip-off to the gallbladder. Instead, the senile write-off was employed, risking the possibility that the patient might experience a fall or accident because of drug-induced dizziness and confusion. If the physician had had a life history that showed the patient was usually stoical in response to stress, her appearance with nonspecific complaints would clearly have called for serious study.*

thorough cardiac evaluation was normal. The complaint really reflected depression over a conflict with a son. We remained in cordial disagreement about his walking ability. I conveyed my judgment that he was unrealistic while putting my arm around him.

However, there are times when apparently sympathetic words and gestures can destroy a good relationship. If the physician is overly protective, he may undercut the patient's self-respect. Equally undermining is bringing in family members without the patient's consent, even when they are important to the patient's management. It is a delicate matter to suggest loss of independence but it can be done – and family members can be brought in – when the patient is treated with respect as well as sympathy. I have taken this approach: "I'm worried about whether you're able to take care of yourself at home. I know you don't want to leave and go into a nursing home. Let's have a frank talk. There are ways to make it possible, like having someone visit you regularly, or to have your son or daughter see you a few times a week to make sure you have dinner. I don't think you're eating properly. You and I discussed this the other day, and you agreed that you're not." If the patient insists that the family not be involved, some other form of assistance should be sought.

When the patient wants the family brought in, the physician can indicate meaningful roles to play – by having them seek out community resources and by involving them in the patient's drug or physical therapy regimens. Their collaboration takes pressure off the physician. Sometimes, families want the physician to take responsibility for a decision when they feel guilty about it. For example, if the physician is convinced that a patient who cannot decide for himself is ready for a nursing home, he may tell the family, "I think you'd feel relieved if I were the one to take responsibility for admission to the home." If they agree, the physician goes ahead.

Not all relationships go smoothly, of course. Among signs of a breakdown are nonpayment of bills and missed appointments. My pattern has been to try to find out why. I encourage the patient to tell me of disappointment or anger about the care he or she is getting. Asking for a consultation is another sign of a deteriorating relationship. I respect the request without hurt feelings, since it is the patient's right. But I will ask if there is a complaint. If it is justified, I must acknowledge it. I realize that, in this era of malpractice litigation, it may be hard to admit that something may not have been handled right, but some way of showing frankness is always feasible. Certainly, a desire to improve the relationship can be expressed, or more information or reassurance can be given about therapy. One must keep in mind that only rarely will older patients simply tell the doctor they do not like him. Typically, they just stop coming.

Also part of a good relationship is an office environment that shows concern for the older patient. Barrier-free access to the office from the street should be assured. Receptionists may need instruction on how to react to patients without putting them down. Scheduled telephone hours may be a big help. Patients can be told what words to use when they feel they must reach the doctor immediately, and the physician who knows the patient well will recognize the degree of urgency.

We professionals have much to learn about the doctor-patient relationship, our part in it, and what makes it go well or badly. The subject deserves scientific study, with feedback into physician training. Among ingredients I have tried to identify as crucial are: 1) getting to know the patient well through a life history; 2) giving the patient a full hearing; 3) being appropriately frank; 4) viewing the older patient as a participant in making decisions about care; 5) recognizing unconscious prejudice and conflicts; 6) adopting approaches that enhance the patient's independence and self-respect and preserve the patient's life-style as much as possible; 7) establishing treatment goals that are realistic; 8) recognizing problems referable to other professionals and the family; 9) dealing with the patient's negative attitudes toward self and physician. In no case should senility be considered other than a diagnosis requiring careful assessment. The key to geriatrics is comprehensiveness of evaluation, which also happens to be a key to improved physician-patient relationships.

Selected References

Index

Illustration and Data Source Credits

Selected References

Chapter 1

Lamy PP, Kitler ME: Drugs and the geriatric patient. J Am Geriatr Soc 19:1:23, 1971

Lamy PP, Kitler ME: The geriatric patient: age-dependent physiologic and pathologic changes. J Am Geriatr Soc 19:871, 1971

Vestal RE, Norris AH, Tobin JD: Antipyrine metabolism in man: influence of age, alcohol, caffeine and smoking. Clin Pharmacol Ther 18:425, 1975

Bender AD: Pharmacodynamic principles of drug therapy in the aged. J Am Geriatr Soc 22:296, 1974

Jelliffe RW: An improved method of digoxin therapy. Ann Intern Med 69:703, 1968

Chan RH, Benner EJ, Hoeprich PD: Gentamicin therapy in renal failure: a nomogram for dosage. Ann Intern Med 76:773, 1972

Bennett WM, Singer I, Golper T: Guidelines for drug therapy in renal failure. Ann Intern Med 86:754, 1977

Smithard DJ, Langman MJS: Drug metabolism in the elderly. Br Med J 2:520, 1977

Altman PL, Dittmer DS: Blood and Other Body Fluids, pp. 492-500. Federation of American Society for Experimental Biology, Washington D.C., 1961

Caranasos GJ, Stewart RB, Cluff LE: Drug-induced illness leading to hospitalization. JAMA 228:713-717, 1974

Gibson RM, Muelle MS, Fisher CR: Age differences in health care spending, fiscal year 1976. Social Security Bulletin 40:3-14, 1977

Richey DP, Bender D: Pharmacokinetic consequences of aging. Annual Review of Pharmacology and Toxicology 17:49-65, 1977

Vestal RE, McGuire EA, Tobin JD: Aging and ethanol metabolism. Clin Pharmacol Ther 21:343-354, 1977

Vestal RE: Drug use in the elderly: A review of problems and special considerations. Drugs (in press).

Chapter 2

Butler RN, Lewis MJ: Aging and Mental Health, 1st ed. The C.V. Mosby Company, St. Louis, 1973

Harris R: The Management of Geriatric Cardiac Disease. J.B. Lippincott Co., Philadelphia, 1970

Rodstein M, Savitsky E, Starkman R: Initial adjustment to a long-term care institution, medical and behavioral aspects. J Am Geriatr Soc 24:65, 1976

Eckstein D: Common symptoms and complaints of the elderly. J Am Geriatr Soc 21:440, 1973

American Medical Association: The Quality of Life–The Later Years. Publishing Sciences Group Inc., Acton, Mass., 1975

Rossman I, Ed: Clinical Geriatrics. J.B. Lippincott Co., Philadelphia, 1971.

Butler RN: Why Survive? Being Old in America. Harper & Row, New York, 1975

Hastings JB: Mass screening for colorectal cancer. Am J Surg 127:228-233, 1974

Albanese AA, Edelson A, Herbert A: Problems of bone health in elderly. Ten-year study. New York State J Med 75:326, 1975

Butler RN: Successful aging and the role of the life review. J Am Geriatr Soc 22:529, 1974

Schouten J: Important factors in the examination and care of old patients. J Am Geriatr Soc 23:180, 1975

Kornzweig AL: The prevention of blindness in the aged. J Am Geriatr Soc 20:383, 1972

Chapter 3

Reichel W: Complications in the care of 500 elderly hospitalized patients. J Am Geriatr Soc 13:973, 1965

Rossman I, Ed: Clinical Geriatrics. J.B. Lippincott Co., Philadelphia, 1971

Brocklehurst JC, Ed: Textbook of Geriatric Medicine and Gerontology. Churchill Livingstone, Edinburgh, 1973

Hodkinson HM: An Outline of Geriatrics. Academic Press, London, 1975

Andres R: Relation of physiological changes in aging to medical changes in disease of the aged. Mayo Clin Proc 42: 674, 1967

Andres R: Aging and diabetes. Med Clin North Am 55:835, 1971

Hall MRP: Drug therapy in the elderly. Br Med J 4: 582, 1973.

Howell TH: Causation of diagnostic errors in octogenarians: a clinicopathological study. J Am Geriatr Soc 14:41, 1966

Howell T: Multiple pathology in nonagenarians. Geriatrics 18:899, 1963

Reichel W, Ed: Clinical Aspects of Aging. Williams and Wilkins, Baltimore, Maryland, 1978.

Rowe J et al: The effect of age on creatinine clearance in men: a cross-sectional and longitudinal study. J Gerontol 31:155, 1976

Chapter 4

Geriatric Psychiatry. Berezin M, Cath S, Eds. International University Press, New York, 1965

Human Aging. Birren J et al, Eds. U.S. Dept. HEW, NIMH, PHS Publ 986

Bond A, Lader M: The use of analogue scales in rating subjective feelings. Br J Med Psychol 47:211, 1974

Folstein M, Luria R: Reliability, validity and clinical application of the visual analogue mood scale. Psychol Med 3:4:479, 1973

Bender AD: Pharmacologic aspects of aging: additional literature. J Am Geriatr Soc 15 (1):68-74, 1967

Butler RN: Clinical psychiatry in late life. Clinical Geriatrics. Rossman I, Ed. J.B. Lippincott Co., Philadelphia, 1971, pp. 439-459

Butler RN: Mental health and aging: life perspectives. Geriatrics 29 (11): 59-60, 1974

Butler RN: Psychiatry and the elderly: an overview. Am J Psychiatry, 132 (9): 893-900, 1975

Comfort A: Sexuality in old age. J Am Geriatr Soc 22 (10); 440-442, 1974

Drugs and the elderly mind. Lancet 2:126, 1972

Freeman JT: Some principles of medication in geriatrics. J Am Geriatr Soc 22:289, 1974

Weinberg J: Some psychodynamic aspects of agedness. Aging and the Brain. Gaitz CM, Ed. Plenum Press, New York, London, 1972

Chapter 5

Wells CE: Dementia, 2nd ed. F.A. Davis Company, Philadelphia, 1977

Poser CM: The presenile dementias. JAMA 233:81, 1975

Kahn RL, Goldfarb AI, Pollack M: Brief objective measures for the determination of mental status in the aged. Am J Psychiatry 117:326, 1960

Epstein LJ, Simon A: Organic brain syndrome in the elderly. Geriatrics 22:145, 1967

Terry RD, Gonatas N, Weiss W: Ultrastructural studies in Alzheimer's presenile dementia. Am J Pathol 44:269, 1964

Adams RD, Fisher CM, Hakim S: Symptomatic occult hydrocephalus with normal cerebrospinal fluid pressure. A treatable syndrome. N Engl J Med 273:117, 1965

Shenkin HS, Greenberg J, Bouzarth WF: Ventricular shunting for relief of senile symptoms. JAMA 225:1486, 1973

Menzer L, Sabin T, Mark VH: Computerized axial tomography—use in the diagnosis of dementia. JAMA 234:754, 1975

Byrd GJ: Acute organic brain syndrome associated with gentamicin therapy. JAMA 238: 53, 1977

Stefoski D et al: Correlation between diffuse EEG abnormalities and cerebral atrophy in senile dementia. J Neurol Neurosurg Psychiatry 39: 751, 1976

Huckman MS et al: Computerized tomography in the diagnosis of degenerative diseases of the brain. Semin Roentgenol 12: 63, 1977

Katzman R, Terry RD, Bick K: Alzheimer's Disease: Senile Dementia and Related Disorders. Raven Press, New York (in press)

Katzman R: The prevalence in malignancy in Alzheimer's disease. A major killer. Arch Neurol 33: 217, 1976

Chapter 6

Wisoff BG, Marvin ML, Aintalian A: Results of open heart surgery in the septuagenarian. J Gerontol 31:275-277, 1976

Barnhorst DA, Giuliani ER, Pluth J: Open heart surgery in patients more than 65 years old. Ann Thorac Surg 18:81-90, 1974

Guthrie RB, Spellberg RD, Benedict JS: Open-heart valve surgery in patients 65 and older. Arch Surg 105:42-43, 1972

Librach G, Schadel M, Seltzer M: The initial manifestations of acute myocardial infarction. Geriatrics 31:41-46, 1976

Harris A, Davies M, Redwood D: Aetiology of chronic heart block: a clinico-pathological correlation in 65 cases. Br Heart J 31:206, 1969

Lewis KB, Criley JM, Nelson RJ: Early clinical experience with the rechargeable cardiac pacemaker. Ann Thorac Surg 18:5:490, 1974

Fischell RE, Lewis KB, Love JW: A long-lived, reliable rechargeable cardiac pacemaker. International Symposium on Advances in Pacemaker Technology, Erlangen-Nurnberg, West Germany,

September 26, 1974. Johns Hopkins Applied Physics Laboratory.

Bedford PD, Caird FL: Valvular Disease of the Heart in Old Age. Little, Brown & Co., Boston, 1960

Burch GE, DePasquale NP: Geriatric cardiology. Am Heart J 78:700, 1969

Harris RH: The Management of Cardiovascular Disease in the Geriatric Patient. J.B. Lippincott Co., Philadelphia, 1970

Rossman I, Ed: Clinical Geriatrics. J.B. Lippincott Co., Philadelphia, 1971

Bhat PK, Watanabe K, Rao DB: Conduction defects in the aging heart. J Am Geriatr Soc 22:517-520, 1974

Chapter 7

Kannel WB, Sorlie P: Hypertension in Framingham in Epidemiology and Control of Hypertension. Paul O, Ed. Symposia Specialists, Miami, Florida, 1975, pp. 553-592

Kannel WB: Some lessons in cardiovascular epidemiology from Framingham. Am J Cardiol 37:269, 1976

Dayton S, Pearce ML, Hashimoto S: A controlled clinical trial of a diet high in unsaturated fats in preventing complications of atherosclerosis. Circulation 40: (Suppl 2) 1, 1969

Castelli WP, Doyle JT, Gordon T: HDL cholesterol and other lipids in coronary heart disease, The Cooperative Lipoprotein Phenotyping Study. Circulation 55: 767-772, 1977

Gordon T, Castelli WP, Hjortland MC: High density lipoprotein as a protective factor against coronary heart disease. The Framingham Study. Am J Med 62: 707-713, 1977

Glueck CJ, Fallat RW, Spadafora M: Longevity syndromes. Circulation 52: II-272, 1975

Gordon T, Castelli WP, Hjortland MC: Predicting coronary heart disease in middle-aged and older persons. The Framingham Study. JAMA 238:497-499, 1977

Gofman JW, Young W, Tandy R: Ischemic heart disease, atherosclerosis and longevity. Circulation 34:679-697, 1966

Miller GJ, Miller NE: Plasma high density lipoprotein concentration and development of ischemic heart disease. Lancet 1:16, 1975

Walker WJ: Changing United States life-style and declining vascular mortality: cause or coincidence? N Engl J Med 297: 163-165, 1977

Cardiovascular diseases: guidelines for prevention and care. Primary Prevention of the Atherosclerotic Diseases. Wright IS, Fredrickson DT, Eds. Washington DC, United States Government Printing Office, 1974, pp. 15-56

VA Cooperative Study: Effect of treatment on morbidity in hypertension. Part I. JAMA 202:116, 1967

Chapter 8

Wylie CM: Death statistics for cerebrovascular disease: a review of recent findings. Stroke 1:184-193, 1970

Wylie CM: The community medicine of cerebrovascular disease. Stroke 1: 385-396, 1970

Whisnant JP, Matsumoto N, Elveback LR: The effect of anticoagulant therapy on the prognosis of patients with transient cerebral ischemic attacks in a community: Rochester, Minn., 1955 through 1969. Mayo Clin Proc 48: 844-848, 1973

Sund TM Jr: Surgical therapy of occlusive vascular diseases of the brain. Surgery Annual, Vol 6. Nyhns LM, Ed. Appleton-Century-Crofts, New York, 1973, 393-411

Sund TM Jr, Sandok BA, Whisnant JP: Carotid endarterectomy, complications and pre-operative assessment of risk. Mayo Clin Proc 50: 301-306, 1975

Levin EB: Use of the Holter electrocardiographic monitor in the diagnosis of transient ischemic attacks. J Am Geriatr Soc 24: 516-521, 1976

Genton E, Gen M, Hirsh J, Harker LA: Platelet-inhibiting drugs in the prevention of clinical thrombotic disease. N Engl J Med 293: 1174-1178, 1975

Fields WS, Lemak NA, Frankowski RF, Hardy RJ: Controlled trial of aspirin in cerebral ischemia. Stroke 8: 301-316, 1977

Hass WK: Aspirin for the limping brain. Stroke 8: 299-300, 1977

Dyken ML et al: Cooperative study of hospital frequency and character of transient ischemic attacks, I. Background, organization and clinical survey. JAMA 237: 882-886, 1977

Haerer AF, Gotschall RA, Conneally PM: Cooperative study of hospital frequency and character of transient ischemic attacks, III. Variations in treatment. JAMA 238: 142-146, 1977

Barnett HJM: Canadian cooperative platelet-inhibiting drug trial in threatened stroke. Abstracts of the 3rd Joint Meeting on Stroke and Cerebral Circulation. Stroke 9: 16-17, 1978

Chapter 9

Wintrobe MM et al: Clinical Hematology, 7th ed. Lea & Febiger, Philadelphia, 1974

Earney MA, Earney AJ: Geriatric hematology. J Am Geriatr Soc 20:174, 1972

Maekawa T: Hematological diseases. The Care of the Geriatric Patient. Cowdry EV, Steinberg FU, Eds. The C.V. Mosby Company, St. Louis, 1971, p. 112

Murphy EA, Abbey H: The normal range – a common misuse. J Chron Dis 20:79, 1967

Botwinick J: Who are the aged? Geriatrics 29:124, July 1974

Thomas JH: Anaemia in the elderly. Br Med J 4:280, 1973

Batata M, Spray GH, Bolton FG: Blood and bone marrow changes in elderly patients, with special reference to folic acid, vitamin B_{12}, iron, and ascorbic acid. Br Med J 2:667, 1967

Mitra ML: Diagnostic significance of high erythrocyte sedimentation rate with iron deficiency anemia in the elderly. J Am Geriatr Soc 20:284, 1972

Caird FI: Problems of interpretation of laboratory findings in the old. Br Med J 4:384, 1973

Lewis R: Anemia – a common but never a normal concomitant of aging. Geriatrics 31:53, 1976

Fernandez G, Schwartz JM: Immune responsiveness and hematologic malignancy in the elderly. Med Clin North Am 67: 1253, 1976

McLennan WJ, Andrews GR, Macleod C: Anaemia in the Elderly. Q J Med 42:1, 1973

Chapter 10

Zboralske FF, Amberg JR, Soergel KH: Presbyoesophagus: cineradiographic manifestations. Radiology 82:463, 1964

Levrat M, Pasquier J, Lambet R, Tissot A: Peptic ulcer in patients over 60. Experience in 287 cases. Am J Dig Dis 11:279, 1966

Andrews GR, Haneman B, Arnold BJ: Atrophic gastritis in the aged. Aust Ann Med 16:230, 1967

Isokoski, Krohn K, Varisk: Parietal cell and intrinsic factor antibodies in a Finnish rural population sample. Scand J Gastroenterol 4:251, 1969

Balacki JA, Dobbin WO: III. Maldigestion and malabsorption: making up for lost nutrients. Geriatrics 29:157, 1974

Sklar M: Functional bowel distress and constipation in the aged. Geriatrics 27:79, 1972

Portis SA, King JC: The gastrointestinal tract in the aged. JAMA 148:1073, 1952

Manousos ON, Truelove SC, Lumsden K: Prevalence of colonic diverticulosis in general population of Oxford area. Br Med J 3:762, 1967

Morgan ZR, Feldman M: Liver, biliary tract and pancreas in aged; an anatomic and laboratory evaluation. J Am Geriatr Soc 5:59, 1957

Sklar M, Kirsner JB, Palmer WL: Symposium on medical problems of aged; gastrointestinal disease in the aged. Med Clin North Am 40:223, 1956

Grodsinsky C, Brush BE, Ponka JL: Management of complicated biliary tract disease in geriatric patients. J Am Geriatr Soc 20:531, 1972

Rosenberg IR, Friedland N, Janowitz HD, Dreiling DA: The effect of age and sex upon human pancreatic secretion of fluid and bicarbonate. Gastroenterology 50:191, 1966

Chapter 11

Andres R: Aging and diabetes. Med Clin North Am 55:835, 1971

Clark OH, Demling R: Management of thyroid nodules in the elderly. Am J Surg 132:615, 1976

Davis PJ, Davis FB: Hyperthyroidism in patients over the age of 60 years. Clinical features in 85 patients. Medicine 53:161, 1974

Finch CE: The regulation of physiological changes during mammalian aging. Quarterly Journal of Biology 51:49, 1976

Gregerman RI, Bierman IL: Aging and hormones. Chapter 27, Textbook of Endocrinology, 5th ed. Williams RH, Ed. W. B. Saunders, 1974

Gregerman RI, Davis PJ: Effects of intrinsic and extrinsic variables on thyroid hormone economy. Werner SC, Ingbar SH, Eds. Chapter 12, The Thyroid: A Fundamental and Clinical Text, 4th ed. Harper & Row, New York, 1978, pp. 223-289

Helderman JH, Vestal RE, Rowe JW, Tobin JD, Andres R, Robertson GL: The response of arginine vasopressin to intravenous ethanol and hypertonic saline in man: the impact of aging. J Gerontol 33:39, 1978

Muggeo M, Fedele D, Tiengo A, Molinari M, Crepaldi G: Human growth hormone and cortisol response to insulin stimulation with aging. J Gerontol 30:546, 1975

Rubenstein HA, Butler VP Jr, Werner SC: Progressive decrease in serum triiodothyronine concentrations with human aging: radioimmunoassay following extraction of serum. J Clin Endocrinol Metab 37:247, 1973

Snyder PJ, Utiger RD: Thyrotropin response to thyrotropin-releasing hormone in normal females over forty. J Clin Endocrinol Metab 34:1096, 1972

Steams EL, MacDonnell JA, Kaufman BJ, Padua R, Lucman TS, Winter JSD, Faiman C: Declining testicular function with age. Hormonal and clinical correlates. Am J Med 57:761, 1974

Weidman P, De Myttenaere-Bursztein, Maxwell MH, de Lima J: Effect of aging on plasma renin and aldosterone in normal man. Kidney Int 8:325, 1975

Chapter 12

Smythe H: Nonsteroidal therapy in inflammatory joint disease. Hospital Practice, 10:9, 1975

Howell DS, Sapolsky AS, Pita JC, Woessner JF: The pathogenesis of osteoarthritis. Semin Arthritis Rheum 5:384, 1976

Jaffe IA: D-penicillamine. Bull Rheum Dis 28:948, 1978

Bluhm GB: The treatment of rheumatoid arthritis with gold. Arthritis Rheum 5:14, 1976

Swezey RL: Essentials of physical management and rehabilitation in arthritis. Semin Arthritis Rheum 3:349, 1974

Primer on the Rheumatic Diseases, 7th ed. Arthritis Foundation, New York, 1973; JAMA (Suppl) 224:5, 1973

Moskowitz RW: Clinical Rheumatology: A Problem Oriented Approach to Diagnosis and Management. Lea & Febiger, Philadelphia, 1975

Hollander JL, McCarty DJ Jr: Arthritis and Allied Conditions, 8th ed. Lea & Febiger, Philadelphia, 1972

Ditunno JF, Ehrlich GE: Rehabilitation of the elderly patient with rheumatoid arthritis. Geriatrics 25:164, 1970

McBeath AA: Osteoporosis and degenerative arthritis. Postgrad Med 57:7:171, June 1975

Jayson MIV: Clinics in Rheumatic Diseases. W.B. Saunders Company, London, April 1976

Kolodny AL, McLoughlin PT: Comprehensive Approach to Therapy of Pain. Charles C Thomas, Publisher, Springfield, Ill., 1966

Chapter 13

Gordan GS, Vaughan C: The role of estrogens in osteoporosis. Geriatrics 32 (9):42-8, 1977

Jowsey J: Osteoporosis: dealing with a crippling bone disease of the elderly. Geriatrics 32 (7): 41-50, 1977

Marshall DH, Crilly RG, Nordin BE: Plasma androstenedione and oestrone levels in normal and osteoporotic postmenopausal women. Br Med J 2 (6096): 1177-9, 5 Nov 77

Marshall DH, Horsman A, Nordin BE: The prevention and management of post-menopausal osteoporosis. Acta Obstet Gynecol Scand (Suppl) (65): 49-56, 1977

Ziel HK, Finkle WD: Increased risk of endometrial carcinoma among users of conjugated estrogens. N Engl J Med 23:1187, 1975

Arthes FG, Sartwell PE, Lewison EF: The pill, estrogens and the breast. Cancer 28:1391, 1971

Friedrich EG: Vulvar Disease. W.B. Saunders Company, Philadelphia, 1976

Leis HP, Black MM, Sall S: The pill and the breast. J Reprod Med 16:5, 1976

Novak E, Woodruff D: Novak's Gynecologic and Obstetric Pathology. W.B. Saunders Company, Philadelphia, 1974

Ryan KJ, Gibson DC: Menopause and Aging. Department of Health, Education, and Welfare, Publication No. (NIH) 73-319. U.S. Government Printing Office, Washington, D.C., 1971

Smith DC, Prentice R, Thompson DJ, Herrmann WL: Association of exogenous estrogen and endometrial carcinoma. N Engl J Med 293:1164, 1975

Taymor ML, Green TH: Progress in Gynecology, Vol VI. Grune & Stratton, New York, 1975

Chapter 14

Krishnamurthy GT, Tubis M, Hiss J: Distribution pattern of metastatic bone disease. JAMA 237:2504, 1977

Silver RT, Young RC, Holland JF: Some new aspects of modern cancer chemotherapy. Am J Med 62:775, 1977

Engel A, Larsson T: Cancer and Aging. Thule International Symposia. Nordiska Bokhandelns Forlag, Stockholm, 1968

Holland JF, Frei E: Cancer Medicine. Lea & Febiger, Philadelphia, 1973

Rubin P: Current Concepts in Cancer. American Medical Association, Chicago, 1974

Greenspan EM, Ed: Clinical Cancer Chemotherapy. Raven Press, New York, 1975

Nealon TF, Ed: Management of the Patient with Cancer. W.B. Saunders Company, Philadelphia, 1976

Krupp PJ, Lee FYL, Bohm JW: Epidermoid cancer of the vulva. CA 26:360, 1976

Silverberg E: Cancer statistics 1977. CA 27:26, 1977

Alexanian R: Plasma cell neoplasms. CA 26:38, 1976

Murphy G: Prostatic cancer. CA 24:282, 1974

Gottlieb JA, Hill CI Jr: Adriamycin therapy in thyroid carcinoma. Cancer Therapy Reports 6, Part 3:223, 1975

Chapter 15

Bruce AW, O'Cleireachain F, Morales A: Carcinoma of prostate. A critical look at staging. J Urol 117:319, 1977

Scott WW, Wade JC: Medical treatment of benign nodular prostatic hyperplasia with cyproterone acetate. J Urol 101:81, 1969

Ray GR, Cassidy JR, Bagshaw MA: Definitive radiation therapy of carcinoma of the prostate. A report of 15 years' experience. Radiology 106:407, 1973

Nicholson TC, Richie JP: Pelvic lymphadenectomy for stage B1 adenocarcinoma of the prostate. Justified or not? J Urol 117:199, 1977

Whitmore WF Jr: Symposium on hormones and cancer therapy; hormone therapy in prostatic cancer. Am J Med 21:697, 1956

Wilson CS, Dahl DS, Middleton RG: Pelvic lymphadenectomy for the staging of apparently localized prostatic cancer. J Urol 117:197, 1977

O'Conor VJ Jr, Bulkey GJ, Sokol JK: Low suprapubic prostatectomy: comparison of results with the standard operation in two comparable groups of 142 patients. J Urol 90:301, 1963

Millin T, McAlister CLO, Kelley PM: Retropubic prostatectomy experience based on 757 cases. Lancet 1:381, 1949

Bergman RT, Turner R, Barnes RW: Comparative analysis of one thousand consecutive cases of transurethral prostatic resection. J Urol 74:533, 1955

McLaughlin AP, Saltstein SL, McCullough DL: Prostatic carcinoma: incidence and location of unsuspected lymphatic metastases. J Urol 115:89, 1977

Kelalis PP, McLean P: The treatment of diverticulum of the bladder. J Urol 98:349, 1967

Nesbit RM, Baum WC: Endocrine control of prostatic carcinoma. Clinical and statistical survey of 1,818 cases. JAMA 143:1317, 1950

Grayhack JT, Sadlowsky RW: Results of surgical treatment of benign prostatic hyperplasia. Benign Prostatic Hyperplasia, 125-134. DHEW Publication No. (NIH) 76:1113

Silverberg E: Urologic cancer: statistical and epidemiological information. American Cancer Society, 1973

Chapter 16

Berezin MA, Stotsky B: The geriatric patient. The Practice of Community Health. Grunebaum H, Ed. Little, Brown & Co., Boston, 1970

Butler RN, Lewis MI: Aging and Mental Health. The C.V. Mosby Co., St. Louis, 1973, pp. 99-104

Butler RN, Lewis MI: Sex After Sixty. Harper & Row, New York, 1976

Finkle AL: Sexual function during advancing age. Chapter 29, Clinical Geriatrics. Rossman I, Ed. J.B. Lippincott Co., Philadelphia, 1971

Irwin T: Sexuality in later years. Physicians World, November, 1973, pp. 53-56

Kaplan HS: The New Sex Therapy. Brunner/Mazel Publication, in cooperation with Quadrangle/The New York Times Book Co., New York, 1974

Martin CE: Marital and sexual factors in relation to age, disease and longevity. Wirt RD, Winokur G, Roff M: Life History Research in Psychopathology, Vol 4. University of Minnesota Press, Minneapolis, 1976

Masters WH, Johnson VE: Human Sexual Inadequacy. Little, Brown & Co., Boston, pp. 316-350

McCary JL: Human Sexuality, 2nd ed. D. Van Nostrand Co., New York, 1973, pp. 256-268.

Oaks WW, Melchiode GA, Ficher I, Eds: Sex and the Life Cycle. Grune & Stratton, New York, 1976

Rubin I: Sexual Life After Sixty. Basic Books, Inc., New York, 1965

Scheingold LD, Wagner NN: Sound Sex and the Aging Heart. Human Sciences Press, New York, 1974

Chapter 17

Fisher AA: Contact Dermatitis, 2nd ed. Lea & Febiger, Philadelphia, 1973

Belisario JC: Cutaneous manifestations associated with internal cancer. Cutis 1:513-522, 544, 569-576, 1965

Cripps DJ, Hegedus S: Protection factor of sunscreens to monochromatic radiation. Arch Dermatol 109:202, 1974

Mohs FE: Chemosurgery in Cancer, Gangrene and Infections. Charles C Thomas, Springfield, Illinois, 1956

Clark WH: Advances in biology of the skin. The Pigmentary System, Vol III. Montagne W Ed. Pergamon Press, New York, 1967, pp. 621-647

Fraser JF: Bowen's disease and Paget's disease of the nipple. Their relation to dyskeratosis. Archives of Dermatology and Syphilis 18:809-828, 1928

Curth HO, Hilberg AW, Machacek GF: The site and histology of the cancer associated with malignant acanthosis nigricans. Cancer 15:433-439, 1962

Bailey BN: Bedsores. Edward Arnold, London, 1967, p. 130

Chapter 18

Kornzweig AL, Feldstein M, Schneider J: Eye in Old Age, IV. Ocular survey of over 1,000 persons with special reference to normal and disturbed visual function. Am J Ophthalmol 44:29, July 1957

Goriu G: Clinical Glaucoma. Vol I, Ophthalmology Series. Henkind P, Ed. Marcel Dekker, Inc., New York, 1977

Feldstein M, Kornzweig AL, Schneider J: Ocular Surgery in the Aged. JAMA 170:1261, 1959

Kahn HA, Liebowitz HM, Ganley JP: Framingham Eye Study. I. Outline and major prevalence findings. Am J Epidemiol 106:17,

July 1977

Jaffe N: Intraocular lens – current status. Ophthalmology 85:52-58, January 1978

Faye EE: The Low-vision Patient. Clinical Experience with Adults and Children. Grune & Stratton, New York, London, 1970

Kornzweig AL: Eye on old age. Chapter 13, Clinical Geriatrics. Rossman I, Ed. J.B. Lippincott Co., Philadelphia, 1971

Weale RA: The Aging Eye. Hoeber Medical Division, Harper & Row, New York, 1963

Seitz R: The Retinal Vessels (translated by Blodi FC). The C.V. Mosby Company, St. Louis, 1964

Kornzweig AL: Senescence of the eye. Modern Ophthalmology, Systemic Aspects, Vol 2, 2nd ed. Butterworth & Co., Ltd., London, 1972

Black RL, Oglesby RB, Von Sallman L, Bunim JJ: Posterior subcapsular cataracts induced by corticosteroids in patients with rheumatoid arthiritis. JAMA 174:166, 1960

Foote FM, Boyce VS: Screening for glaucoma. J Chronic Dis 2:247, 1955

Chapter 19

Tucker HM: Conservation laryngeal surgery in the elderly patient. Laryngoscope 87:1955-1999, 1977

Chandler JR: Malignant external otitis: further considerations. Ann Otol Rhinol Laryngol 86: 417-428, 1977

Nager GT: Paget's disease of the temporal bone. Ann Otol Rhinol Laryngol 84: Suppl 22:1-32, 1975

Gapany-Gapanavicius B: Otosclerosis: Genetics and Surgical Rehabilitation. J. Wiley & Sons, New York, 1975

Henderson D, Hamernik RP, Dosanjh DS, Mills JH, Eds: Effects of Noise on Hearing. Raven Press, New York, 1976

Pollack MC: Amplification for the Hearing Impaired. Grune & Stratton, New York, 1975

Paparella M, Shumrick D: Otolaryngology, Vol I, II, III. W.B. Saunders Company, Philadelphia, 1973

Conley J: Concepts in Head & Neck Surgery. Grune & Statton, New York, 1970

Fine P, Ed: Deafness in Infancy & Early Childhood. Williams & Wilkins, Baltimore, 1974

Oyer HJ, Oyer EJ: Communication and Aging. University Park Press, Baltimore, 1976

Worthington EL, Lunin LF, Heath M, Catlin FI, Eds: Index-Handbook of Ototoxic Agents 1966-1971. The Johns Hopkins University Press, Baltimore, 1973

Davis H, Silverman SR: Hearing and Deafness, 2nd ed. Holt, Rinehart, and Winston, New York, 1966

Chapter 20

Ziffren SE, Hartford CE: Comparative mortality for various surgical operations in older versus younger age groups. J Am Geriatr Soc 20: 485, 1972

Santos AL, Gelperin A: Surgical mortality in the elderly. J Am Geriatr Soc 23: 42, 1975

Williams J, Hale H: The advisability of inguinal hernioplasty in the elderly. Surg Gynecol Obstet 12: 100, 1966

Siegel JH, Chodoff P, Eds.: The Aged and High Risk Surgical Patient: Medical, Surgical, and Anesthetic Management. Grune & Stratton, New York, 1976

Jake RJ: Analysis of geriatric surgical experience in a veterans home. J Am Geriatr Soc 24: 8, 1976

Alexander S: Surgical risk in the patient with arteriosclerotic heart disease. Surg Clin North Am 48:513, 1968

Knapp RM, Topkins MJ, Artusio JF: The cerebrovascular accident and coronary occlusion in anesthesia. JAMA 182:332, 1962

Kozell D, Mittelpunkit A, Meyer KA: Laboratory findings in obstructing gastroduodenal ulcer. Arch Surg 91:347, 1965

Mattingly TW: Patients with coronary arteriosclerotic disease as a surgical risk. Am J Cardiol 12:279, 1963

Greenfield LJ: Surgery in the Aged. W.B. Saunders Company, Philadelphia, 1975

Mitty WF Jr: Surgery in the Aged. Charles C Thomas, Springfield, Ill., 1966

Schein J, Dardik H: A selective approach to surgical problems in the aged. Clinical Geriatrics. Rossman I, Ed. J.B. Lippincott Co., Philadelphia, 1971, p. 405

Chapter 21

Pindborg JJ: Atlas of Diseases of the Oral Mucosa, 2nd ed. The C.V. Mosby Co., St. Louis, 1973

Scopp IW: Oral Medicine, 2nd ed. The C.V. Mosby Co., St. Louis, 1973

Ten-State Nutritional Survey in the United States, 1968-1970. I, II, DHEW Pub. No. (HSM) 72-8130; III, 72-8131; IV, 72-8132; V, 72-8133; Highlights, 72-8134. Center for Disease Control, Atlanta, Ga., Health Services and Mental Health Administration, 1972

Current Estimates from the Health Interview Survey. United States - 1975. Data from the National Health Survey. DHEW Pub. No. (HRA) 77-1543

Hartsook EI: Food selection, dietary adequacy and related dental problems of patients with dental prosthesis. J Prosthet Dent 32:32-40, 1974

Miller EL: Types of inflammation caused by oral prosthesis. J Prosthet Dent 30:380-384, 1973

Wical KE: Studies of residual ridge resorption. Part I and Part II. J Prosthet Dent 32:13-22, 1974

Rissin L, Garcia DA, Chauncey HH, House JE: The effects of age and prosthetic appliances on food selection in adult males. J Dent Res 56:735, 1977

House JE, Rissin L, and Kapur KK: Analysis of the interrelationships between masticatory performance and food preference. J Dent Res 56:736, 1977

Suomi JD, Doyle J: Oral hygiene and periodontal disease in an adult population in the United States. J Periodontal 43:677-684, 1972

Enwonwu CO, Edozien JC: Epidemiology of periodontal disease in Western Nigerians in relation to socioeconomic status. Arch Oral Biol 15: 1231-1244, 1970

Chiranjeevi K, Wade AB: Periodontal effects of a national health service on an immigrant population. J Periodontol 43: 718-722, 1972

Kapur KK, Glass RL, Loftus ER: The Veterans Administration longitudinal study of oral health and disease. Aging and Human Development 3:125-137, 1972

Virtanen KK, Makinen KK, Oksala E: Palatal stomatitis: a histochemical and biochemical study. J Dent Res 35:674-684, 1977

Chapter 22

Anderson WF: The Practical Management of the Elderly. Blackwell Scientific Publications, London, 1977, p.90

Coni N, Davison W, Webster S: Rehabilitation Lecture Notes on Geriatrics. Blackwell Scientific Publications, 1977, pp. 72-82

Judge TG, Caird FI: Drug Treatment of the Elderly Patient. Pitman Medical, Kent, England, 1978, pp. 47-48

Hunt TE, Crichton RD: One third of a million days of care at home: 1959-1975. Can Med Assoc J 116: 1351, 1977

Smyer MA: Differential Usage and Differential Effects of Services for Impaired Elderly. Advances in Research, Duke University, for the Study of Aging and Human Development, 1: 4, 1977

Krusen FH, Kottka FJ, Ellwood PM: Handbook of Physical Medicine and Rehabilitation, 2nd ed. W.B. Saunders Company, Philadelphia, London, Toronto, 1971

Rush HA: Rehabilitation Medicine. The C.V. Mosby Company, St. Louis, 1971

Peszczynski M: Rehabilitation in hemiplegia. Rehabilitation and Medicine, Licht S. Elizabeth Licht Publishing Co., New Haven, Conn., 1968

Handbook of Rehabilitation Nursing Techniques in Hemiplegia. Kenny Rehabilitation, Chicago, 1964

Lowen EW, Rush HA: Self Help Devices (Monograph XXI). Institute of Physical Medicine and Rehabilitation, New York, 1962

Stokoo W, Silverman DR: Stroke Rehabilitation. Videotape or film in three parts with supplementary booklet produced by Washington/Alaska Regional Medical Program, Seattle

Patient education brochures: Up and Around, Strike Back at Stroke, Do It Yourself Again, Heart of the Home. Available from American Heart Association and its affiliates.

Chapter 23

Kane RL, Jorgensen LA, Teteberg B: Is good nursing-home care feasible? JAMA 235:516, 1976

Positive Approaches to Selecting Alternative Living Arrangements for the Elderly. Sandoz Pharmaceuticals, East Hanover, New Jersey, 1975

Williams TF, Hill G, Fairbank ME, Knox KG: Appropriate placement of the chronically ill and aged. A successful approach by evaluation. JAMA 226:1332, 1973

Guidelines for a Medical Director in a Long-Term Care Facility. Committee on Aging, American Medical Association, 1974

Fonrose HA: The medical director in an extended care facility. J Am Geriatr Soc 24:92, 1976

Solon A, Greenawalt L: Physicians participating in nursing homes. Med Care 12:486, 1974

Chapter 24

Rossman I: Environments of geriatric care. Postgrad Med 49:215, 1971

Rossman I: Newer options for the elderly patient other than institutionalization. Chapter 42, Clinical Aspects of Aging. Reichel W, Ed. Williams & Wilkins Co., Baltimore, 1978

Brocklehurst JC, Ed: Geriatric Care in Advanced Societies. University Park Press, Baltimore, 1975, p. 155

Lurie E, Kalish RA, Wexler R, Ansak M: On Lok Senior Day Health Center, a case study. Gerontologist 16:39, 1976

Forced idleness, impoverishment, ill health, isolation. 1973 Symposium, Problems of Older People, New York Academy of Medicine. Bull NY Acad Med 49:12, 1973

Rossman I: The after care project: a viable alternative to home care. Med Care, 12:534, 1974

Barriers to Health Care for Older Americans. Hearings before the Senate Subcommittee on Health of the Elderly, July 9, 1974, Washington, D.C. U.S. Government Printing Office, Washington, D.C., 1975

Rossman I, Ed: Clinical Geriatrics. J.B. Lippincott Co., Philadelphia, 1971, p. 525

Adult Day Facilities for Treatment, Health Care, and Related Services. Working paper for Senate Special Committee on Aging. U.S. Government Printing Office, Washington, D.C., September 1976

Reichel W: Complications in the care of five hundred elderly hospitalized patients. J Am Geriatr Soc 13:11:973, 1965

Mather HG, Morgan DC, Pearson NG: Myocardial infarction: a comparison between home and hospital care for patients. Br Med J 1(6015): 925, 1976

CHAPTER 25

Our Future Selves: A Research Plan Toward Understanding Aging. U.S. Government Printing Office, Washington, D.C., 1977

Spence DC, Feigenbaum EM, Fitzgerald F: Medical attitudes toward the geriatric patient. J Am Geriatr Soc 16:976, 1968

Birren JE, Butler RN, Greenhouse SW: Human aging: a biological and behavioral study. U.S. Public Health Service Publication No. 986, Washington D.C. U.S. Government Printing Office, 1963, reprinted 1971, 1974

Butler RN, Lewis MI: Aging and Mental Health, 2nd ed. The C.V. Mosby Company, St. Louis, 1977

Butler RN: Ageism: another form of bigotry. Gerontologist 9:243, 1969

Lewis MI, Butler RN: Life review therapy. Geriatrics 29:165, 1974

Index

A

Acanthosis nigricans
    and gastrointestinal neoplasms, 139
Accidents
    and injuries in hospital, 18, *21*
    prevention of falls in retirees, 16
    in unfamiliar institutional environment, 18
Acetaminophen
    absorption, age differences, 5
Acetazolamide
    therapy of wide-angle glaucoma, 145
Acetylcholine
    therapy of retinal artery occlusion, 147-148
Achalasia of esophagus
    incidence, 74
Achlorhydria
    affecting drug absorption, 5
Acne
    secondary, in rhinophyma and rosacea, 136
Acoustic nerve
    involvement in vertigo, 155
Acoustic trauma, 154-155
ACTH (*see* Corticotropin)
Activities of daily living
    rehabilitation goals and measures, 150, 172, 178, 182
Adaptation, psychological, 24-25, *173*
Addison's disease
    contraindication of fluorohydrocortisone in, 87-88
    contraindication of parenteral saline in the elderly, 87
    replacement glucocorticoid therapy in, 87-88
Adenocarcinoma
    prostate, adrenalectomy and hypophysectomy in, 124
    prostate, causing urinary tract problems, 118
    prostate, diagnosis, 123
    prostate, estrogen therapy, 123, 124
    prostate, increased incidence with age, *122*
    prostate, metastases in, *123*
    prostate, postradiotherapy impotence, 124
    prostate, prognosis as related to stage, 123-124
    prostate, radiotherapy, *123*, 124
    prostate, staging, *123*, 124
    prostate, treatment methods, *123*, 124
Adipose tissue
    changes in proportion of with age, *3*, 4
Adrenal cortex
    pituitary-adrenocortical axis, functional changes with age, 83
Adrenal gland hyperfunction
    incidence, age factor in, *87*
Adrenal gland hypofunction, *87*
Adrenalectomy
    in prostatic adenocarcinoma, *123*, 124
After care, 196-197
    in hospital physical therapy department, *193*
    recreation therapy in hospital department, *193*
    transport of patients in wheelchair-adapted van, *192*, 196
Aged
    population trends in U.S., *182*, *183*, *200*, *203*
    proportion of geriatric population living in institutions, *184*
Aging
    body composition and weight changes in, *3*, 4
    cardiac output decrease in response to demand in, 41
    and decline in physiological processes, 17, *18*
    of the skin, 134
    VA Normative Aging Study, 169
    visual acuity decline and retention in, 141, *142*
Alcohol, ethyl
    and effect of age on antipyrine metabolism, *8*
    effect on drug metabolism, 4-5
Alcoholism, 11, 14, 28
    in evaluation of dementia, 35
    incidence in psychiatric admissions, *24*
Aldosterone
    blood level decline with age, 83, *84*
    renin-aldosterone system, decreased responsiveness with age, 83
Allopurinol
    therapy of gout, indications and dosage, 101
Alzheimer's disease (*see also* Dementia, senile)
Alzheimer's disease
    cerebral atrophy in, *32*, *33*
    diagnostic features, 33-34
    differentiation from depression with secondary dysfunction, 37
    NIH workshop-conference on, 34
    senile dementia of Alzheimer type, recommended terminology, 34
American Dental Association (ADA)

Page number in italics indicates illustration

oral health education programs, 167
Aminopyrine
  metabolism by liver, decrease with age, *5*
Amitriptyline
  therapy of depression, dosage, 29
Amobarbital
  metabolism by liver, decrease with age, *5*
Amyl nitrate
  therapy of retinal artery occlusion, 147-148
Analgesics
  dosage in osteoarthritis, *93*
  evaluation in mild and severe pain, *116*, 117
  therapy of rheumatoid arthritis, dosage, *96*
Analgesics, anti-inflammatory
  dosage in osteoarthritis, *93*
Androgen antagonists
  therapy of benign prostatic hypertrophy, 119
Androgens
  production decline with age, 90
Anemia
  complicated, as indication for transfusion in elderly, *67*
  diagnosis, unnecessary workups in, 191
  drug-induced, *70*
  normocytic-normochromic, etiologic diagnosis, 70
Anemia, aplastic
  drug-induced, *70*, *71*
  as indication for transfusion in elderly, *67*
Anemia, hemolytic
  in hypoplastic crises, as indication for transfusion in elderly, *67*
Anemia, hypochromic, 67-68
  initial workup in diagnosis, 67
  microcytic, 67-68
  microcytic and macrocytic, blood smears, *67*
  in vitamin B 12 deficiency, blood smear, *68*
Anemia, macrocytic
  in folic acid or vitamin B 12 deficiency, diagnosis, 68-70
  Schilling test in, possible errors, 69-70
Anemia, pernicious
  bone marrow specimen in, *69*
  causing chronic brain syndrome, 34
  diagnosis, 69
Anemia, sideroblastic
  diagnosis, 67-68, *69*
  drug therapy, pyridoxine, 68
Anesthesia, spinal
  in prostatectomy, 121
Aneurysm
  surgery, indications, *164*
Angina pectoris, 42-43
  coitus in, 130
  differentiation from neuritic intercostal pain in spinal osteoporosis, 98
  hypertension control in, 53-55
  in thyroxine replacement therapy of hypothyroidism, 86
Angiography
  in carotid and subclavian occlusions, risks, 60
  in mesenteric and celiac arteriosclerosis, 164
  in subclavian steal syndrome, *61*
Aniline compounds
  occupational exposure to and bladder cancer incidence, 113

Antacids
  adverse reactions to, 2
  therapy of peptic ulcer, 77
  therapy of reflux esophagitis, pitfalls, 75-76
Antibiotics
  causing altered oral microbial balance, *Candida albicans* overgrowth in, 170
  causing cochlear damage, 154, *155*
  therapy of senile ectropion, 149
Anticholinergic agents *(see* Parasympatholytics)
Anticoagulants
  and surgery in transient cerebral ischemia, hospital comparative study, 62
Antidepressive agents
  causing depression of libido, *129*
  therapeutic use in primary care, *29*, 30
Antidiabetics *(see* Sulfonylurea compounds*)*
Antidiuretic hormone *(see* Vasopressin*)*
Antihypertensive agents
  causing depression of libido, *129*
Antineoplastic agents
  combination therapy of metastatic liver melanoma, result, *115*
  combination therapy of multiple myeloma of skull, results, *112*
Antiprotozoal agents
  toxic potential and cochlea, *155*
Antipyrine
  metabolism changes with age, *5, 7, 8*
Antispasmodics *(see* Parasympatholytics*)*
Antiseptics
  therapy of skin ulcer, 140
Anxiety
  after cataract extraction, counseling, 205
  concerning sexual function in Peyronie's disease, counseling, 205
  drug therapy, minor tranquilizers, 29
  of elderly in hospital, preventive measures, 192
  in evaluation of senile dementia, 36-37
  in hearing disorders, 157
  in sexual maladjustment, counseling, 27-28
Aortic aneurysm
  abdominal, relation of life expectancy to benefit of surgery in, *161*
Aortic rupture
  of abdominal aneurysm, elective surgery in impending rupture, 165
Aortocoronary bypass, 43
Appendicitis, 79, 164
  as symptom of right colon cancer, 164
Appendix
  histologic change with age, 79
Appetite
  adverse effects of maxillary denture, 167-168
Aqueous humor
  dynamics in narrow- and wide-angle types of glaucoma, *146*
Arrhythmia
  age factor in therapeutic approach, 44
  etiologic diagnosis, 43-44
  evaluation, portable ECG tape recorder in, 44
  incidence, increase with age, 43
Arterial occlusive diseases
  subclavian artery, causing stroke, *58*

surgery, least-harmful procedure rule in, 165
  vertebral artery, causing stroke, *58*
Arteriosclerosis
  mesenteric arteries and celiac axis, 164
  retinal arterioles in, *144*
  risk factors, 47-55
Arthritis
  self-help devices, *97*, 98
Arthritis, rheumatoid, 96-97 *(see also* Rheumatoid nodule*)*
  counseling of family by primary physician, 97
  diagnosis, 93-95, *100*
  drug therapy, *95*, *96*
  of hand, differentiation from osteoarthritic deformities, *94*
  incidence, 93, *100*
  interphalangeal involvement, x-ray, *98*
  referral to specialists, 95
  sex ratio in, *100*
  treatment by family physician, 95
  x-ray of hand and carpal bone involvement, *98*
Aspirin
  adverse reactions, 2
  causing neurosensory hearing loss, 154
  dosage in rheumatoid arthritis, blood salicylate monitoring in, 95
  evaluation in pain control, *116*,117
  interactions with prescribed drugs, 7
  therapy of transient cerebral ischemia, 62
Astringents
  therapy of senile ectropion, 149
Atropine
  -containing drugs, hazard in glaucoma patients, 143
Attitude of health personnel
  medical students' negative attitude toward elderly, 202
  of physicians, toward death in cancer, 117
  physician's attitude toward chronic disease, 201-202
  physician's attitude toward elderly, 199, 201-203, 205
  physician's attitude toward geriatric rehabilitation, 172-173
Attitude to death
  of family, counseling, 28
  of physicians, in relation to cancer, 117
Attitude to health
  patients' fatalism concerning aging, 199, 201
  patients' fears concerning disease, 201
Auditory threshold
  in decline of hearing acuity with age, sex factor in, *154*
Aurothioglucose
  dosage in rheumatoid arthritis, *96*

B

Backache
  caused by spinal cancer and injuries, 174
Bacteremia
  in catheterized prostatic hypertrophy patient, 122-123
  in prostatism, 118, 122

Bacterial infections
    conjunctivitis, etiologic diagnosis, 149
    precipitating congestive heart failure, 42
Baisden, R.: Hematologic Problems, 65-72
Balanitis
    causing urethral stenosis, 118
Basilar artery
    occlusion in stroke, diagnosis, 59
Basso, A.: The Prostate in the Elderly Male, 118-124
Baths
    aggravation of pruritus hiemalis, 134-135
Behavior
    change, in diagnosis of physical illness, 15
Behavior disorders, functional
    counseling by primary physician in, 26-27
    evaluation by primary physician, 25-26
    management by primary physician, 23-30
    and senile dementia, differentiation, 36-37
    and sex disorders, 130
    therapeutic alternatives, 28, *29*, 30
Belladonna alkaloids
    in over-the-counter drugs, interactions with prescribed drugs, 7
17-Beta estradiol
    therapy of postmenopausal osteoporosis, *108*
Bile duct neoplasms
    Klatskin tumor *79*, *80*
Biliary tract diseases, 79-81
    surgery, indications, *164*
Biofeedback
    in treatment of reflux esophagitis, 75
Bladder, neurogenic
    diagnosis and drug therapy, 121
Bladder diseases
    diverticula, 118
    incompetence of neck after prostatectomy, 121
Bladder neoplasms
    diagnosis, 113-114
    incidence and etiology, 113
    surgical approach, 165
    therapy, 114
    transitional cell carcinoma, 118
Blindness
    caused by diabetic retinopathy, 147
    low-vision aids, 150
    low-vision clinic in home for the aged, 150
    self-help methods taught by volunteer aides, 150
Blood cells
    in chloramphenicol-induced anemia, leukopenia, and thrombocytopenia, *71*
Blood pressure
    in prediction of cardiovascular morbidity, 48
Blood proteins
    drug-binding, decrease with age, 4, *5*
Blood transfusion
    indications and contraindications, 66, *67*
Blood volume
    excessive expansion, avoidance in elderly, 66
    lack of change in with age, 66
Body composition
    changes in with age, *3*
Body water
    changes in with age, *3*, 4

Body weight
    reduction in hypertension control, 50
Bone diseases, 91-101, 107
Bone marrow examination
    in anemia of various types, 67, *69*, *71*
Bone neoplasms
    metastatic from breast, therapy, 111-112
    metastatic from prostate, *113*, *123*
    multiple myeloma, 114
Bone resorption
    in dental ridge, and chewing ability in denture wearers, 167
Boric acid
    therapy of conjunctivitis, 149
Bouchard's nodes, 93, *94*
Braces
    and supports in stroke rehabilitation, 179
Brain
    atrophy, in evaluation of dementia, 35
    atrophy in Alzheimer's disease, *32*, *33*
    tomography, computerized axial, in etiologic differentiation of stroke, *62*
Brain stem
    ischemia in stroke, diagnosis, 59-60
Brain syndromes, organic, 31-37 (*see also* Confusion, Dementia, senile, *and* Hydrocephalus, normal pressure)
Brain syndromes, organic
    acute, 31-33, *36*, 37
    Alzheimer type of senile dementia, recommended terminology, 34
    chronic, 33-37
    etiological evaluation, 35
    incidence in psychiatric admissions, *24*
    mixed, 35, 37
    paintings by nursing home patients, *194*
Breast neoplasms
    diagnosis in primary practice, 11
    incidence, 11, *110*
    metastases in, age-related differences, 111-112
    mortality, increase with age, 109
    Paget's disease of nipple, 139
    prognosis in elderly, 111-112
Bromides
    adverse reactions to, 2
Butler, R. N.: The Doctor and the Aged Patient, 199-206

C

Caffeine
    effect on antipyrine metabolism, age factor, *8*
    effect on drug metabolism, 4-5
Calcium, dietary
    supplements in treatment of osteoporosis, 98
Canadian Cooperative Platelet-Inhibiting Drug Trial in Threatened Stroke, 62
Cancer (*see* Neoplasms)
Carbonic anhydrase inhibitors
    therapy of glaucoma, 145, 147
Carcinogens, occupational
    aniline dye exposure and bladder cancer, 113
    causing lung cancer, delayed development after exposure, 109-110

Carcinoma
    thyroid gland, age factor in incidence, *87*
Carcinoma, basal cell
    diagnosis and therapy, 138
    of face, chemosurgery and excision, *137*
    occurrence, 10
    vulva, histopathology, *104*
Carcinoma, bronchogenic
    occupational carcinogen-induced, 109-110
Carcinoma, epidermoid
    skin, *137*, 139
Carcinoma, papillary
    thyroid gland, prognosis, 112
Carcinoma, squamous cell
    lip, *137*
    and precancerous skin conditions, 138
    of scalp, cervical metastases in prognosis, 116
Carcinoma, transitional cell
    bladder, diverticula as sites of, 118
Cardiac output
    age-related changes affecting pharmacokinetics, 5
    decrease in response to demand with age, 41
Cardiovascular diseases
    estrogen-induced, 124
    eye diseases and manifestations in, 149
    occurrence, 9
    primary care in, 9-10
    risk factors, 47-55
Carotid artery diseases
    angiography in occlusion, risks, 60
    occlusion, age as operability factor, 61-62
    occlusion, angiography and radionuclide imaging, *63*
    occlusion, benefits and risks of surgery, 61
    occlusion, causing stroke, *58*, 59
    ophthalmodynamometry in diagnosis, 147
    in polymyalgia rheumatica, diagnosis, 100
    surgical and nonsurgical management, 61
Carpal bones
    involvement in rheumatoid arthritis, x-ray, *98*
Castelli, W.P.: CHD Risk Factors, 47-55
Castration
    in prostatic adenocarcinoma, 123, 124
    in treatment of benign prostatic hypertrophy, 119
Cataract, 19, 143, 144
Cataract extraction, 143
    postoperative anxiety, counseling in, 205
Catheter, indwelling
    in prostatic hypertrophy, nonoperated, 122-123
Cerebral aneurysm
    diagnosis, ocular auscultation in, 143
Cerebral angiography
    in internal carotid stenosis, 63
Cerebral arteriosclerosis, 19, 34, 147
Cerebral embolism and thrombosis
    causing stroke, *58*, *59*
Cerebral hemmorhage
    causing stroke, *58*, *59*
Cerebral ischemia, transient, 57, 61, 63-64
    anticoagulants as alternative to surgery, 62
    diagnosis, 59
    drug therapy, aspirin, Canadian cooperative study, 62

219

sulfinpyrazone, Canadian cooperative
  study, 62
drug therapy versus surgery, hospital
  comparative study, 62
internal carotid narrowing in, diagnosis by
  ophthalmodynamometry, 147
prediction of functional loss in further
  episodes, 63
in previous history of stroke, according to
  etiology, *59*
subclavian steal syndrome in, 60
surgery, 60-62
surgical and nonsurgical management,
  comparative survival in, 61
Cerebral ventricles
  in normal pressure hydrocephalus,
    radionuclide imaging, 34
Cerebrovascular disorders
  in central vertigo, diagnosis, 155
  eye diseases and manifestations in, 149
  incidence, 9
  as surgical risk factor, 162
Cerumen, 152
Cervix neoplasms
  diagnosis, 105-106
Chauncey, H. H., and House, J. E.: Dental
  Problems, 166-171
Cheilitis
  angular, 167, 170, *171*
Chenodeoxycholic acid
  therapy of cholelithiasis, possibilities, 79
Chloramphenicol
  -induced bone marrow hypoplasia, *71*
Chlordiazepoxide
  dosage, 29
Chlorpropamide
  -induced hyponatremia, 90
Cholelithiasis
  cholecystectomy in, 79, 164-165
  differential diagnosis from Klatskin tumor,
    79
  drug therapy, chenodeoxycholic acid, 79
  drug therapy and surgery in, 79
  elective surgical approach, 164-165
  emergency and elective cholecystectomy,
    comparative mortality in, 164
  incidence, increase with age, 79
Cholesteatoma
  and otitis media in hearing loss, 153
  middle ear, surgery, 153-154
Cholesterol
  blood, and age as cardiovascular risk
    factors, *53, 54, 55*
  blood levels, dietary control, 50
Cholesterol, dietary
  age factor in prescription of
    anti-atherogenic diet in elderly, 45-46
Chondrocalcinosis, *100*
  pseudogout, differentiation from gout,
    100-101
Chronic disease
  institutionalization in, 181
Clothing
  dyes in, causing contact dermatitis, 135
  in skin protection, 135, 136
Cochlea
  drug-induced damage, 154, *155*
Cognition
  mental status examination, 203-204

status as prognostic indicator in stroke, *173*
Coitus
  in angina pectoris patients, 130
  after myocardial infarct, 130
  stress level of exertion in, 130
Colchicine
  therapy of gout, dosage and side effects,
    101
Colon
  changes in function and morphology with
    age, 77-78
Colonic neoplasms
  diagnosis, 11, 81, 164
  incidence, 11, 81
  and ventral hernia, differential diagnosis,
    163
Colostomy, 162
Coma
  occurrence in stroke, according to etiology,
    59
Community health services
  potential care resources for aged, *179*
  role in caring for senile dementia patient,
    35
Conditioning, operant
  in treatment of reflux esophagitis, 75
Confusion, 13-14 (*see also* Brain syndromes,
  organic)
  acute confusional state, *36*
  causes of confusional reactions, 15, 32-33
  drug-induced confusional reaction, 31,
    32-33
  physical disease presenting as acute
    confusional reaction, *18*
Conjunctivitis
  drug therapy, boric acid and
    sulfacetamide, 149
  etiologic diagnosis, bacterial cultures in,
    149
Constipation, 16, 77-78
  paradoxical diarrhea and incontinence in,
    78-79
  stool softeners, adverse effects, 78
Coronary care units
  as environment detrimental to patient, 194
  mortality in, comparison with home care,
    194
Coronary disease
  age factor in bias favoring diagnosis of, 39
  coitus in, 130
  risk, diabetes as factor, 47
Corticotropin (ACTH)
  ectopic production in cancer, 88
  ectopic secretion, age factor in incidence,
    87
  pituitary capacity for release, with age, 83
Cortisol
  blood level stability with age, *84*
Cortisone
  therapy of Addison's disease, 88
  therapy of vulvar moniliasis, 103
Cost-benefit analysis
  in cancer treatment in elderly, 116
Counseling
  in anxiety concerning sex problems, 27-28
  in anxiety following cataract extraction,
    205
  in depression, *29*
  of family of rheumatoid arthritis patient,
    97

of family on attitude to death, 28
in functional behavior disorders, 26
in heart disease management, 45-46
in hypochondriasis, 28
in paranoia, 28
of patient and family for anxiety
  concerning hospitalization, 191-192
in retirement community primary care,
  11-15
in retirement-related alcoholism, 28
in retirement-related depression, 28
sex counseling, 125-133
in situational behavior disorders, 27
in stroke, 63
in suicide prevention, 27
in visual loss, 142
Creatinine
  clearance, normal values with aging, 4
Creatine phosphokinase
  blood levels in hypothyroidism, 86
Cripps, D. J.: Skin Care and Problems,
  134-140
Cyproterone
  therapy of benign prostatic hypertrophy,
    119
Cystocele
  and postmenopausal vaginal relaxation,
    106
Cytodiagnosis
  of uterine neoplasms, technics and
    apparatus, 106

D

Davis, P. J.: Endocrines and Aging, 82-90
Day care, 197-198
Deafness, 15, 153-154 (*see also* Acoustic
  trauma)
  caused by acoustic neuroma, 155
  causing anxiety, physician's approach in
    reassuring patient, 157
  in cholesteatoma and otitis media, 153
  drug-induced neurosensory loss, 154
  in otosclerosis, 153
Decubitus ulcer, *21*, 140
Deglutition disorders, 75
Dehydration
  prevention in rehabilitative measures, 173
Dementia
  as prognostic indicator in stroke, *173*
Dementia, senile (*see also* Alzheimer's disease,
  Brain syndromes, organic, *and* Cerebral
  Arteriosclerosis)
  and alcoholism, 35
  Alzheimer type, diagnosis, 37
  Alzheimer type, recommended
    terminology, 34
  and anxiety, 36-37
  case summary, 31
  causes, diagnosis and therapy, 34-35
  cerebral and cerebellar atrophy in, 35
  definition, differential diagnosis and
    treatment, *36*
  differential diagnosis, 35-37
  etiological evaluation, 35-36
  and functional behavior disorders,
    differentiation, 36-37

220 *Page number in italics indicates illustration*

hazards of psychotropic drugs in, 35
and hepatic encephalopathy, 35
home care services, 35
and hypertension, with pseudobulbar palsy, 34
incidence, 12
maintenance of patient in community, 35
mixed brain syndromes, 35
NIH workshop-conference on, 34
and paranoia, 36-37
tests of intellectual ability in evaluation, 35-36
vascular (multi-infarct) type, 34
and Wernicke-Korsakoff syndrome, 35
Dental prosthesis
care of dentures of nursing home patients, 171
causing diminished flavor perception, 167
chewing ability in wearers, 167-169
examination by primary physician, 170, 171
food preferences in wearers, age-related changes in, 167
"home repair" of, risks, 170
needs of elderly, 166-167
Dental ridge
bone resorption in, and chewing ability in denture wearers, 167
Depression
appraisal of current emotional status in, 26
drug therapy in primary care, 29, 30
ECT in, 30
GI manifestations, 74
hospitalization in, 29, 30
with hypochondriasis, 19
incidence in psychiatric admissions, 24
primary care, self-rating scale in, 26
prognosis, 24, 37
relation to maladaptive life style patterns, 25
retirement-related, counseling by primary physician, 28-29
with secondary dysfunction, differentiation from Alzheimer type dementia, 37
therapeutic alternatives, 29, 30
Dermatitis
stasis, leg ulcer in, 139
Dermatitis, contact
caused by dyes in clothing, 135
Dermatitis medicamentosa, 135
Dermatomyositis
clinical features, 100
diagnosis, in exclusion of rheumatoid arthritis, 94
incidence, increase with age, 100, 139
and internal cancer, 139
sex ratio in, 100
Diabetes mellitus
and age as cardiovascular risk factors, 47, 51-52, 53, 54, 55
causing pruritus, 140
diet, insulin and sulfonylurea compounds in management, 89
as etiologic factor in vulvar moniliasis, 103
glucose tolerance test, age-adjusted criteria, 88, 89
incidence and complications in elderly, 88-89
management, influence of University Group Diabetes Program, 88-89
and myocardial infarct, 43
sulfonylurea therapy, increased mortality from myocardial infarct and stroke in, 89
as surgical risk factor, 162
Diabetic retinopathy, 147
macular exudates and hemorrhages in, 144
photocoagulation in, 147
vitrectomy in, 147
Diagnosis
adverse effect of workups on elderly, 190-191
differential, in problem-oriented approach, 22
hospital workup, explanations to patient concerning procedures, 192
missed diagnoses in senile "write-off," 205
pitfalls in geriatric diagnosis, 17-22
restraint in evaluative studies, 21, 22
signs and symptoms, interpretation in elderly, 17, 18
subjective and objective findings, assessment in primary care, 20
unnecessary workups, as protection against malpractice litigation, 191
Diagnosis, laboratory
in systematic approach to geriatric drug prescribing, 6, 7-8
test results, significance of age-related physiological changes in, 17
Diagnosis, oral
Triage assessment of patient needs, 171
Diarrhea
paradoxical, in constipation with fecal impaction, 78-79
Diazepam
dosage, 29
metabolism, changes with age, 5
Dichloracetic acid
in chemosurgery of basal cell carcinoma, 137
Diet
anti-atherogenic, age factor in prescription for heart patients, 45-46
in management of gout, 101
Diet, salt-free
in hypertension and heart failure, counseling, 46
Dietary fats
in blood lipid control, 49-50
Dietary fiber, 78-79
Diethylstilbestrol
therapy of postmenopausal osteoporosis, dosage, 108
Digoxin
adverse reactions to, 2
dosage estimation in elderly, 4
half-life, age-related differences, 7
renal excretion, decrease with age, 4, 5
Dihydrostreptomycin
blood levels, age-related differences, 7
renal excretion, decrease with age, 5
Diphenylhydantoin
causing gingival proliferation, 170, 171
plasma binding capacity, decrease with age, 5
Diuretics
prescription on "as needed only" basis in heart patients, 46
toxic potential and cochlea, 155
Diverticulitis, colonic
medical management, 164
surgery, indications, 164
Diverticulosis, colonic
dietary fiber and drug therapy in, 79
incidence, 73, 74
Dizziness
orthostatic, 19
Drug detoxication, metabolic
changes with age, 4, 5, 80
Drug hypersensitivity
insulin allergy, at-risk group of elderly, 89
pharmacy drug history in prevention of reactions from multiple prescriptions, 7
Drug interactions
between over-the-counter and prescribed drugs, 7
monitoring in geriatric prescribing, 6
Drug prescriptions (see Prescriptions, drug)
Drug therapy, 1-8
adverse effects of various drugs on eye, 143
adverse reactions, 2, 3, 6, 7-8, 18, 21
adverse reactions, role of pharmacy drug history in prevention, 7
age factor in dosage, 1
causing aplastic anemia, diagnosis, 70
causing depression of libido, 131
causing thrombocytopenia, 66-67
causing untoward hematologic reactions, 70
drug forgetfulness precipitating acute heart failure, 41-42
enhanced drug effect in elderly, 18
geriatric prescribing, systematic approach, 5, 6, 7-8
instructions to patient in, 22
overdosage from multiple prescriptions, prevention, 7
patient compliance, monitoring, 5-7
renal function testing in dosage, 4
restraint in, 22
Drug therapy, combination
causing confusional reaction, 31-33
overprescribing, 2-3
Drug utilization
expenditures by elderly in U. S., 2
Drugs
causing cochlear damage, 154
causing depression of libido, 129
sensitivity to, changes with age, 5
storage and toxicity in obese elderly, 4
toxicity, age factor in, 1
toxicity in emaciated elderly, 4
Drugs, over-the-counter
adverse reactions to, 2
interactions with prescribed drugs, 7
Duodenal ulcer
diagnosis, symptom variation with age, 77
drug therapy, antacids, 77
incidence, 74, 77
surgery, correlation of mortality with advancing age in, 162
Dyes
contact dermatitis from clothing dyes, 135
Dysphasia
as prognostic indicator in stroke, 173
Dyspnea, exertion, 19

221

E

Ear, external
  tumors, and otitis media, 154
Ear, internal (*see* Labyrinth)
Ear, middle
  tumors, and otitis media, 154
Ear diseases
  cholesteatoma, surgery, 153-154
  tympanosclerosis, causing hearing loss, 153
Ear neoplasms
  and otitis media, 154
Echocardiography
  in mitral stenosis with heart failure and pulmonary edema, *41*
Eckstein, D.: Common Complaints of the Elderly, 9-16
Economics, dental
  dental care restrictions in Medicare and Medicaid, 166
  public funding of dental care for elderly, 171
  Triage programs and expenditures, 171
Ecothiopate iodide
  therapy of wide-angle glaucoma, 145
Ectropion
  senile, *148*, 149
Edentulous state
  change in facial appearance of person lacking dentures, *167*, *168*
  incidence in elderly, 166-167, *168*, 169
Ejaculation
  retrograde, after prostatectomy, 121
Elbow
  tophus elbow in gout, differentiation from rheumatoid arthritis nodules, 92
Electric countershock
  decision to use in arrhythmia in elderly, 44
Electrocardiography
  in complete heart block, *42*
  portable tape recorder in evaluation of arrhythmia, 44
Electroconvulsive therapy (ECT)
  in depression, 30
Emaciation
  drug toxicity increase in, 4
Emergencies
  in geriatric surgery, 160
Emotional disorders
  combined with physical complaints in elderly, 15
  occurrence, 11
Emotions
  appraisal of current emotional status in depression, 26
  emotional behavior as prognostic indicator in stroke, *173*
Employment
  home care patients' commercial handicrafts, *195*
Endarterectomy
  in carotid artery occlusion, benefits and risks, 61
Endocrine diseases
  iatrogenic, 89-90
  incidence, age factor in, 87
Endocrine glands
  changes in function with age, 82-83, *84*

Endoscopy
  esophagogastroduodenoscopy in peptic ulcer hemorrhage, 77
Enterocele
  with tenesmus, 105
Entropion
  senile, *148*, 149
Environment
  change causing agitation and confusion in elderly, 15
Enzymes
  liver, changes with age, 80
Erythrocyte count
  standard values in elderly, 65, *66*
Erythrocyte sedimentation
  in polymyalgia rheumatica, 100
Erythrocytes
  in acquired sideroblastic anemia, blood smear, *69*
  in macrocytic-hypochromic anemia, blood smear, *67*, *68*
  in microcytic-hypochromic anemia, blood smear, *67*
Erythropoiesis
  in normocytic-normochromic anemia, reticulocyte count, 70
Eserine
  therapy of narrow-angle glaucoma, 147
Esophageal diseases, 74, *75*, 76
Esophagitis, reflux
  drug therapy, antacids, pitfalls in, 75-76
  anticholinergics, contraindications, 76
  urecholine, 75
  positional therapy, 75
  therapy, biofeedback and operant conditioning, 75
Esophagus
  change in function with age, 74-75
Estrogenic substances, conjugated
  therapy of postmenopausal osteoporosis, *108*
Estrogens
  blood level decline with age, *84*
  carcinogenic potential, monitoring of endometrial changes during osteoporosis therapy, *108*
  deficiency, postmenopausal, complications of vaginal relaxation in, 104
  prevention of osteoporosis, carcinogenic potential, 107-108
  side effects, cardiovascular, 124
  therapy of postmenopausal vaginal mucosa atrophy, 104, *105*
  therapy of postmenopausal osteoporosis, 98, 107, *108*
  therapy of prostatic adenocarcinoma, *123*, 124
  therapy of senile vaginitis, 104
  therapy of stress urinary incontinence, 104-105
Estrone
  therapy of postmenopausal osteoporosis, dosage, *108*
Ethinyl estradiol
  therapy of postmenopausal osteoporosis, dosage, *108*
Eustachian tube
  block by nasopharyngeal tumor, and infection, *152*, 154

dysfunction in otitis media, neurogenic aspect, 154
  involvement in chronic paranasal sinus infection, *153*
Exercise therapy
  prevention of dehydration and hyperthermia in, 173
Exertion
  during coitus, stress level of, 130
  in heart patients, counseling by physician, 46
  precipitating congestive heart failure, 42
Expenditures, health
  geriatric, 166, *167*, 181, 198, *202*
Extracellular fluid
  changes in with age, *3*, 4
Eye
  adverse effects of drugs on, 143
  adverse effect of hydroxychloroquine on, 95-96
  auscultation in diagnosis of cerebral aneurysm, 143
Eye diseases, 141-150
  diagnosis, family physician's role, 149
  etiology, 149
Eye manifestations, 149
Eye movements
  testing in regular physical checkup, 142
Eyeglasses
  expenditures of elderly on, *202*

F

Facial dermatoses
  acne, secondary, in rhinophyma and rosacea, *136*
Facial expression
  change in edentulous person lacking dentures, *167*, *168*
Facial neoplasms
  basal cell carcinoma, chemosurgery and excision, *137*
Fallopian tube neoplasms, 107
Family
  attitude to death, counseling, 28
  of hospitalized patient, counseling, 191-192
  negative attitudes toward nursing homes, 185-186
  of patient requiring institutionalization, 185-186
  of patient requiring surgery, negative attitudes of, 160
  role in heart patient-physician communication, 46
  of stroke patient, role in rehabilitation, 178
  of surgical patient, surgeon's advice to, 161
Fatigue
  causes, 14-15
Fecal incontinence
  paradoxical, in constipation, 78-79
Feces, impacted
  occurrence in hospital, *21*
  with paradoxical diarrhea and incontinence, 78-79
Femoral neck fractures
  occurrence, 10
  surgery and postoperative therapy, 10
Fenoprofen

therapy of rheumatoid arthritis, dosage, 95
Ferris, P.: Surgical Management of the Elderly, 159-165
Financing, government
   public spending for geriatric health care, 202
Finger joint
   osteoarthritic, x-ray, *99*
   osteoporotic, in rheumatoid arthritis, x-ray, *98*
Fluorescein angiography (*see* Fundus fluorescence photography)
Fluorides
   therapy of osteoporosis, 98-99
Fluorohydrocortisone
   contraindication in elderly Addisonian patients, 87-88
Folic acid deficiency
   with macrocytic anemia, diagnosis, 69-70
Food preferences
   of denture wearers, age factor, 167-168
   shift to easily chewed foods by elderly, 168-169
   shift to salty or sweet foods by elderly, 168
Fractures
   occurrence, 10
   thoracic vertebrae, in osteoporosis, *107*
Fractures, spontaneous
   in osteoporosis, 98-99
Framingham Study
   26-year follow-up, 47-55
Fundus fluorescence photography, 148
Furosemide
   adverse reactions to, 2
   inducing hyperglycemia, 89

G

Gallbladder diseases
   incidence, *74*
Gastrectomy
   in gastric ulcer, methods, 163
   mortality correlation with advancing age in, *163*
   partial, in peptic ulcer with obstruction, mortality in, 163
Gastric juice
   acid and pepsin secretion, decrease with age, 77
Gastric mucosa
   changes with age, 76
Gastritis, atrophic, 76
Gastrointestinal diseases, 73-81
   functional, age factor in, 73, *74*
   incidence, 11, 73, *74*
Gastrointestinal neoplasms
   and acanthosis nigricans, 139
   diagnosis, 81
   incidence, 73, *74*
   mortality, 81
   surgery, postop. mortality, 81
Genitalia, female
   postmenopausal atrophy, *103*
Geriatric nursing
   in nursing homes, 186-187
Geriatrics
   diagnosis and care as a challenge in, 199-200

diagnosis and treatment plan in problem-oriented approach, 20
diagnostic evaluations, restraint in, 21, 22
drug therapy, multiple, restraint in, *22*
evaluation units, assessment of patients' care needs, 183-184
in-hospital hazards and complications, 18, 20
life history-taking in comprehensive examination, 203-204
multidisciplinary approach, 22
multiple problems in elderly, 17-22
physician-patient relations in, 199-206
pitfall of "wastebasket" diagnosis, 20
10-point treatment chart, *22*
primary care in retirement community, 9-16
public spending for geriatric health care, 202
research and training support, 203
as a specialty of growing importance, 200
treatment difficulties in patients with multiple problems, 21
Gerontological treatment centers
   short-term evaluation and treatment of disturbed patients, 183-184
Gerontology
   evaluation and treatment in gerontological centers, *183*, 184, *185*
   nursing home placement decisions by evaluation unit, 184, *185*
   research and training support, 203
Gingival diseases
   diphenylhydantoin-induced proliferation, management, 170, *171*
Gingivitis, 19
Glaucoma
   aqueous humor dynamics in, *146*
   diagnostic difficulties, 145
   drug therapy, 145, 147
   hazards of atropine-containing drugs in, 143
   incidence, increase with age, 145
   iridectomy, peripheral, in narrow-angle type, *146*
   narrow-angle, 145, 147
   narrow-angle and wide-angle types, determination, 145
   screening for in regular physical checkup, 142
   trabeculotomy in wide-angle type, *146*, 147
   wide-angle, drug therapy, 145, 147
Glover, B. H.: Sex Counseling, 125-133
Glowacki, G.: Postmenopausal Gyn Problems, 102-108
Glucocorticoids
   blood levels, maintenance with age, 83
   causing cataract, 143
   dosage in rheumatoid arthritis, 96
   intra-articular, in osteoarthritis, caution in use, *93*
   replacement therapy in Addison's disease, 87
   side effects in arthritis therapy, 96
   with thyroxine replacement therapy in severe hypothyroidism, 86
Glucocorticoids, topical
   contraindications in dendritic keratitis, 149
   fluorinated, in therapy of pruritus, 136

therapy of kraurosis vulvae, 104
Glucose tolerance test
   age-adjusted criteria in diagnosis of diabetes, 88, *89*
Gold sodium thiomalate
   dosage in rheumatoid arthritis, *96*
   side effects, 96
Gout
   causing pruritus, *140*
   clinical features, 100
   diagnosis, urate crystals in, 101
   diet restriction in, 101
   differentiation from pseudogout, 100-101
   drug therapy, 101
   incidence, age peak of occurrence, *100*
   management of acute attacks, 101
   sex ratio in, *100*
   tophus elbow, differentiation from rheumatoid arthritis nodules, *92*
Guanethidine
   contraindication in thyrotoxicosis with mild heart failure, 85
Gynecologic diseases
   history taking of perimenopausal and postmenopausal patients, 102
   postmenopausal, 102-108
Gynecologic neoplasms
   incidence, increase with age, 112

H

Hand
   in osteoarthritis, x-ray, *99*
   in rheumatoid arthritis, x-ray, *98*
Hand deformities, acquired
   in osteoarthritis and rheumatoid arthritis, differentiation, *94*
Handicapped
   sex behavior of, counseling, 130-131
   toothbrushing aids and devices for the disabled, 170-171
Head and neck neoplasms, 156
   squamous cell carcinoma of scalp, cervical metastases in prognosis, 116
   surgical possibilities, 156-157
Headache
   occurrence in stroke, according to etiology, *59*
Health education, dental
   ADA programs, 167
Health facilities
   nursing facility in retirement community, 9, *10*
Health services accessibility
   dental, cost and practitioner availability in, 171
Health services needs and demand
   oral health needs, assessment by Triage, 171
Hearing
   acuity decline with age, 152, *154*
Hearing aids, 155-156
Hearing disorders
   caused by tympanosclerosis, 153
   cerumen accumulation in, 152
   importance of early diagnosis and therapy, 151

incidence, 11, 151
referral to specialist, 151
Hearing tests
in hearing aid candidates, 156
Heart block (*see also* Pacemaker, artificial)
complete, ECG before and after pacemaker, *42*
etiologic diagnosis, 43-44
incidence, increase with age, 43
Heart defects, congenital
congestive heart failure in, 41
Heart disease, hypertensive
congestive heart failure in, 40
Heart diseases
age factor in differential diagnosis, 39
age factor in evaluation and treatment, 39-46
counseling in management, 45-46
patient involvement in care measures, 46
as surgical risk factor, 162
Heart enlargement
in atrial septal defect, causing heart failure, *42*
as cardiovascular risk factor, age differences, 47, *53, 54, 55*
as myocardial infarct risk factor, 51
Heart failure, congestive
acute, caution in treatment of elderly, 42
causes, 39, *40, 41, 42*
diuretic prescription on "as needed only" basis, 46
drug forgetfulness precipitating acute episodes, 41-42
etiologic diagnosis, 39-42
hypertension as risk factor with age, 49
in hypertensive heart disease, 40
salt restriction in, counseling, 46
in thyrotoxicosis, 85
Heart injuries
congestive heart failure in, 41
Heart septal defects, atrial
cardiomegaly and heart failure in, 41, *42*
Heberden's nodes, 93, *94*
Hemangioma
cherry angioma, 136
Hematocrit
standard values in elderly, 65, *66*
Hematologic diseases, 65-72
causing pruritus, *140*
with chronic infection, 65
diagnosis, 65
occult blood loss determination in, 65
Hemiplegia
bed positions and supports in, *177, 178*
rehabilitation, walking aid in, *176*
Hemoglobin
standard values in elderly, 65, *66*
Hemorrhage
as indication for transfusion in elderly, 67
postmenopausal vaginal bleeding, 104
Hemorrhage, gastrointestinal, 68
Heparin
inducing reversible hypoaldosteronism and hypokalemia, 90
Hepatic duct
Klatskin tumor, *79*, 80
Hepatic encephalopathy
in evaluation of dementia, 35

Hepatitis
differential diagnosis, 81
mortality, increase with age, 80
Hernia, 162-163
Herpes simplex, ocular (*see* Keratitis, dendritic)
Hiatal hernia
causes and incidence, 76
Hip fractures
in osteoporosis, 98, 99
rehabilitation goals and choice of surgical procedure in, 174
Hodgkin's disease
pruritus in, 139
Home care services
as alternative to institutionalization, 189
availability nationwide, 195-196, *197*
cost comparison with nursing homes, 198
and hospitalization, comparison of physician-patient relations in, 195
and hospitalization, cost comparison, 181
illustrative examples, *191*
initial evaluation of candidate for care, 194
patients' commercial handicrafts, *195*
program of Montefiore Hospital, N.Y.C., 194-196
public support for, 193-194
for senile dementia patient, 35
social worker's evaluation of patient acceptability, 194-195
for stroke patients, 179-180
types of disorders managed in, *190*
for typical "nursing home" type patient, 195
Homes for the aged
low-vision clinic in, 150
proportion of geriatric population living in, *184*
self-help methods taught to blind by aides, 150
Hormones
blood levels, changes and stability in with age, *84*
Hormones, ectopic
ACTH secretion, age factor in incidence, *87*
ACTH secretion in cancer, 88
parathyroid hormone secretion, age factor in incidence, *87*
parathyroid hormone secretion in cancer, 88
vasopressin secretion in cancer, 88
Hospital infections, 18, *21*
Hospital nursing staff
role in basic stroke rehabilitation measures, 178
Hospitalization
adaptation of hospital procedures to elderly, 192
adverse effects of diagnostic workups on elderly, 190-191
alternatives to institutionalization, 189-198
anxiety of elderly in hospital, prevention, 192
care expenditures of elderly, *202*
in depression, *29*, 30
evaluation of patient's need for, *185*
geriatric overutilization of hospitals, 190
and home care, comparison of physician-patient relations in, 195

and home care services of nursing homes, cost comparison, 181
overemphasis of institutionalization, contributory factors, 190
patients' negative reactions to, 189-192
risks in hospital for geriatric patients, 189
in stroke, versus home care, 63-64
unnecessary diagnostic workups in hospital, 191
Hospitals
care resources for aged, *179*
drug prescribing in, precautions, 8
Hospitals, psychiatric
leading causes of first admissions, *24*
proportion of geriatric population living in, *184*
House, J. E. (*see* Chauncey, H. H.)
Housing
European geriatric housing projects, *196*, 198
in retirement community, patient furnishing of units, *14*
specialized housing for elderly, 198
Humidity
in control of pruritus hiemalis, 134
Hunt, T. E.: Rehabilitation of the Elderly, 172-180
Hydrocephalus, normal pressure (*see also* Brain syndromes, organic)
cisternal radionuclide imaging in, 34
diagnosis and surgery, 34
evaluation, clinical judgment in, 34
Hydrochloric acid, gastric
secretion, decrease with age, 77
Hydrochlorothiazide
adverse reactions to, 2
Hydrocortisone, topical
therapy of pruritus, 135-136
therapy of rosacea, 136
therapy of skin ulcer, 140
Hydronephrosis
in prostatism, 118
Hydroxychloroquine
dosage in rheumatoid arthritis, 96
therapy of rheumatoid arthritis, adverse effect on eye, 95-96
Hypercalcemia
in diagnosis of hyperparathyroidism, 87
thiazide diuretic avoidance in, 88
Hypercorticism (*see* Adrenal Gland Hyperfunction)
Hyperglycemia
furosemide-induced, 89
thiazide diuretic-induced, 89-90
Hyperkalemia
heparin-induced, 90
Hyperparathyroidism
diagnosis, 87
incidence, age factor in, *87*
with significant hypercalcemia, avoidance of thiazide diuretics in, 87
Hypertension
and age as cardiovascular risk factors, 47, *48*
control in angina pectoris, 53-55
and dementia, with pseudobulbar palsy, 34
as heart failure risk factor with age, 49
retinal arterioles in, *144*
as risk factor in myocardial infarct and

stroke, *49*
  as risk factor in stroke, 58
  salt restriction in, counseling, 46
  treatment goal, 48
Hypertension, pulmonary
  congestive heart failure in, diagnosis and treatment, 40
Hyperthermia
  induced by heat applications in dehydrated patient, 173
Hyperthyroidism
  causing high output heart failure, 41
  diagnosis in elderly, 83-85
  drug therapy, 85
  with heart failure, contraindication of guanethidine, 85
  with heart failure, propranolol therapy, 85
  incidence, 83, *87*
  radioiodine therapy, 85
  severe, therapy, 85
Hyperuricemia
  as cardiovascular risk factor, 47, 52
Hypoaldosteronism
  heparin-induced, 90
Hypochondriasis
  counseling by primary physician in, 28
  with depression, 19
Hyponatremia
  chlorpropamide-induced, 90
Hypophysectomy
  in prostatic adenocarcinoma, *123, 124*
Hypothalamo-hypophyseal system
  pituitary response to TRH, changes with age in males, 82-83
Hypothyroidism
  causing chronic brain syndrome, 31, 34
  causing marked memory loss, 31
  causing pruritus, 140
  creatine phosphokinase blood levels in, 86
  diagnostic problems, 86
  diagnostic value of radioiodine uptake test, 85-86
  incidence, increase with age, 85, *87*
  severe, thyroxine replacement dosage, 86
  severe, value of glucocorticoids with replacement thyroxine, 86
  thyroxine blood levels in hypothyroid and euthyroid patients, 85
  thyroxine replacement therapy, inducing angina pectoris, 86
  TRH test in elderly, sex differences in TSH response, 86
  triiodothyronine blood levels in euthyroid and hypothyroid patients, 85
  TSH blood levels in diagnosis, 86

I

Iatrogenic disease
  endocrine, 89-90
  reactions to procedures in hospital, 18, *21*
Ibuprofen
  therapy of rheumatoid arthritis, dosage, 95
Idoxuridine
  therapy of dendritic keratitis, 149
Imipramine
  dosage, 29
Immobilization
  incapacitating effect, 174
Immunity
  reduced resistance, relation to increased cancer incidence with age, 110
Immunoglobulins
  abnormal pattern in multiple myeloma, result of combination chemotherapy, *112*
Immunosuppressive agents
  therapy of rheumatoid arthritis, *96*
Impotence, 126
  caused by prostatic hypertrophy, 127
  contraindication of psychotropic drugs in sexual depression, 127
  etiologic diagnosis, drug history in, 127-128
  management by primary physician, 125-128
  medical history taking in, 126-128
  after prostatectomy, 121-122, 124, *127*
  after prostatectomy, penile prosthesis in, 122
  psychogenic, 121, 127
  after radiotherapy of prostatic adenocarcinoma, 124
  referral to specialists in, 131-132
Indomethacin
  dosage in rheumatoid arthritis, 95
Infarction
  intestinal, preventive measures and surgery, 163-164
Infection
  chronic, in patient with blood disorder, 65
Insomnia, 14-15
  and aggravation of pruritus, 135
Insulin
  allergy, at-risk group of elderly, 89
  blood level stability with age, *84*
  control of blood sugar, complications in, 89
  output changes with age, 83
Insurance, health
  annual expenditures by elderly, 167
  prepaid primary care in retirement community, 9
Intestinal absorption
  drug absorption in achlorhydria, 5
Intestinal diseases
  angina, angiography in, 164
  infarction, preventive measures and surgery, 163-164
  ischemia, angiography in, 164
Intestinal neoplasms
  as common cancer type in elderly, 110
Intestinal obstruction
  surgical approach, 163
Intestine, small
  changes in function and morphology with age, 77
Intraocular pressure
  testing in regular physical checkup, 142
Intrinsic factor
  deficiency, causes, 69
Iodine radioisotopes
  therapy of thyrotoxicosis, 85
  thyroid uptake, diagnostic value in hypothyroidism, 85-86
  thyroid uptake, suppression testing, 84-85
Iris
  iridectomy, peripheral, in glaucoma, 146
Iron
  body stores, evaluation in anemia, 67-68
  iron-enriched vitamins masking iron loss caused by GI hemorrhage, 68

J

Jaundice
  causes in elderly, 80-81
Jaundice, obstructive
  caused by Klatskin tumor, *79, 80*
Jejunum
  Roux-en-Y jejunostomy in palliative treatment of Klatskin tumor, *80*
Joffe, J. R.: Functional Psychiatric Disorders 23-30
Joint diseases, 91-101
  referred pain in, 173-174

K

Keratitis, dendritic
  diagnosis, 149
  drug therapy, corticosteroids, contraindications, 149
  idoxuridine, 149
Keratoconjunctivitis sicca
  diagnosis, objective test in, 149
  drug therapy, methylcellulose solution, 149
Keratosis
  actinic, *135*
  actinic, precancerous aspect, 138
Kidney
  digoxin excretion, decrease with age, 4
  drug excretion, decrease with age, 4, *5*
  functional changes with age, 17, *18*
Kidney function tests
  in estimating drug dosage in elderly, 4
Kidney tubules, distal
  responsiveness to vasopressin, decrease with age, 83
Klatskin tumor, *79, 80*
Kleh, J.: When to Institutionalize, 181-188
Klipper, A. R. (*see* Kolodny, A. L.)
Kolodny, A. L., and Klipper, A. R.: Bone and Joint Diseases, 91-101
Kornzweig, A. L.: Visual Loss in the Elderly, 141-150
Kraurosis vulvae, *104*

L

Labyrinth
  in systemic diseases affecting hearing, 154
Labyrinth diseases
  drug-induced cochlear damage, 154
  and hearing loss, 154
  toxic potential of common medications, 155
Lamy, P. P., and Vestal, R. E.: Drug Prescribing for the Elderly, 1-8
Language
  ability as prognostic indicator in stroke, *173*
Laryngeal neoplasms
  post-laryngectomy speech rehabilitation, 157

225

referral to specialist in, 156
Laxatives
  abuse and dependency, 78
  Ex Lax, adverse reactions, 2
Leg ulcer
  drug therapy, topical antiseptics, 140
  topical hydrocortisone, 140
  in stasis dermatitis, *139*
  Unna's boot in, 140
Length of stay
  reduction by utilization review, 181
Lenses
  intraocular implant after cataract extraction, 143
Lentigo
  senile, *135*
Leukemia, lymphocytic, chronic
  benign nature in elderly, 70-71, *72*
  complications, immunologic aspects, and therapy, 114-115
  diagnosis, 70
  incidence, increase with age, sex factor in mortality, 114
  management by family physician, 71
  survival time after onset of symptoms, *72*
Leukemia, myelocytic, chronic
  diagnosis, 72
  diagnosis and therapy, 114
Leukocyte count
  standard values in elderly, 65, *66*
Leukopenia
  drug-induced, *70, 71*
Leukoplakia, oral, *137, 170*
  incidence, correlation with smoking, 169, 170
Lewis, K. B.: Heart Disease in the Elderly, 39-46
Libido
  suppression by drugs, *129*, 131
Life style
  history, role in defining rehabilitation goals, 26
  independent living, unrealistic patient attitude concerning, 185
  maladaptive life style patterns, 25
Lip neoplasms
  squamous cell carcinoma, *137*
Lipids
  blood, as cardiovascular risk factor, 47, 49
  blood, dietary control, VA study, 49
Lipoproteins, high-density (HDL)
  blood level determination in older patients, 50
  as cardiovascular risk factor in older age groups, 49-50, *51*
Liver
  drug metabolism, changes with age, 4, *5*
  enzyme changes with age, 80
  functional, morphologic and weight changes with age, 80
  functional changes with age, 17, *18*
Liver diseases
  causing pruritus, *140*
Liver neoplasms
  metastatic melanoma, result of combination chemotherapy, *115*
Long term care
  alternatives to institutionalization, 189-198
  functional and psychosocial assessments of patient in care planning, 182
  institutionalization of chronically ill, 181
  patients' negative reactions to institutionalization, 189-192
  role of geriatric evaluation units in assessing patient needs in, 183
  triage application in, 181-182
Longevity
  longer survival of elderly population, *203*
Lung neoplasms
  incidence, increase with age, sex factor in, *111*
  metastatic from leg sarcoma, result of combination chemotherapy, *115*
  mortality, increase with age, 109
  occupational carcinogen-induced, delayed development after exposure, 109-110
Lupus erythematosus, systemic, *100*
  diagnosis, in exclusion of rheumatoid arthritis, 94
Lymphatic metastasis
  from prostatic adenocarcinoma, *123*, 124
Lymphoma
  pruritus in, 139

M

Macroglobulinemia
  diagnosis, 71-72
Macula lutea
  pigmentary changes in macular degeneration, *144*
  retinal hemorrhage in diabetic retinopathy *144*
  in retinal vascular occlusions, 147
Macular degeneration
  causes and treatment, 144-145
  with pigmentary changes in macular region, *144*
Malnutrition
  pharmacological significance in elderly, 4
Malpractice
  trends, contributing to unnecessary diagnostic workups, 191
Mannitol
  therapy of narrow-angle glaucoma, 147
Mastication
  and bone resorption in denture wearers, 167
  problems in denture wearers, 168-170
  shift to easily chewed foods by elderly, 168-169
Masturbation
  by elderly women, 128
Medicaid
  for nursing home patients, 187-188
Medicare
  dental care restrictions in, 166
Medical history taking, 203-204
  drug history in sexual problems, 127-128, *130*
  in impotence, 126-128
  of perimenopausal and postmenopausal patients, 102
  in systematic approach to geriatric drug prescribing, *6*, 7-8
Medical records
  drug utilization (Medicaid), 7
  medication flow sheet for problem-oriented patient record, 20, *22*
  nursing home procedures as factor in home selection, 187
  pharmacy drug history, role in preventing adverse reactions, 7
  problem-oriented patient chart, 18, *19*, 20, *22*
Melanoma
  liver metastasis, result of combination chemotherapy, *115*
  postmenopausal recurrence, 112
  skin, surgery in, 139
  therapeutic approaches, 112-113
Memory disorders, 13-14
  drug forgetfulness precipitating acute heart failure, 41-42
  reversible, in hypothyroidism, 31
Menopause
  medical history of perimenopausal and postmenopausal patients, 102
  postmenopausal atrophy of genital tract, *103*
  postmenopausal cortical bone calcium loss, 107
  postmenopausal decline in urethral competence, 104
  postmenopausal gynecologic problems, 102-108
  postmenopausal vaginal mucosa atrophy, topical estrogen therapy, 104, *105*
  postmenopausal vaginal relaxation, complications, 104, *106*
Mental disorders
  with clinical onset in later life, 25
  in geriatric patients, *18*, 23
  management by primary physician, 23-30
  recurrence in later life, 25
  urgent conditions, referral to specialists, 26
Mental health services
  availability for senior citizens, 28
Mesenteric vascular occlusion
  arteriosclerosis, angiography in, 164
Methimazole
  therapy of thyrotoxicosis, 85
Methylcellulose
  therapy of keratoconjunctivitis sicca, 149
Metronidazole
  therapy of trichomonal vulvitis, 103
Miconazole
  therapy of vulvar moniliasis, 103
Microsomes, liver
  drug-degrading enzyme activity, decrease with age, 4
Mineral oil
  in control of pruritus hiemalis, 135
Miotics
  long-acting, in glaucoma treatment, 145
Mitral valve stenosis
  congestive heart failure in, *40, 41*
Moniliasis, oral
  in antibiotic-altered oral microbial balance, 170
  causing angular cheilitis, 170, *171*
  role in denture stomatitis, 170
Moniliasis, vulvovaginal
  drug therapy, 103
  etiology, diabetes as factor, 103
Morphine

serum levels, increase with age, 5
Mouth
  microbial balance, Candida albicans overgrowth in antibiotic-induced change, 170
Mouth neoplasms
  incidence, increase with age, 170
Mouth neoplasms
  premalignant aspect of leukoplakia, *170*
Mucin
  gastric, age-related change in secretion, 77
Multiphasic screening
  annual, in retirement community, 11
Multiple myeloma, 114
  diagnosis, 71-72
  immunoglobulin abnormal pattern in, result of combination chemotherapy, *112*
  of skull, result of combination chemotherapy, *112*
Muscle cramp
  nocturnal, in leg, 19
Muscles
  histochemistry in polymyalgia rheumatica, 100
Musculoskeletal diseases
  primary care in, 16
Myelofibrosis
  idiopathic, diagnosis, 72
Myocardial diseases, primary
  congestive heart failure in, 41
Myocardial infarct
  age factor in low-cholesterol diet prescription, 45-46
  age factor in treatment options, 43
  in diabetics, presenting symptoms, 43
  home care versus coronary care unit, comparative mortality in, 194
  incidence in sulfonylurea-treated diabetics, 89
  morbidity, systolic pressure in prediction of, 48
  mortality, comparison of coronary unit and home care, 194
  occurrence without pain in elderly, 173
  precipitating stroke, 43
  risk factors, 47, *48*, *49*, 50-52, *53*, *54*, *55*
  sexual activity after infarct, 130
  "silent" infarct, diagnosis and prognosis, 51
  as surgical risk factor, 162
Myocarditis
  congestive heart failure in, 41

N

Naproxen
  therapy of rheumatoid arthritis, dosage, 95
Narcotics
  causing depression of libido, *129*
Nasopharyngeal neoplasms
  blocking eustachian tube, infection in, *152*, 154
Nasopharynx
  involvement in middle ear infection, 154
National Institute of Mental Health
  Center for Studies of the Mental Health of the Aging, 203
National Institute on Aging, 203
Neoplasm recurrence, local
  postmenopausal, of melanoma, 112
Neoplasm staging
  prostatic adenocarcinoma, *123*, 124
Neoplasms, 109-117
  causing pruritus, *140*
  and dermatomyositis, 139
  diagnosis, 110-111
  diagnosis, rheumatic disease as symptom, 92
  diagnosis by palpation or x-ray, number of cell mass doublings before detection, *114*
  ectopic hormone-secreting, 88
  high-risk sites in elderly, 110
  incidence, 109, *110*, *111*
  incidence increase with age, relation to carcinogen exposure, 109-110
  pain control, evaluation of analgesics in, *116*, 117
  physician's attitude to death in, 117
  prognosis, age-related differences in, 111
  skin manifestations, 139
  terminal care, death with dignity in, 117
  therapy, 116-117
Neurologic examination
  at gerontological treatment center, *183*
Neurologic manifestations
  as prognostic indicator in stroke, *173*
  of stroke, *58*
Neuroma, acoustic, 155
Neuroses
  incidence in psychiatric admissions, *24*
Nevus, 137
Nitroglycerin
  therapy of esophageal spasm, 75
Norethindrone
  adverse reactions to, 2
Nursing homes
  acceptability and certification, 187
  alternatives to, 189-198
  cost comparison with home care, 198
  drug prescribing in, precautions, 8
  in Europe and U.S., comparison, 193
  expenditures by elderly on care in, 202
  family physician's periodic review of patient's progress in, 188
  and home care in stroke, 63-64
  and hospitalization, cost comparison, 181
  institutionalization of chronically ill, 181-188
  Medicaid for patients, 187-188
  negative attitudes concerning, 185-186, 192-193
  nursing staff, appraisal of, 187
  oral hygiene deficiencies in, 171
  overutilization, 190
  placement, decision making, 181-183, *185*, 186
  placement, preparing the patient, 185
  quality of care in, 181
  recreational therapy in Netherlands home, *194*
  risks for geriatric patients in, 189
  selection factors, 186-187
  utilization by elderly, 181
Nursing services
  in after care, 196
Nutrition
  as affecting pharmacokinetics, 4
Nutrition disorders
  management by family physician, 74
Nystatin
  therapy of vulvar moniliasis, 103

O

Obesity
  increased drug storage and toxicity in, 4
Occult blood, 65, 68
Occupational therapy
  patient evaluation by therapist in gerontological treatment center, *183*
  referral of stroke patient for testing, 176
  therapist's role in basic stroke rehabilitation measures, 178
Ophthalmoscopy
  in regular physical checkup, 142
Oral health
  access to dental treatment, 171
  annual expenditures for care by elderly, 166, *167*
  dental problems of elderly, 166-171
  improved current oral health picture, 167
  primary physician's role in, 166, 170
  semiannual examination by primary physician, 170
  Triage assessment of patient needs, 171
  VA dental longitudinal study, 169-170
Oral hygiene
  in nursing homes and chronic care hospitals, deficiencies in, 171
Osteoarthritis, 19, 92-93
  Bouchard's and Heberden's nodes, 93, *94*
  clinical features, 93, *100*
  differentiation from rheumatoid arthritis, 95
  drug therapy, *93*
  of hand, x-ray, *99*
  hand deformities in, differentiation from rheumatoid arthritis, *94*
  incidence, 10, 93, *100*
  interphalangeal joint involvement, x-ray, *99*
  sex ratio in, *100*
  surgery, 93
Osteoarthropathy, hypertrophic pulmonary
  in bronchial or pleural cancer, 139
Osteoporosis
  clinical characteristics, 98, *100*
  collapsed vertebrae in, differentiation of costal pain from coronary pain, 98
  drug therapy, 98-99, 107, *108*
  hip fractures in, 98-99
  incidence, 10, 98, *100*
  of interphalangeal joints in rheumatoid arthritis, 98
  management, basic approach in, 98
  prevention, carcinogenic potential of estrogens, 107-108
  primary care in, 10
  sex ratio in, *100*
  spontaneous fractures in, 98, 99
  of thoracic vertebrae, with compression fractures, *107*
Otitis externa
  malignant, 152-153
Otitis media

and cholesteatoma in hearing loss, 153
chronic, 154
and chronic paranasal sinus infection, 154
and eustachian tube dysfunction, 154
in nasopharyngeal tumor blocking eustachian tube, *152*, 154
and tumors of external or middle ear, 154
Otorhinolaryngologic diseases, 151-157
Otosclerosis
causing hearing loss, 153
Ovarian neoplasms
diagnosis, methods, 106-107
prognosis, 106
Ovary
endocrine function decline with age, 83

P

Pacemaker, artificial
anchorage and replacement in heart block, 45
in complete heart block, ECG, *42*
elimination of age barrier to insertion, 44-45
implantation in nonagenarian, *43*, 44-45
problems in elderly, 45
pulse generator drift, *44*, 45
recharging power cell, 45
Paget's disease, extramammary
vulva, histopathology, *104*
Paget's disease of breast, 139
Pain
analgesic evaluation in, *116*, 117
painless myocardial infarct occurrence in elderly, 173
referred, 173-174
perception abnormalities, hindering geriatric rehabilitation, 173-174
thoracic, causes in elderly, 42-43
Palatal diseases
leukoplakia incidence, correlation with smoking, *169*, 170
Pancreas
histologic changes with age, 81
Pancreatic neoplasms
incidence, increase with age, *111*
mortality, increase with age, 109
Paralysis
of limbs in stroke, 59
Paralysis, pseudobulbar
and dementia, in hypertensive patient, 34
diagnostic features, 34
Paranoia
counseling by primary physician in, 28
in evaluation of senile dementia, 36-37
prognosis, 37
Papaverine
therapy of retinal artery occlusion, 147-148
Parasympatholytics
causing depression of libido, *129*
contraindications in reflux esophagitis, 76
in management of neurogenic bladder, 121
precipitation of urinary retention in prostatism, 118
Parathyroid hormone
blood level decline with age, 83, *84*

in diagnosis of hyperparathyroidism, 87
ectopic secretion, *87*, 88
Parotid neoplasms
skin metastases in, *138*
Parotitis
occurrence in hospital, *21*
Patient acceptance of health care
of after care program, 196-197
negative reactions to nursing homes, 189-193
patient's right to decide concerning institutionalization, 204-205
patient care planning, 181-182, 184, *185*, 186-187
Patient compliance
in geriatric drug prescribing, monitoring, 5, *6*, 7
Penicillamine
therapy of rheumatoid arthritis, 96
Penicillin
half-life, age- and sex-related differences, 7
renal excretion, increase with age, 5
Penis
prostheses creating erection in impotence, 122
Pepsin
secretion, decrease with age, 77
Peptic ulcer
obstructive, mortality in partial gastrectomy and vagotomy, 163
surgery, indications, 163
Peptic ulcer hemorrhage
complications, decreased tolerance with age, 77
localization, esophagogastroduodenoscopy in, 77
mortality, increase with age, 77
surgery, mortality correlation with advancing age, *162*
surgical approach, age factor in, 163
urgency in diagnosis and surgery, 77
Peptic ulcer perforation
surgery, mortality correlation with advancing age, 162
surgical approach, age factor in, 163
Perception
as prognostic indicator in stroke, *173*
Perceptual disorders
pain perception abnormalities as hindrance to geriatric rehabilitation, 173-174
test of perceptual loss, *174*
Periarteritis nodosa, *100*
Pericardial effusion
congestive heart failure in, diagnosis, 40-41
Perphenazine
dosage and adverse effects, 30
Personality
change in as sign of dementia, 12-14
Personality disorders
incidence in psychiatric admissions, 24
Petrolatum
in control of cutaneous xerosis, 135
in control of pruritus hiemalis, 134
Peyronie's disease
sexual function in, counseling, 205

Pharmacies
drug history maintenance in prevention of adverse reactions from multiple prescriptions, 7
Pharmacokinetics
changes with age, 3-4, *5*
effect of alcohol, 4-5, *8*
effect of caffeine, 4-5, *8*
effect of malnutrition in elderly, 4
effect of smoking, 4-5, *8*
effect of reduced cardiac output, 5
intestinal absorption in achlorhydria, 5
plasma half-life, age-related differences, 7
protein binding decrease with age, 4
renal excretion, decrease with age, 4, *5*
Phenothiazine tranquilizers
adverse effects, 29-30
dosage, 30
Phenylbutazone
absorption, age-related differences, 5
half-life, age-related differences, 7
therapy of gout, dosage, 101
therapy of rheumatoid arthritis, dosage and side effects, 96
Physical examination
eye examination in, 142
in systematic approach to geriatric drug prescribing, *6*, 7-8
Physical therapy
after care in hospital department, *193*
prevention of dehydration and hyperthermia in, 173
referral of stroke patient for testing, 176
role in stroke rehabilitation, 178
thermal, testing patient's temperature sensation in, 174
Physician-patient relations, 22, 199-206
in home care and hospital, comparison, 195
patient and family hostility toward physician, 185
physicians' negative attitudes toward elderly, 201-203
in retirement community primary care, 11-12, 14
Pilocarpine
therapy of glaucoma, ocusert method, 145, 147
Pituitary gland, anterior
ACTH release capacity, retention with age, 83
pituitary-adrenocortical axis, functional changes with age, 83
pituitary-thyroid axis, changes with age, 82
TRH testing, misleading results in elderly men, 82-83
Plasma volume
changes in with age, *3*, 4
Pneumoencephalography
of cerebral atrophic changes in Alzheimer's disease, *32*
Pneumonia, aspiration
occurrence in hospital, *21*
Polyarteritis nodosa (*see* Periarteritis nodosa)
Polycythemia vera
diagnosis, 72
Polymyalgia rheumatica, *100*
Polymyalgia rheumatica
complicated by giant cell arteritis, 100

diagnostic errors in, 99
differentiation from Takayasu syndrome, 100
drug therapy, prednisone, dosage, 100
histochemistry of muscle fibers in, 100
Polymyositis, *100*
Polyps
gastric, risk in atrophic gastritis, 76
Povidone-iodine
therapy of trichomonal vulvitis, 103
Precancerous conditions (*see also* Leukoplakia, oral)
actinic keratosis, diagnosis and therapy, 138
gastritis, atrophic, 76
Prednisone
adverse reactions to, 2
therapy of polymyalgia rheumatica, dosage, 100
Prescriptions, drug
drug expenditures of elderly, *167, 202*
hazards in geriatric prescribing, 1-8
inappropriate prescribing, 2
medication flow sheet for problem-oriented patient record, 20, *22*
multiple, role of pharmacy drug history in preventing adverse reactions, 7
systematic approach to geriatric prescribing, 5, *6*, 7-8
tranquilizers prescribed in senile "write-off," 205
Probenecid
therapy of gout, dosage, 101
Proctoscopy
frequency necessary in cancer detection, 111
Progestational hormones
challenge in estrogen therapy of osteoporosis, *108*
Propranolol
contraindication in thyrotoxicosis with mild heart failure, 85
therapy of thyrotoxicosis, 85
Proprioception
as prognostic indicator in stroke, *173*
Propylthiouracil
therapy of thyrotoxicosis, 85
Prostate, 118-124
Prostatectomy
abdominal approach, potency impairment in, *127*
in adenocarcinoma, *123, 124*
fiberoptic resectoscope, *120*
perineal approach, potency impairment in, *127*
postop. complications, 121-122, 124
postop. impotence, penile prosthesis for creating erection in, 122
retropubic, suprapubic, and transurethral approaches, *120,* 121
spinal anesthesia in, 121
transurethral, 121-122, *127*, 165
Prostatic hypertrophy
and bladder diverticula, in prostatism, 118
causing impotence, 127
causing urinary tract problems, 118
drug therapy, antiandrogens, 119
drug therapy, cyproterone acetate, 119
etiology, 119
and hydronephrosis, in prostatism, 118
hypertrophic median lobe causing symptoms of prostatism, *119*
kidney damage in, 165
nonoperated, risk of infection and bacteremia in catheterized patient, 122-123
therapy, castration in, 119
Prostatic neoplasms
adenocarcinoma, diagnosis, 123
adenocarcinoma, increased incidence with age, *122*
adenocarcinoma, metastases in, *123*
adenocarcinoma, postradiotherapy impotence, incidence, 124
adenocarcinoma, prognosis as related to stage, 123-124
adenocarcinoma, radiotherapy, *123,* 124
adenocarcinoma, staging of, *123,* 124
adenocarcinoma, treatment methods, *123,* 124
and bladder diverticula, in prostatism, 118
causing urinary tract problems, 118
as common cancer type in elderly, 110
and hydronephrosis, in prostatism, 118
incidence, increase with age, 113
management, 113
metastatic to bone, site percentages, *113*
mortality, increase with age, 113
skin metastases in, *138*
Prostatitis
causing symptoms of prostatism, 118
Prosthesis
intraocular lens implant after cataract extraction, 143
penile, for impotence after prostatectomy, 122
Protein binding
of drugs, decrease with age, 4, *5*
Pruritus
aggravation in insomnia, 135
caused by stress, 135
causes, 140
drug therapy, topical fluorinated glucocorticoids, 136
topical hydrocortisone, 135-136
environmental humidity in control of, 134
hiemalis, 134-135
as manifestation of internal cancer, 139
occurrence in elderly, 134
and vulvitis, drug therapy, 103
Pseudogout (*see under* Chondrocalcinosis)
Psychological tests
in depression, 26
mental status examination of geriatric patient, 203-204
of perceptual loss, *174*
in senile dementia, 36
Psychosomatic disorders, 14-15
gastrointestinal, age factor in, 73, *74*
Psychotropic drugs
contraindication in sexual depression, 127
hazards in senile dementia, 35
Pulmonary edema
in mitral stenosis with heart failure, 40, *41*
Pulmonary embolism
occurrence in hospital, 18, *21*
Purpura
senile, 72, 138

Pyridoxine
therapy of sideroblastic anemia, 68

Q

Quality of health care
in nursing homes, 181, 187

R

Radionuclide imaging
and angiography in evaluation of operability of internal carotid stenosis, *63*
cisternal, in normal pressure hydrocephalus, *34*
Receptors, hormone, 83
Recreation
in after care in hospital department, *193*
recreational therapy in Netherlands nursing home, *194*
Rectal diseases
diagnosis in primary practice, 16
Rectal neoplasms
diagnosis, required frequency of proctoscopy, 111
Rectocele, 105, *106*
Referral and consultation, *22*
in head and neck tumors, 156
in hearing disorders, 151
in laryngeal tumors, 156
to occupational therapist for testing in stroke, 176
to physical therapist for testing in stroke, 176
psychiatric referral in depression, *29*
in rheumatoid arthritis, 95
in sexual problems, *130,* 132
to speech therapist for testing in stroke, 176
in untreated venereal diseases related to sexual depression, 131-132
Rehabilitation, 172-180
aims of geriatric therapy, *180*
commercial handicrafts of home care patients, *195*
denial of services because of age, 173
goals, relation to choice of surgical procedure, 174-175
goals, relation to life style history of patient, 26
independence in activities of daily living as goal in, 172
mobilization of elderly patient, approach, 174
pain perception abnormalities as hindrance in, 173-174
physicians' attitudes toward geriatric rehabilitation, 172-173
pitfalls in geriatric rehabilitation, 172-173
primary physician's role in, 172
special features and realities of geriatric rehabilitation, 172
in stroke, 63, *175,* 176-180
in stroke, prognostic indicators, *173*
Reichel, W.: Multiple Problems in the Elderly,

17-22
Reichel, W.: Organic Brain Syndromes, 31-37
Renin
  renin-aldosterone system, decreased responsiveness with age, 83
Research support
  in geriatrics and gerontology, 203
Respiratory tract diseases
  incidence, 11
  smoking as causative factor in elderly, 52
Retinal artery
  arteriosclerotic and hypertensive arterioles, *144*
  occlusion, 147-148
Retinal diseases
  fluorescein angiography in, contraindications, 148
Retinal hemorrhage
  in diabetic retinopathy, *144*
  in occlusion of central retinal vein branch, *144*
Retinal vein
  occlusion, *144,* 147-148
Retirement
  alcoholism and depression in, counseling, 28
Retirement communities
  counseling in primary care in, 11-15
  multiphasic screening in, 11
  patient furnishing of units in, *14*
  primary care in N.J. community, 9, *10,* 11-16
  skilled nursing facility in, 9, *10*
  social contact between residents, *12*
Rheumatic heart disease
  congestive heart failure in, 39-40
Rheumatism
  clinical features of rheumatic diseases, *100*
  diagnosis, 91-92
  incidence, 91, *100*
  management by primary physician, 91-92
  sex ratio in rheumatic diseases, 100
  as symptom of cancer, 92
Rheumatoid nodule, 92, 95
Rhinophyma
  and rosacea, with secondary acne, *136*
Robbins, S.: Stroke in the Geriatric Patient, 57-64
Rosacea
  drug therapy, 136
  and rhinophyma, with secondary acne, *136*
Rossman, I.: Options for Care of the Aged Sick, 189-198
Ruben, R. J.: Otolaryngologic Problems, 151-157

S

Salicylates
  blood level monitoring in aspirin therapy of rheumatoid arthritis, 95
Saline
  contraindication in elderly Addisonian patients, 87
Saliva
  diminished production induced by tranquilizing agents, 170
  lowered pH and buffering capacity induced by tranquilizing agents, 170
Sarcoma
  lung metastases in, result of combination chemotherapy, *115*
Schilling test
  in macrocytic anemia, possible errors, 69-70
Schizophrenia
  incidence in psychiatric admissions, *24*
Schlemm's canal
  and aqueous humor dynamics in glaucoma, *146*
Schuster, M. M.: Disorders of the Aging GI System, 73-81
Scleroderma, systemic
  clinical features, *100*
  diagnosis, in exclusion of rheumatoid arthritis, 94
  incidence, increase with age, *100*
  sex ratio in, *100*
Sebaceous cyst
  milia, 137-138
Sebaceous glands
  hypertrophy in rhinophyma and rosacea, *136*
Seborrhea, 136
Sedatives
  causing depression of libido, *129*
Self-help devices
  practical aids for the arthritic, *97, 98*
  quadriped walking aid for hemiplegic, *176*
  Saskapole, *177, 178*
  toothbrushing aids for the disabled, 170-171
Sensation
  as prognostic indicator in stroke, *173*
Sensory aids
  low-vision aids, 149-150
Septicemia
  risk in indwelling urinary catheter in nonoperated prostatic hypertrophy, 122-123
Serpick, A. A.: Cancer in the Elderly, 109-117
Serum albumin
  reduced albumin and drug binding sites with age, 4
Sex behavior
  coital potency retention in elderly men, *126*
  counseling, 125-133, 205
  in elderly women, psychological aspects, 128-129
  maladjustment causing anxiety, 27-28
  normal desire and expression in elderly, 125
  of physically disabled, counseling, 130-131
Sex disorders, 125-129, *130,* 131-133 (see also Impotence)
Sex hormones
  production in elderly, 90
Sinusitis
  chronic, with eustachian tube involvement, 153
  and otitis media, 154
Sleep disorders
  drug therapy, minor tranquilizers in primary care, *29*

Skin
  aging of, 134
  care of in elderly, 134-140
Skin diseases, 10-11, 134-140
  actinic keratosis, precancerous aspect, 138
  milia, 137-138
  solar degeneration, 136
  spider angiomas, 137
  xerosis, 19, *134,* 135
Skin diseases, bullous
  as manifestation of internal cancer, 139
  pemphigoid, *139*
Skin neoplasms
  basal cell carcinoma, *137,* 138
  cherry angioma, 136
  as common cancer type in elderly, 110
  diagnosis in primary practice, 10-11
  epidermoid carcinoma, *137,* 139
  incidence, 10, 115-116
  melanoma, 112-113, 139
  metastatic, *138,* 140
  radiotherapy, 116
  squamous cell carcinoma, 138
Skin ulcer, 140
Skull neoplasms
  multiple myeloma, result of combination chemotherapy, *112*
Smoking
  and age as cardiovascular risk factors, *53, 54, 55*
  and bladder cancer, positive correlation, 113
  as cardiovascular risk factor, 47, 52
  causing respiratory diseases, 52
  correlation with incidence of oral leukoplakia, *169,* 170
  and effect of age on antipyrine metabolism, *8*
  effect on drug metabolism, 4-5
Soaps
  aggravation of pruritus hiemalis, 135
Social adjustment
  problems related to depression, 24-25
Social behavior
  contact between retirement community residents, *12*
Social welfare
  community services for senior citizens, 204
Social work
  worker's evaluation of patient acceptability for home care, 194
  worker's involvement in after care, 196
Sodium bicarbonate
  aggravation of cutaneous xerosis, 135
Soft tissue neoplasms
  metastatic, from breast, therapy, 111-112
Somatotropin
  secretion, age-related changes, 83
Speech therapy
  referral of stroke patient for testing, 176
Spinal diseases
  cervical, secondary to osteoarthritis, 19
  osteoporosis, differentiation of costal pain from coronary pain in, 98
  osteoporosis, with compression fractures, *107*
Spinal injuries
  diagnosis, back pain in, 174
Spinal neoplasms
  diagnosis, back pain in, 174

Sterility, male
    caused by prostatectomy, 121
Stimulants
    causing depression of libido, *129*
Stomach
    changes with age, *76*, 77
Stomach neoplasms
    incidence, increase with age, *110*
    mortality, 109
    risk in atrophic gastritis, 76
    skin manifestations of metastasis, *138*
    surgical approach, 163
Stomach ulcer, 19
    diagnosis, symptom variation with age, 77
    drug therapy, antacids, 77
    gastrectomy in, methods, 163
    incidence, *74*, 77, 163
    incidence of malignancy in, 163
Stomatitis
    caused by tranquilizing agents, 170
Stomatitis, denture
    role of moniliasis in, 170
Stress
    as factor in pruritus, 135
    and functional GI disorders, 73
    individual differences in dealing with, 24-25
Stroke, 57-64
    and arteriosclerotic dementia, 34
    assessment of brain damage in, 175-176
    avoidance of excess care in, 64
    brain stem ischemia in, diagnostic signs, 59-60
    caused by carotid artery occlusion, diagnosis, 59
    compensating for functional loss in, 63
    convincing patient of recovery potential in, 178
    counseling by primary physician, 63
    diagnosis, signs and symptoms, *58*, 59
    encouragement of patient and family in, 63
    etiologic differentiation by computerized axial tomography, *62*
    functional recovery in, 179-180
    with hemiplegia, bed positions and supports in, *177*, 178
    home care services in, 179-180
    hospitalization or nursing home versus home care in, 63-64
    incidence, increase with age, 58, *60*
    incidence after transient ischemic attack, 57, 61
    incidence in sulfonylurea-treated diabetics, 89
    intracranial and extracranial vascular lesions in, *58*
    management and rehabilitation, stages in, *175*, 176-180
    morbidity, systolic pressure in prediction of, 48
    mortality, 57
    paralysis of limbs in, 59
    patient's reactions to disability, effect on rehabilitation, 176, 178
    precipitated by myocardial infarct, 43
    primary physician's examination of patient, 176
    prognosis, 62-63, *173*
    referral to therapists for testing, 176
    rehabilitation, 62-63, 178-179, *180*
    rehabilitation, Saskapole in, *177*, 178
    risk factors, 47-52, *53*, *54*, *55*, 58
    symptoms, according to etiology, *59*
    vertigo as manifestation of brain stem ischemia in, 59
Students, medical
    negative attitudes toward elderly, 202
Subclavian artery
    occlusion causing stroke, *58*, 60
Subclavian steal syndrome, 60, *61*
Suicide
    counseling in prevention, 27
    occurrence, 23, *25*
Sulfacetamide
    therapy of conjunctivitis, 149
Sulfamethizole
    absorption and excretion, age factor, *5*
Sulfinpyrazone
    therapy of gout, dosage, 101
    therapy of transient cerebral ischemia, Canadian cooperative study, 62
Sulfonylurea compounds
    in control of diabetes complications, 88-89
    incidence of myocardial infarct and stroke in treated diabetics, 89
Sulfur
    in hydrocortisone cream, therapy of rosacea, 136
Sunscreening agents
    prevention of solar cutaneous degeneration, 136
Surgery, operative, 159-165
    choice of procedure in relation to rehabilitation goals, 174-175
    decision-making in geriatric surgery, 159, *160*
    emergency and urgent conditions in, 160
    patient-family attitudes, 160
    patient's right to know in, 161-162
    preop. evaluation, 159, *160*, 161-162
    preop. reassurance of patient, 162
    risk, 162
    surgeon's advice to patient and family, 160-161
    surgical stress precipitating congestive heart failure, 42
Surgical instruments
    fiberoptic resectoscope for transurethral prostatectomy, *120*
Sweating
    decrease with age, 173
Sympathomimetics
    in over-the-counter preparations, interactions with prescribed drugs, *7*

T

Takayasu syndrome
    differentiation from polymyalgia rheumatica, 100
Tape recording
    portable recorder in evaluation of arrhythmia, 44
Taste
    shift to salty or sweet foods by elderly, 168
Telangiectasis
    spider angiomas, 137
Temperature sense
    testing prior to thermal treatments, 174
Temporal arteritis
    in polymyalgia rheumatica, importance of early diagnosis, 100
Tenesmus
    and enterocele or rectocele, 105
Testosterone
    blood level decline with age, 83, *84*
    therapy of kraurosis vulvae, 104
    therapy of osteoporosis, 98
Tetracycline
    blood levels, age-related differences, *7*
    renal excretion, decrease with age, *5*
Thiazide diuretics
    avoidance in hyperparathyroidism with hypercalcemia, 87
    inducing hyperglycemia, 89-90
Thioridazine
    dosage and adverse effects, 30
Thirst
    reduction with age, 173
Thoracic diseases
    pain, causes in elderly, 42-43
Thoracic vertebrae
    osteoporosis, with compression fractures, *107*
Thrombocytopenia
    chloramphenicol-induced, blood smear, *71*
    drug-induced, 66-67, 70
Thyroid antagonists
    therapy of thyrotoxicosis complicated by heart failure, 85
Thyroid function tests, 82-83, 85-86
Thyroid gland
    pituitary-thyroid axis, changes with age, 82
    radioiodine uptake, adverse effects of triiodothyronine suppression testing, 84-85
Thyroid hormones
    blood levels, changes with age, 82
Thyroid neoplasms
    incidence, age factor in, *87*
    mortality, increase with age, 86
    prognosis, age-related differences, 112
    surgery, effect on survival in elderly, 86-87
    undifferentiated anaplastic carcinoma, prognosis, 112
Thyroid nodules, 86-87
Thyrotoxicosis (*see* Hyperthyroidism)
Thyrotropin (TSH)
    blood level stability with age, *84*
    blood levels in diagnosis of hypothyroidism, 86
    TSH stimulation test in hypothyroidism, 86
Thyrotropin-releasing hormone (TRH)
    diagnosis of hypothyroidism in elderly, sex differences in TSH response, 86
    testing with, misleading results in elderly men, 82-83
Thyroxine
    blood level changes with age, 82
    blood level stability with age, *84*
    replacement therapy, 86
Tinnitus
    causes, diagnostic difficulties, 155
Tolmetin
    therapy of rheumatoid arthritis, dosage, 95
Tomography, computerized axial
    of brain, in etiologic differentiation of stroke, *62*

of brain atrophy in Alzheimer's disease, *33*
Tongue neoplasms, *170*
Tooth abrasion, *163*
Toothbrushes
    aids and devices for the disabled, 170-171
Trabecular meshwork
    trabeculotomy in wide-angle glaucoma, *146*, 147
Training support
    in geriatrics and gerontology, 203
Tranquilizing agents
    causing depression of libido, *129*
    causing lowered salivary pH and buffering capacity, 170
    causing stomatitis and angular cheilitis, 170
    precipitating urinary retention in prostatism, 118
    prescription in senile "write-off", 205
    reducing rate of saliva production, 170
Tranquilizing agents, minor
    dosage, 29
    therapy of anxiety and sleep disorders, *29*
    therapy of functional behavior disorders, 28, *29*, 30
Transport of patients
    wheelchair-adapted van in after care, *192*, 196
Triage
    application to long-term care, 181-182
Trichomonas vaginitis
    vulvar, metronidazole therapy, 103
    vulvar, povidone-iodine gel therapy, 103
Trifluoperazine
    dosage and adverse effects, 30
Triiodothyronine
    adverse effects in thyroid suppression testing, 84-85
    blood level changes with age, 82, *84*
    blood levels in euthyroid and hypothyroid patients, 85

U

University Group Diabetes Program, 88-89
Urea
    therapy of narrow-angle glaucoma, 147
Urecholine
    therapy of reflux esophagitis, 75
Urethra
    postmenopausal decline in competence, 104
Urethral stricture, 118, 121
Uric acid
    crystal detection in diagnosis of gout, 101
Uricosuric agents
    therapy of gout, criteria of use, 101
Urinary catheterization
    in diagnosis of urethral stricture, 121
    indwelling catheter in nonoperated prostatic hypertrophy patient, 122-123
Urinary incontinence
    after prostatectomy, incidence, 122
Urinary incontinence, stress, 19, 104-105
Urinary tract infections
    bladder diverticula as reservoirs of, 118
    in prostatism, 118
    risk in indwelling catheter in nonoperated prostatic hypertrophy, 122-123
Urination disorders
    bladder outlet obstruction in men, 118
    in prostatic adenocarcinoma, 118, 123
    in prostatic hypertrophy, 118, *119*
    prostatism, 118-119, 121
    retention, occurrence in hospital, *21*
    in urethral stricture, 118
Urogenital neoplasms
    causing hypochromic anemia, 63
Urologic diseases, 11
Urticaria
    as manifestation of internal cancer, 139
Uterine hemorrhage
    postmenopausal, causes, 106
Uterine neoplasms
    diagnosis, 106
    estrogen-induced, monitoring of endometrial changes during osteoporosis therapy, 107, *108*
    incidence, increase with age, 109
Uterine prolapse
    and postmenopausal vaginal relaxation, *106*
Utilization review
    hospital utilization review committees, 181
    in reduction of length of stay, 181

V

VA blood lipid control study, 49
VA dental longitudinal study, 169-170
VA Geriatrics Research and Educational Clinical Centers, 203
VA Normative Aging Study, 169
Vagina
    postmenopausal atrophic changes in mucosa, topical estrogen therapy, 104, *105*
    postmenopausal relaxation, complications, 104, *106*
Vaginal diseases
    postmenopausal bleeding, 104
    prolapse, surgical procedures, 105
Vaginal neoplasms
    diagnosis, 105
Vaginitis
    postmenopausal, 104
Vagotomy
    in peptic ulcer with obstruction, 163
Vasopressin
    ectopic production in cancer, 88
    responsiveness of distal renal tubules to, decrease with age, 83
    secretion, lack of change with age, 83
Venereal diseases
    untreated, in sexual depression, referral in, 131-132
Venous insufficiency
    stasis skin ulcer in, 140
Ventral hernia
    and colonic cancer, differential diagnosis, 163
Vertebral artery
    occlusion, causing stroke, *58*, 59
Vertigo, 16, 19, 155
    as manifestation of brain stem ischemia in stroke, 59
    in stroke, diagnostic importance, 59
Vestal, R. E. (*see* Lamy, P. P.)
Vestibular apparatus
    in peripheral vertigo, 155
Vincristine
    adverse reactions to, 2
Vision disorders, 15-16, 141-150
    counseling by primary physician in, 142
    incidence, 11
    low-vision aids, 149-150
    primary physician's role in management, 141
    in stroke, diagnostic relevance, 59
Vision tests
    by primary physician, 141-142
    in regular physical checkup, 142
Visual acuity
    decline and retention with age, 141, *142*
Vitamin A
    tretinoin gel, therapy of rosacea, 136
Vitamin B_{12} deficiency, 69, 74
    diagnosis in macrocytic anemia, Schilling test, 69
    hypochromic anemia in, blood smear, *68*
    with macrocytic anemia, diagnosis, 68-70
    macrocytic hypochromic anemia in, blood smear, *67*
Vitamin C deficiency
    diagnosis, 74
Vitamin D
    and calcium treatment of osteoporosis, 98
Vitamins
    iron-enriched, masking iron loss caused by GI hemorrhage, 68
Vitreous body
    vitrectomy in diabetic retinopathy, 147
Volunteer workers
    teaching self-help methods to blind, 150
Vulvar neoplasms
    basal cell carcinoma, histopathology, *104*
    diagnosis, 103-104
    Paget's disease, histopathology, *104*
Vulvitis
    with pruritus, drug therapy, 103

W

Waldenstrom's macroglobulinemia (*see* Macroglobulinemia)
Warfarin
    adverse reactions to, 2
    plasma binding capacity, decrease with age, 5
Wernicke-Korsakoff syndrome
    in evaluation of dementia, 35
Wheelchairs
    transport of patients in especially adapted van, *192*, 196
Workmen's compensation
    in acoustic trauma, 154-155
Wound healing
    slow and less complete healing in elderly, 174
Wounds and injuries
    occurrence in hospital, 18, *21*

Z

Zinc
    Unna's boot in therapy of skin ulcer of leg, 140
Zinc chloride
    in chemosurgery of basal cell carcinoma, *137*

Illustration Credits

CHAPTER 1: 2, Albert Miller, data summarized by Caranasos; 3, Lyn Van Eyck; 6, 8, Albert Miller; 7, Albert Miller, data summarized by Bender

CHAPTER 3: 19, Irwin Kuperberg; 20 (bottom), 21 (bottom), Albert Miller

CHAPTER 4: 24, Albert Miller, adapted from Redick, Kramer, & Taube, "Epidemiology of Mental Illness and Utilization of Psychiatric Facilities Among Older Persons," reprinted from *Mental Illness in Later Life*, Busse & Pfeiffer, Eds., American Psychological Association, 1973; 25, Albert Miller (U.S. National Center for Health Statistics); 26, 27, 29, Albert Miller

CHAPTER 6: 42 (bottom), Albert Miller

CHAPTER 7: 48, 49, 51, Albert Miller

CHAPTER 8: 58, Carol Donner; 60, Albert Miller, adapted from Wylie, CM: "Death statistics for cerebrovascular disease; a review of recent findings." Stroke: Journal of Cerebral Circulation: 187, 1970

CHAPTER 9: 66 (bottom), 72, Albert Miller

CHAPTER 10: 74, 77, Albert Miller; 80, Neil O. Hardy

CHAPTER 11: 84, Albert Miller, adapted from Gregerman, RI, Bierman, EL, "Aging & Hormones," in *Textbook of Endocrinology*, 5th edition, Williams, RH, Ed., © W.B. Saunders Co., Philadelphia, 1974; 85, 87, 89, Albert Miller

CHAPTER 12: 94, Albert Miller

CHAPTER 13: 103, 106, Carol Donner

CHAPTER 14: 110-112, 116, Alan Iselin; 113, Nancy Lou Gahan (data from Krishnamurthy, GT, et al, "Distribution pattern of metastatic bone disease," Journal of the American Medical Association, 237:2504, 1977); 114, Alan Iselin (data from Silver, et al, "Some new aspects of modern chemotherapy," American Journal of Medicine, November 1977, pg. 775, modified from Collins, et al, "Observations on growth rates of human tumors," American Journal of Roentgenology, 76:988, 1956)

CHAPTER 15: 119, 123, Neil O. Hardy; 120, Carol Donner; 122, Albert Miller

CHAPTER 16: 126, Albert Miller (data from Martin, Baltimore Longitudinal Study); 127, Carol Donner; 130, Albert Miller

CHAPTER 18: 142, Albert Miller; 146, Neil O. Hardy

CHAPTER 19: 152, 153, Neil O. Hardy; 154, Albert Miller (National Health Survey)

CHAPTER 20: 160, Irwin Kuperberg; 161, Albert Miller, adapted from Drs. Baker & Roberts, Univ. of Pennsylvania, "Survival in Abdominal Aneurysms," Journal of the American Medical Association, 212(3), April 20, 1970, pg. 445; 162-163, Albert Miller, data from Mitty, WF, Jr., "Surgery in the Aged," Charles C. Thomas, Publisher, 1966, and Schein and Dardik, "A Selective Approach to Surgical Problems in the Aged," Isadore Rossman, Ed., *Clinical Geriatrics*, J.B. Lippincott Co., Philadelphia, 1st edition, 1971, pg. 405

CHAPTER 21: 167, 168, 169, Albert Miller

CHAPTER 22: 179, Albert Miller

CHAPTER 23: 182, 183 (top), Albert Miller

CHAPTER 24: 197, Albert Miller (National Health Survey)

CHAPTER 25: 200, 203, Albert Miller; 202, Albert Miller (National Center for Health Statistics)

Data and Photo Sources

CHAPTERS 9, 14, 25, © 1978

CHAPTERS 11, 13, 15, 16, 17, 18, 19, 21, 22, 23, 24, © 1977

CHAPTERS 1, 2, 3, 4, 5, 6, 7, 8, 10, 12, 20, © 1976

CHAPTER 2: 10, Meadow Lakes Retirement Community; 11-14, Frank Ritter

CHAPTER 5: 32-33, courtesy Dr. Leon Menzer, Sabin & Marck, P.C., Brookline, Mass.; 34-35, courtesy Dr. Pablo E. Dibos

CHAPTER 7: 53, 54, 55, adapted from the Framingham Heart Study, Section 28, Probability of developing certain cardiovascular diseases in eight years at specified values of some characteristics, Daniel McGee, DHEW, Publication 74-618

CHAPTER 8: 61-63, courtesy Radiology Department, Franklin Square Hospital; 63, courtesy Dr. Pablo E. Dibos

CHAPTER 10: 75, 79, courtesy Department of Radiology, Baltimore City Hospitals; 76, micrograph courtesy of Dr. R. Garcia Bunuel, Baltimore City Hospitals

CHAPTER 14: 110-111 (top), 1975 data from American Cancer Society

CHAPTER 23: 183 (bottom), 186, 187, photos, Dan Bernstein